# Physical Therapy of the Low Back
## Second Edition

# CLINICS IN PHYSICAL THERAPY

EDITORIAL BOARD

Already Published

**Hand Rehabilitation**
Christine A. Moran, M.S., R.P.T., guest editor

**Sports Physical Therapy**
Donna Bernhardt, M.S., R.P.T., A.T.C., guest editor

**Pain**
John L. Echternach, Ed.D., guest editor

**Therapeutic Considerations for the Elderly**
Osa Littrup Jackson, Ph.D., guest editor

**Physical Therapy Management of Arthritis**
Barbara Banwell, M.A., P.T., and Victoria Gall, M.Ed.,
P.T., guest editors

**Physical Therapy of the Cervical and
Thoracic Spine**
Ruth Grant, M.App.Sc., Grad.Dip.Adv.Man.Ther.,
guest editor

**TMJ Disorders: Management of the
Craniomandibular Complex**
Steven L. Kraus, P.T., guest editor

# Physical Therapy of the Low Back

**Second Edition**

**Edited by**

**Lance T. Twomey, Ph.D.**

Deputy Vice-Chancellor
Professor of Physiotherapy and Clinical Anatomy
Curtin University of Technology
Perth, Western Australia
Australia

**James R. Taylor, M.D., Ph.D.**

Associate Professor
Department of Anatomy and Human Biology
University of Western Australia
Medical Faculty
Nedlands, Western Australia
Research Fellow
Department of Neuropathology
Clinical Assistant
Sir George Bedbrook Spinal Unit
Royal Perth Hospital
Perth, Western Australia
Spinal Physician
Perth Pain Management Centre
Applecross, Western Australia
Australia

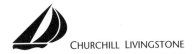
CHURCHILL LIVINGSTONE

New York, Edinburgh, London, Madrid, Melbourne, San Francisco, Tokyo

**Library of Congress Cataloging-in-Publication Data**

Physical therapy of the low back / edited by Lance T. Twomey, James R.
  Taylor. — 2nd ed.
        p.  cm. — (Clinics in physical therapy)
    Includes bibliographical references and index.
    ISBN 0-443-08894-2
    1. Backache—Physical therapy. 2. Backache.  I. Twomey, Lance T.
  II. Taylor, James R., Ph.D.  III. Series.
    [DNLM: 1. Physical Therapy.  2. Back Pain—rehabilitation.  WE
  755 P578 1994]
  RD771.B217P49  1994
  617.5′64062—dc20
  DNLM/DLC
  for Library of Congress                                                  93-43152
                                                                                   CIP

Distributed in the United Kingdom by Churchill Livingstone, Robert Stevenson
House, 1–3 Baxter's Place, Leith Walk, Edinburgh EH1 3AF, and by associated companies, branches, and representatives throughout the world.

The Publishers have made every effort to trace the copyright holders for
borrowed material. If they have inadvertently overlooked any, they will be
pleased to make the necessary arrangements at the first opportunity.

Acquisitions Editor: *Carol Bader*
Copy Editor: *Katharine Leawanna O'Moore-Klopf*
Production Supervisor: *Patricia McFadden*

Printed in the United States of America

First published in 1994      7  6  5  4  3  2

*To our wives,*
*Meg and Mamie*

# Contributors

**Nikolai Bogduk, M.D., Ph.D., B.Sc.(Med.), F.A.C.R.M.(Hon.)**
Professor, Department of Anatomy, University of Newcastle Faculty of Medicine; Director, Cervical Spine Research Unit, Mater Misericordiae Hospital, Newcastle, New South Wales, Australia

**Margaret I. Bullock, Ph.D., F.T.S.**
Professor, Department of Physiotherapy, The University of Queensland, Brisbane, Queensland, Australia

**Joanne E. Bullock-Saxton, Ph.D.**
Lecturer, Department of Physiotherapy, The University of Queensland, Brisbane, Queensland, Australia

**Caroline Drye, M.S., P.T.**
Clinical Instructor, Kaiser Hayward Physical Therapy Residency Program in Advanced Orthopaedic Physical Therapy, Hayward, California; Private Practitioner, Redwood Orthopaedic Physical Therapy, Castro Valley, California

**Brian C. Edwards, B.Sc., B.App.Sc., Grad.Dip.Man.Ther.**
Specialist Manipulative Physiotherapist and Honorary Fellow, Curtin University of Technology; Principal, Brian C. Edwards and Associates, Perth, Western Australia, Australia

**Joe Farrell, M.S., P.T.**
Senior Clinical Instructor, Kaiser Hayward Physical Therapy Residency Program in Advanced Orthopaedic Physical Therapy, Hayward, California; Private Practitioner, Redwood Orthopaedic Physical Therapy, Castro Valley, California

**Ruth Grant, M.App.Sc., Grad.Dip.Adv.Man.Ther.**
Professor, Department of Physiotherapy, and Dean, Faculty of Health and Biomedical Sciences, University of South Australia, Adelaide, South Australia, Australia

**Gwendolen A. Jull, M.Phty., Grad.Dip.Man.Ther., F.A.C.P.**
Senior Lecturer, Department of Physiotherapy, The University of Queensland; Specialist Manipulative Physiotherapist, Private Practice, Brisbane, Queensland, Australia

**Mike Koury, M.S., P.T.**
Clinical Instructor, Kaiser Hayward Physical Therapy Residency Program in Advanced Orthopaedic Physical Therapy, Hayward, California; Private Practitioner, Redwood Orthopaedic Physical Therapy, Castro Valley, California

**Colleen B. Liston, A.U.A., Grad.Dip.Hlth.Sc., M.App.Sc., M.A.P.A., M.C.S.P.**
Senior Lecturer, School of Physiotherapy, Curtin University of Technology;
Consultant Physiotherapist, Cerebral Palsy Association, and Consultant
Physiotherapist, Community Health Services, Western Australia Department of
Health, Perth, Western Australia, Australia

**Geoffrey D. Maitland, M.B.E., A.U.A., F.C.S.P., F.A.C.P.(Monog.), F.A.C.P.,
M.App.Sc.**
Visiting Specialist Lecturer for the Graduate Diploma in Advanced Manipulative
Therapy, School of Physiotherapy, University of South Australia, Adelaide, South
Australia, Australia

**Robin A. McKenzie, O.B.E., F.C.S.P., F.N.Z.S.P.(Hon.), Dip.M.T.**
Consultant and Director, Spinal Therapy and Rehabilitation Centre, The McKenzie
Institute International, Pauatahanui, New Zealand; Director, Clinical Services, The
McKenzie Institute International Clinics, Wellington, New Zealand

**Carolyn A. Richardson, Ph.D., B.Phty.(Hon.)**
Senior Lecturer, Department of Physiotherapy, The University of Queensland,
Brisbane, Queensland, Australia

**Nils Schönström, Ph.D.**
Head, Department of Orthopaedic Surgery, Ryhov Hospital, Jönköping, Sweden

**M. Scott Sullivan, M.S., P.T.**
Assistant Professor, Department of Physical Therapy, Virginia Commonwealth
University Medical College of Virginia, Richmond, Virginia

**James R. Taylor, M.D., Ph.D.**
Associate Professor, Department of Anatomy and Human Biology, University of
Western Australia Medical Faculty, Nedlands, Western Australia, Australia; Research
Fellow, Department of Neuropathology, and Clinical Assistant, Sir George Bedbrook
Spinal Unit, Royal Perth Hospital, Perth, Western Australia, Australia; Spinal
Physician, Perth Pain Management Centre, Applecross, Western Australia, Australia

**Patricia H. Trott, M.Sc., Grad.Dip.Adv.Man.Ther., F.A.C.P.**
Associate Professor and Head, School of Physiotherapy, University of South
Australia; Specialist Manipulative Physiotherapist, Adelaide, South Australia,
Australia

**Lance T. Twomey, Ph.D.**
Deputy Vice-Chancellor and Professor of Physiotherapy and Clinical Anatomy,
Curtin University of Technology, Perth, Western Australia, Australia

# Preface

In the seven years that have passed since the publication of the first edition of *Physical Therapy of the Low Back,* the general demographic statistics on low back pain have remained virtually unaltered. Thus, 80 percent of us will still suffer at least one disabling episode of low back pain during our life, while within any large group 30 to 35 percent will have some degree of backache at any point in time. However it is measured, low back pain remains the most costly musculoskeletal disorder in Western society, and it is depressing to have to report that recent evidence has shown that when back clinics are opened in developing agricultural societies, large numbers of people seek treatment.[1]

There have been very considerable advances in the knowledge of the structure and function of the vertebral column in recent years, and a considerable body of further evidence has been gathered to help develop a better understanding of the pathogenesis of low back pain. This additional information is reflected in changes to the first four chapters of this book, where morphology, pathology, and biomechanics are considered in detail. There has also been a considerable advance in our understanding of the effects of the physical therapies on low back pain. In particular, we are now much more aware of the importance of mobility and exercise in the treatment of back pain, while the use of analgesics and rest as treatment of choice has been shown to have little effect.[2,3] The use of intensive exercise programs for the treatment of chronic back pain allied with better measurement tools remains an avenue for further progression in the future.[4]

This second edition has expanded the book from 12 to 16 chapters—indeed, there are six new chapters in this edition. They include chapters on exercise (Ch. 15) and intensive rehabilitation (Ch. 10), on ergonomics (Ch. 12) and lifting (Ch. 13), on back pain in children and adolescents (Ch. 14), and on surgery for intractable low back pain (Ch. 11). While all chapters show progression and change from the first edition, Chapters 6, 8, and 9 contain entirely new material. Similarly, the final chapter—which attempts to gather together the information and provide a rationale for physical therapy for low back pain—has been entirely rewritten based on contemporary knowledge.

Low back pain remains an almost universal condition. There have been improvements in public health education in a number of countries in recent years, and certainly there is a better understanding of how this disabling condition can be effectively managed and treated. Back education, changes in lifestyle that emphasize mobility and exercise, and a more intelligent approach to working and leisure activities are still important measures in the prevention and management of back pain. The physical therapist remains a most important element in this equation.

*Lance T. Twomey, Ph.D.*
*James R. Taylor, M.D., Ph.D.*

## REFERENCES

1. Frymoyer JW, Cats-Baril WL: An overview of the incidences and costs of low back pain. Orthop Clin North Am 22:263, 1991
2. Waddell G: A new clinical model for the treatment of low back pain. Spine 12:632, 1987
3. Deyo RH, Diehl AK, Rosenthal M: How many days of bed rest for acute low back pain? N Engl J Med 315:1064, 1986
4. Twomey LT: A rationale for the treatment of back pain and joint pain by manual therapy. Phys Ther 72:885, 1992

# Contents

# 1 | The Lumbar Spine from Infancy to Old Age

James R. Taylor
Lance T. Twomey

The human lumbar spine, balanced on the pelvis by its muscles and ligaments, supports the whole length of the spine above it in the erect posture. The human lumbar spine is unique in its fully erect posture. In four-footed animals where the tasks of weightbearing and locomotion are shared by four limbs, the thoracolumbar spine forms an upwardly convex bridge between the forelimbs and the hindlimbs. In humans, the erect posture adopted in infancy develops a secondary curve or lordosis in the lumbar spine, which is generally maintained throughout life.

In this erect column, the lowest parts bear the highest loads. This functional requirement is reflected in the large size of the lumbar vertebrae and in the thickness and high proteoglycan content of lumbar intervertebral discs. In addition, the lumbar spine has wide ranges of flexion, extension, and lateral bending. These dual functions of this strong dynamic organ should be maintained over a life span of 70 to 80 years or more. The nature of this dynamic structure varies according to familial characteristics, growth and maturity, gender, and long-term responses to wear and tear. Unfortunately the flexibility and bounce of youth are usually replaced by the stiffness and slow movement of old age, but vertebral osteophytes and degenerate discs, with backache and stiffness, are not inevitable accompaniments of aging. This chapter describes how the complex structure of the lumbar spine varies throughout life and how it is designed to cope with its diverse functions. This chapter begins with a descrip-

1

tion of the normal adult lumbar spine and then describes the development and growth of the spine before dealing with age-related changes in spinal structure and function. Finally, it examines how structure and function influence the common types of injury to the lumbar spine.

## FUNCTIONAL ANATOMY OF THE ADULT LUMBAR SPINE

The spine is the central skeletal axis of the body. The musculoskeletal and visceral structures of the head, neck, upper limbs, and torso are supported by it or hung from it. This axis is strong but not static; it provides wide ranges of bending and twisting in different directions. The contrary requirements of strength and mobility are met by combining strong individual intervertebral joints allowing limited movement, with a large number of motions segments, which collectively give large ranges of movement.

Considering the lumbosacral spine in particular, its strength, resilience, and mobility are essential to normal human posture and activity. Its position affects the posture of the whole spine and head (e.g., pelvic obliquity results in lumbar scoliosis and a whole variety of compensatory changes at higher levels.[1,2] Stiffness in the lumbosacral spine restricts mobility in locomotion, bending, and lifting, and many other normal, everyday activities. Lumbar spinal osteoporosis and shortening with aging allow the rib cage to abut on the pelvis, further restricting movement and respiration.

A thorough knowledge of the normal adult anatomy of the lumbar spine is necessary for a good understanding of the effects of age-related changes.

The anatomy of the lumbar spine is described below in the following sequence: the functional anatomy of the vertebrae and spinal ligaments; the spinal and intervertebral canals and their contents; the biomechanics of injuries; and the functional anatomy of intervertebral discs and zygapophyseal joints. These descriptions are based on our own studies of large series of lumbar spines[3-7] and on other authorities as referenced.

## Weightbearing

The vertebral bodies and intervertebral discs bear over 80 percent of the static compressive load in erect posture.[8] The progressive increase in the surface area of the vertebral end-plates from C2 to the lower lumbar spine reflects the progressive increase in loading from above down. According to Davis,[9] vertebral body end surface area is maximal at L4. The end surface of L5 can be smaller because its forward tilt transfers a larger part of its load to the vertebral arches through the very thick pedicles and transverse processes that characterize L5.

Except for the bony rim a few millimeters wide, each vertebral end-plate is covered by a plate of hyaline cartilage about 1 mm thick. The outer fibrous annulus is attached to the bony rim and the inner fibrocartilaginous annulus is attached to the peripheral parts of the cartilage plate,[3] forming an elliptical envelope for the incompressible "fluid" nucleus pulposus (Figs. 1-1 and 1-2). The average height of adult male lumbar vertebral bodies is about 25 mm and the discs are from 10 to 12 mm thick at their centers. Their average anteroposterior diameter is from 30 to 35 mm. Their transverse dimensions increase from about 40 mm at L1 to about 50 mm at L5. Female vertebral dimensions are on average about 15 percent smaller.[3,4] The girth of the column is dependent in part on the effect of muscular forces during growth, and the female vertebral column is more slender than the male column.

Each vertebral body is kidney-shaped and covered by a thin shell of compact bone. Its internal body architecture reflects its weight-bearing function (Fig. 1-2). A lateral x-ray shows the predominantly vertical orientation of its trabeculae, with cross-ties, particularly numerous near the upper and lower end-plates. The vertical bony trabeculae are quite rigid but they can bend slightly when loaded. Unsupported vertical columns might bend beyond their elastic capacity and fracture, if they did not have the support of the transverse cross-ties, which increase their rigidity. Red hemopoetic marrow fills the honeycombed interstices of this trabecular scaffolding. This composite structure provides both strength and resilience with a small amount of "give" in response to loading, but the main shock absorbers are the intervertebral discs, whose structure and function will be described in detail later.

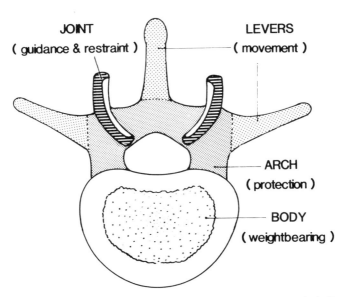

**Fig. 1-1.**  Relationship of the structures of vertebral parts to their functions.

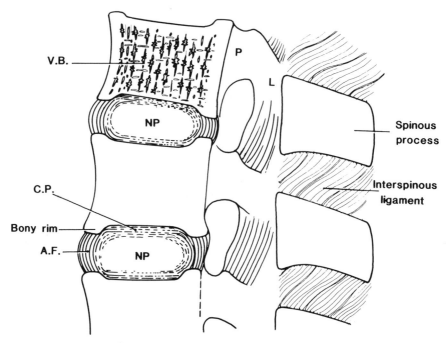

**Fig. 1-2.**   A median sagittal section shows the internal structure or "architecture" of a vertebral body and an intervertebral disc. The vertebral body has vertically oriented weightbearing, trabeculae, and cross-ties formed by transverse trabeculae. The intervertebral disc has a lamellar outer annulus fibrosus *(AF)*. The inner lamellae of the annulus are continuous with the lamellar structure of the cartilage plates *(CP)* as revealed by polarized light. The annulus and cartilage plates form an envelope enclosing the nucleus pulposus (NP). Fusion of the ring apophysis with the centrum forms the bony rim. *P*, pedicle; *L*, lamina; the interlaminar ligaments are the ligamenta flava.

## Protection of Neural Structures

The vertebral arches protect the neural structures in the spinal canal and intervertebral foramina. In contrast to the direct continuity of the anterior elements, specialized for loadbearing, the protective arches are only in contact through their articular processes, the gaps between them being bridged by the elastic ligamenta flava (Fig. 1-2). Each arch is formed by two pedicles, which project backwards from the upper outer margins of a vertebral body and by two laminae, which meet in the midline behind the spinal canal. The pedicles are oval in section with a thick cortex, which is why surgeons use them as points of fixation for metal plates, inserting transpedicular screws through the plates, above and below an unstable segment in a spinal fusion.

The lumbar laminae are flat plates of bone that cover the posterior aspect of the spinal canal, containing the lower part of the spinal cord and the cauda equina within the dural sac. In spinal stenosis, parts of the laminae are removed

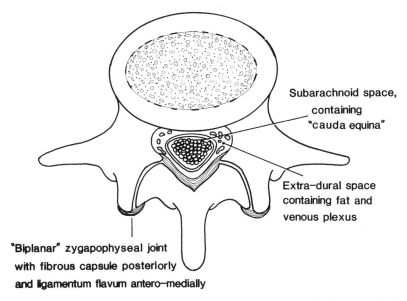

Subarachnoid space,
containing
"cauda equina"

Extra–dural space
containing fat and
venous plexus

"Biplanar" zygapophyseal joint
with fibrous capsule posteriorly
and ligamentum flavum antero–medially

**Fig. 1-3.** The appearance of the zygapophyseal (facet) joints is shown in horizontal section. The cancellous bone of the vertebral body can be seen within the compact bony ring. The contents of the vertebral canal in the lower lumbar region include the cauda equina within the dural sac. The extradural veins form a valveless venous plexus that connects regional veins outside the vertebral column with basivertebral veins at the center of each vertebral body.

by surgeons to "decompress" the cauda equina, in the procedure known as laminectomy. The canal can be entered by a needle inserted in the gap between the adjacent laminae of lower lumbar vertebrae, below the level of the spinal cord. The epidural space is entered first, by passing the needle through the ligamentum flavum into the vascular epidural fat, without piercing the dura. This space surrounds the dura and is traversed by the spinal nerves on their way to the intervertebral foramina. When the needle is passed through the fibrous dura and its membranous inner lining of arachnoid, it enters the subarachnoid space containing the cerebrospinal fluid containing the cauda equina.

## Control of Movements: Levers and Joints

Each vertebral arch has a number of processes that act as levers for movement and as guides and restraints of different types of movements. For each arch there are two transverse processes and one spinous process to which muscles and ligaments are attached; they act like levers. Two superior articular processes project upward from the arch and two inferior articular processes project downward. The articular facets on these processes form zygapophyseal joints (Fig. 1-3) that act like guide rails for movement in flexion, extension, and lateral bending; they also resist axial rotary movements.

The transverse processes are mostly long flat and "spatulate"; those of L3 are longest and those of L1 are shortest, but those of L5 are rounded, stout, and strong. Occasionally the transverse processes of L1 are enlarged with joints, forming lumbar ribs. Their anterior surfaces form parts of the attachments of psoas major and quadratus lumborum. The tips of the L5 transverse processes are attached to the iliac crests by iliolumbar ligaments, which contribute to the stability of the lumbosacral junction.

Lumbar transverse processes are costal elements; on the back of the base of each process is an accessory tubercle from which a small ligament bridges over the medial branch of a dorsal ramus to the mamillary process of the superior articular process. This forms a small tunnel for the nerve as it descends to supply the inferior part of a zygapophyseal joint and the superior recess of the next zygapophyseal joint.

The lumbar spinous processes are large and hatchet-shaped, projecting straight backward from the junction of the right and left laminae at a level 1 cm or more below the corresponding vertebral bodies. The wide gutter-shaped hollow on each side of the spinous processes, between the spinous and transverse processes, is filled by the postspinal muscles, the longitudinal erector spinae and the oblique multifidus. These are enclosed in a strong envelope formed by the posterior and middle layers of the lumbodorsal fascia, which take attachment from the tips of the spinous and transverse processes (Fig. 1-4). These muscles, within their fascial envelope, cover the backwardly projecting lumbar zygapophyseal joints, the laminae, and the ligamenta flava. All these muscles are extensors, but the deepest fascicles of the lumbar multifidus muscles also play an important role as stabilizers of the zygapophyseal joints. Detailed descriptions of all the muscles appear in Chapter 4.

## Spinal Ligaments

The anterior and posterior longitudinal ligaments form long ribbonlike ligaments that line the anterior and posterior surfaces of the vertebral bodies and intervertebral discs of the whole vertebral column. They form contrasting shapes: the broad ribbon of the anterior longitudinal ligament has parallel margins and the posterior longitudinal ligament is dentate in outline, widest at the discs and narrowest at the middle of each vertebral body. The anterior ligament is quite firmly attached to both the anterior vertebral periosteum and to the anterior annulus of each disc, but the posterior ligament is only attached to the discs. Its narrow part bridges over a slight concavity behind each vertebral body, which contains the anterior epidural veins where they connect to the basivertebral veins within each vertebral body. These longitudinal ligaments are continuous, in contrast to the ligaments of the vertebral arches. They are important structures because their fibers may bridge over several segments.

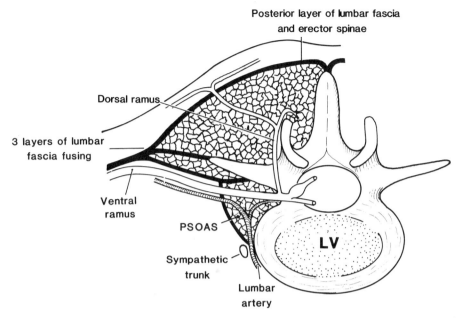

**Fig. 1-4.**   The three layers of the lumbar fascia enclosing the quadratus lumborum in a lateral compartment and the dorsal spinal muscles in a posterior compartment (showing erector spinae and multifidus as one muscle mass). The psoas is enclosed by its own psoas fascia. The division of the spinal nerve into dorsal and ventral rami and of the dorsal ramus into medial and lateral branches is shown. (Modified from Last,[79] with permission.)

While they are thinner than the anterior and posterior annulus of the disc, in the cervical spine they may form the last line of defense against instability, in severe flexion and extension injuries causing avulsion of a disc from an adjacent vertebral body.

The spaces between the laminae are bridged by ligamenta flava, which also form the anterior capsules of the zygapophyseal joints. The spinous processes are connected by oblique interspinous and supraspinous ligaments. So-called intertransverse ligaments are parts of the middle layer of the lumbar fascia.

## Ligamenta Flava

Ligamenta flava are yellow, elastic ligaments that are thickest in the lumbar region, where they are 2 to 3 mm thick. Medial to the zygapophyseal joints, their elastic fibers pass vertically between adjacent laminae and with the laminae they form the posterior boundary of the spinal canal. There may be a narrow midline cleft between the right and left halves of each ligamentum flavum. Over the anterior aspect of each zygapophyseal joint, the lateral fibers of the ligamentum flavum are directed obliquely upward and laterally to form the anterior capsule of the joint and the posterior boundary of the intervertebral foramen. The elasticity of these ligaments maintains the smooth regular contour of the spinal canal in all postures of the spine and they maintain congruity in the anterior parts of the zygapophyseal joints by holding the articular surfaces together. They are stretched by flexion and contract and thicken during extension, without buckling, in the healthy spine. If an intervertebral disc loses its normal thickness or a vertebral body loses its normal height with aging, the ligamentum flavum will thicken as it shortens and may lose its elasticity with aging.[10,11] The more fibrous ligamentum flavum of an elderly person may buckle forward on extension, narrowing the spinal canal. Apparent thickening of the ligamentum flavum is sometimes due to underlying bony hypertrophy in the superior articular process of the zygapophyseal joints. These ligaments help to resist excessive flexion of the spine, but they are less important in restraining excessive flexion than the integrity of congruous zygapophyseal articular facets.[12]

### Supraspinous and Interspinous Ligaments

The supraspinous ligaments and most of the interspinous ligaments are fibrous or collagenous structures, reinforced by the most medial fibers of the erector spinae and by the interspinales. They extend down to L5 but not below L5, except as fibrous muscle insertions. The fibers of each interspinous ligament run upward and backward from one spinous process to the next, as a double layer with a narrow interval between them.[13] Anteriorly they are continuous with the ligamentum flavum on each side. These ligaments appear designed to limit flexion but posterior release experiments[12] suggest that their role in this respect is less than that of other posterior element structures.

## The Spinal Canal and the Intervertebral Foramen

The lumbar spine doubles as a mobile supporting structure and as a conduit for the lower end of the spinal cord and the cauda equina. The lower part of the spinal cord is a vital part of the central nervous system, containing control centers for reflex activity in the lower limbs, bladder, bowel, and reproductive organs. It is also a pathway for motor and sensory communication between the brain and the lower parts of the body. The lumbar enlargement of the cord lies in the thoracolumbar region of the spinal canal and it tapers to a point (the conus), which generally terminates at the level of the L1–L2 disc. Occasionally, it ends slightly higher or some distance lower in the range between T12 and L3; in spina bifida, an abnormal cord may terminate lower than normal if it is tethered to the meninges. The cauda equina is an important part of the peripheral nervous system, collecting the motor and sensory roots into the lumbar and sacral spinal nerves to supply the lower limbs, bladder, and bowel, as well as other pelvic and perineal structures. The cord and cauda equina are contained within the dural sac, which is lined on its inner aspect by the arachnoid membrane containing the cerebrospinal fluid in the subarachnoid space. The dural sac containing the subarachnoid space terminates at the S2 level, marked by the posterior superior iliac spines (Fig. 1-5). Above this level, there is an angled hollow at the lumbosacral junction and the lumbar spinous processes can be readily palpated.

The nerve rootlets that form the spinal nerves arise in parallel continuous lines along the front and along the back of the spinal cord. Sets of these anterior or posterior rootlets converge to form single anterior and posterior roots, which in turn unite to form a spinal nerve. The posterior roots contain about three times as many axons as the anterior roots. The anterior roots transmit the somatic motor fibers from the anterior horn cells (lower motor neurons) and sympathetic preganglionic fibers, from the lateral horn of gray matter in the spinal cord, to the sympathetic ganglia. The dorsal roots transmit a variety of sensory fibers. Those parts of the nerves within the dural sac do not have the strong connective tissue coverings, which they will receive as they pierce the dura to enter the intervertebral foramina. Therefore, the rootlets are not as strong as the spinal nerves and are more vulnerable to injury. The cerebrospinal

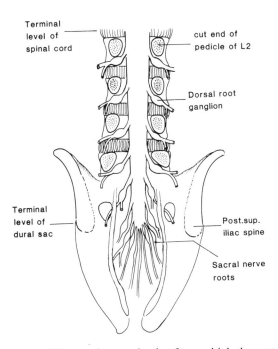

**Fig. 1-5.** A dorsal view of the lumbosacral spine from which the vertebral arches have been removed shows the spinal canal containing the dural sac, which terminates opposite the posterior superior iliac spines. The dura fuses with the outer fibrous covering (epineurium) of each spinal nerve as it exits the dural sac.

fluid that bathes the roots supplies some nutrition to the nervous tissue of the cord and provides some protection from mechanical forces. When the nerve roots pierce the arachnoid and the dura they are surrounded by a short funnel-shaped extension of the arachnoid into the medial end of the foramen. This contains cerebrospinal fluid and can be outlined in a myelogram. The sleeves of arachnoid end in the intervertebral foramina, but the dura continues as a connective tissue sleeve along each spinal nerve, forming its epineurium. Peripheral nerves are tough structures because a high proportion of each nerve is connective tissue. They also contain many small vessels and can become red, swollen, and edematous when "irritated" by noxious mechanical or chemical stimuli. Within the foramen, or in the lateral recess of the spinal canal, each dorsal nerve root forms a fusiform swelling (the dorsal root ganglion). This contains the cell bodies of all sensory neurons, both somatic and visceral, whether they be from skin, muscle, bone, viscera, blood vessels, or the dura itself.

The dimensions and shape of the spinal canal vary according to spinal level and age.[14] At L1, the canal is usually oval in transverse section; at this level, the average sagittal diameter of the bony canal is 20 mm and the average coronal (interpedicular) diameter is 25 mm.[15] Below L1 the canal changes to a triangular outline. It becomes trefoil in shape in older people, especially at lower lumbar levels,[16,17] due to facet hypertrophy and osteophytosis bulging the lateral part of the ligamentum flavum forward. At the same time as these age changes in the facets, there is likely to be some age-related shortening of the osteoligamentous column. These common changes, together with posterior disc bulging or herniation, and lordotic posture with anterior buckling of the ligamentum flavum, collectively or individually reduce the space in the nerve root canals and may produce spinal stenosis, with compression of the nerves. In young adults, nucleus pulposus tissue is soft enough to be extruded from a ruptured disc, when it may impinge on and deform the subarachnoid space. This would be visible on a myelogram as a "filling defect."

**Vessels**

The dural sac, containing the cauda equina, is circular in cross section and only occupies the central part of the triangular spinal canal. The epidural or extradural space contains fat, the spinal nerves descending obliquely to their foramina, and a rich plexus of valveless veins. This internal vertebral venous plexus has widespread connections. It receives at least two veins through each intervertebral foramen and connects to the central marrow of each vertebral body by a basivertebral vein. Within the anterior epidural space the venous plexus forms a ladder pattern of veins. Two longitudinal channels (one on each side) have lateral communications through each intervertebral foramen and a cross communication to each basivertebral vein. At the upper end of the spinal canal the longitudinal veins are continuous with intracranial venous sinuses;

below, they are connected by sacral veins to pelvic venous plexuses. At each intervertebral foramen the plexus is connected to the regional segmental veins: the lumbar, posterior intercostal, and vertebral veins. Blood can flow in any direction in the plexus, according to regional differences in pressure, affected by respiration, coughing, and straining. If a vena cava is blocked, it can form a bypass route for the venous return to the heart. Cancer cells may spread by it from a primary tumor (e.g., in the breast or prostate) to the vertebral spongiosa, giving vertebral metastases, with the possibility of pathologic fracture.

Small arteries also enter the spinal canal from each intervertebral foramen to supply the vertebrae, meninges, and cauda equina. These are mostly very small, but they divide into three branches,[18] one to supply the vertebral body, one to follow the nerve roots (radicular branch), and one to supply the posterior elements. Like the veins they form a ladder pattern of anastomosis with their neighboring vessels in the anterior epidural space. The radicular branches supply the nerve roots and follow them through the dura and arachnoid into the subarachnoid space. One of the radicular arteries, in the thoracolumbar region, is very important because it supplies the lower thoracic and lumbosacral parts of the spinal cord. This "great spinal artery" of Adamkiewicz usually arises from a lower thoracic posterior intercostal artery (most often T10 on the left), and it anastomoses with the anterior and posterior spinal arteries of the spinal cord.[19,20] Because its origin is variable, it may be at risk in operations on aortic aneurysms. If it is inadvertently damaged, paraplegia is the likely result.

The intervertebral foramina are regularly spaced lateral openings from the spinal canal. Each lies between the pedicles above and below, with a vertebral body and intervertebral disc in front, and a zygapophyseal joint, covered by the ligamentum flavum, behind. The average adult foramen is oval and measures 15 mm in height and 8.5 mm in its widest anteroposterior extent, except at L5–S1, which is more rounded and is 12 mm from front to back and 13 mm in height. The space is widest above where it contains the nerve; the lower part is relatively narrow and occupied by veins, which may be separated from the upper part by a small transforaminal ligament. In addition to a spinal nerve, each lumbar foramen transmits a small branch of segmental artery, two or more quite large veins, and a small recurrent branch of the spinal nerve called a sinuvertebral nerve. The sinuvertebral nerves supply the dura and posterior longitudinal ligament, and participate in the supply of the outer lamellae of the posterior annulus fibrosus. In the sacrum there are anterior and posterior foramina that separately transmit the ventral and dorsal rami of the sacral nerves. The anterior sacral foramina also transmit small lateral sacral arteries and veins.

The lumbar foramina are short canals, which range in length from 9 mm at L1–L2 to 2 cm at L5–S1,[14] in proportion to the thickness of the pedicles above and below. Each nerve-root canal receives the spinal nerve roots in their dural sheath, in the lateral recess of the spinal canal, and passes obliquely downward and laterally below the pedicle, into the upper part of the intervertebral foramen. In the medial part of the foramen, the anterior root and the posterior root (with its ganglion) unite to form a mixed spinal nerve and the sleeve of dura becomes continuous with the epineurium of the spinal nerve.[21] This nerve, containing motor, sensory, and sympathetic fibers, passes out through the wide upper part of the foramen, behind the lower part of the vertebral body and above the level of the intervertebral disc. It immediately divides into ventral and dorsal rami. The lumbar ventral rami form a plexus in the psoas muscle and participate with sacral ventral rami in the lumbosacral plexus, forming femoral, obturator, gluteal, and sciatic nerves to supply lower limb structures. The ventral rami of S1–L3 groove the anterior aspect of the sacrum as they pass laterally from their anterior foramina to join the lumbosacral trunk (L4–L5), which descends over the ala of the sacrum. These nerves are stretched fairly taut over the ala and anterior surface of the sacrum as they form the sciatic nerve, which passes out of the pelvis through the greater sciatic notch, then down behind the hip joint. When L4, L5, or S1 is entrapped, combined hip flexion and knee extension stretches the sciatic nerve and pulls on the entrapped nerve and its dural sheath, eliciting pain and reflex muscle spasm. The slump test is a more general test for dural irritation, depending on the same biomechanical principles.

Each dorsal ramus divides into medial and lateral branches: the lateral branch supplies spinal muscles and become cutaneous, supplying the skin of the low back and gluteal region; the medial branch winds around the articular pillar of the superior articular process and supplies two zygapophyseal joints.

The intervertebral foramen may be reduced in size by the same age-related and pathologic processes that affect the spinal canal. These include motion segment instability, with retrolisthesis of the upper vertebra,[5] disc thinning or vertebral end-plate collapse, lordotic posture, and osteophytosis of the zygapophyseal joint. The combination of Z joint osteophytes and reduction in height of the intervertebral foramen are the changes most likely to put the spinal nerve at risk of entrapment (Fig. 1-6). A herniated disc is likely to affect the nerve

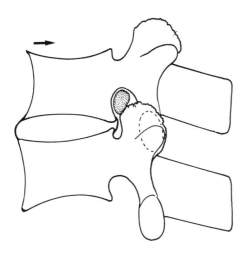

**Fig. 1-6.** Lower lumbar intervertebral foramen, with the narrowing that results from shortening of the column (whether from osteoporostic bowing of the endplates or thinning of the disc) and retrolisthesis of the upper vertebra associated with instability.

descending to the next intervertebral foramen, in the lateral recess of the spinal canal.

## Common Injuries to the Lumbosacral Spine

From our experience of sectioning over 200 lumbar spines and over 100 cervical spines from autopsies, a substantial proportion of them from acute injuries, we have observed a wide variety of bone and soft-tissue injuries. It is interesting to contrast the injuries in the two regions, because their different biomechanical behaviors result in different regional patterns of injury.[22]

The 45° orientation of cervical facets contrasts with the orientation of lumbar facets almost parallel to the long axis of the spine. Cervical movements, around a center of motion in the vertebral body below, are inevitably accompanied by translation between adjacent vertebrae, but the vertical lumbar facets severely limit translation, protecting the disc from shearing. Lumbar flexion and extension are mainly rocking movements of one vertebral body on another, accompanied by upward and downward gliding between the facets. The thickness of the disc can accommodate the very small amount of translatory movement. The relatively large forward slide of one cervical vertebra on the next vertebra, which accompanies cervical flexion, produces shearing forces within the disc. These forces of everyday life produce transverse fissures in the discs, first at the uncovertebral joints, formed during adolescence, and then extending transversely through the whole posterior half of the disc in young adults. Fissuring in lumbar discs is seldom present in young adults. When it appears in later life it is less universal, and usually less obvious, than in cervical discs.

The results of trauma to the lumbar or cervical spines, in high speed acceleration or deceleration injuries, are influenced by the different regional biomechanics described. In very rapid flexion of the neck, the facets slide freely to end range, leaving only a small part of their articular surfaces in contact, and most of the bending and translatory force in the motion segment is absorbed by the discs. At the same time, the posterior muscles and the posterior ligamentous complex are strained. In severe flexion injuries, the posterior muscles tear, the facets may be dislocated, and the disc may be avulsed from the adjacent vertebra, with a high risk of cord damage. Quite frequently there is no bony injury. In less severe flexion injuries, an incomplete transverse tear appears at the discovertebral junction, without damage to the longitudinal ligaments, and ligamentous and muscular strains, short of tearing, occur in zygapophyseal capsules, adjacent ligaments, and postvertebral muscles. The neck is less well protected by muscles in cervical extension, but the likelihood of fracture is even less than with flexion, except at end range, where the tips of articular processes may be broken. The main injuries are to the discs, which tear, and to the vascular synovial folds within the facet joints, which are bruised. Extension injuries are often multilevel injuries.

By contrast, thoracic or lumbar injuries more frequently result in fractures. In deceleration-flexion, the vertical lumbar facets absorb the first force. Small facet fractures, with avulsion of the mamillary process or infraction of the articular surface of the superior articular process, are common. In more severe injuries a facet may fracture across its base, or through the pars interarticularis, as in spondylolysis. If the facets are not severely fractured in the flexion injury, the motion segment "hinges" on the facets and the anterior elements are compressed. This often results in a wedge compression fracture, most frequently of T12 or L1; alternatively, there is a compression fracture of a vertebral endplate, with intradiscal bleeding or a compression injury to the intervertebral disc itself, with disc contusion or traumatic herniation, but the disc is protected from severe disruption as long as the facets remain intact. Disc tears are less frequent than in the cervical region because there is less translation. Extension injuries to the lumbar spine are uncommon in motor vehicle accidents, but they may occur as a result of occupational or sporting injuries. The inferior facets are driven down against the lamina below and may cause spondylolysis through the isthmus of the pars interarticularis. This injury may occur either as an acute injury (e.g., in Australian football) or as a result of a repeated sporting activity that consistently stresses the low back, such as fast bowling in cricket, or gymnastics.[23]

## Muscles and Fasciae

The lumbar postvertebral muscle masses (erector spinae or multifidus) are larger than the space between the spinous and transverse processes. Thus the tips of the spinous processes are palpated in a longitudinal midline groove between the two muscle masses, and the tips of the transverse processes lie deep to the lateral parts of the muscles. The middle layer of the lumbar fascia passes laterally from the tips of the transverse processes, separating quadratus lumborum from erector spinae, and the posterior layer of the lumbar fascia extends laterally from the tips of the spinous processes, the two layers enclosing the erector spinae and multifidus muscles (see Fig. 1-4). The term *erector spinae* is reserved for the superficial, longitudinally running fibers that span many segments. The muscle erector spinae forms a compact mass in the lumbar region and splits into three columns (the spinalis, longissimus, and iliocostalis), as it ascends into the thoracic region. Multifidus lies deep and medial to erector spinae. The fascicles of multifidus run in an oblique direction and only span two or three segments as they ascend or descend. The deeply placed zygapophyseal joints are covered by the fascicles of multifidus, which are in turn covered by the erector spinae and the posterior, aponeurotic lumbar fascia. The deeper parts of multifidus may play an important role in stabilizing the zygapophyseal joints.[24,25] Detailed descriptions of spinal musculature appear in Chapter 4.

## Sacrum and Sacroiliac Joints

The central part of the bony sacrum is formed by the fusion of five centra but the adult sacrum still contains remnants of intervertebral discs within the bone. The transverse elements fuse to form the alae and lateral masses. The adult sacrum is triangular with its broad base directed upward and forward and its apex directed downward and joined to the coccyx below. Its anterior surface is smooth, with transverse ridges where the discs would have been, with four pairs of anterior sacral foramina between the fused bodies and the lateral masses, opposite the transverse ridges (Fig. 1-7). The rough posterior surface shows a midline spinous crest, and two lateral articular crests with the posterior sacral foramina between the central and lateral crests. Inferiorly, above the joint with the coccyx, the posterior wall of the spinal canal is deficient in an inverted V shape called the sacral hiatus. This gives access to the lower end of the spinal canal, which is filled by fat and veins, the dural sac ending at the S2 level.

On each lateral sacral surface, two areas can be distinguished: a smooth articular area in front and a rough ligamentous area behind. The rough posterior area is for the attachment of the enormously strong sacroiliac ligaments, which suspend the sacrum between the two ilia. The smooth articular surface of the sacroiliac joint is auricular in shape. It may be described as having two "limbs": an upper shorter limb directed upward and backward and a longer lower limb

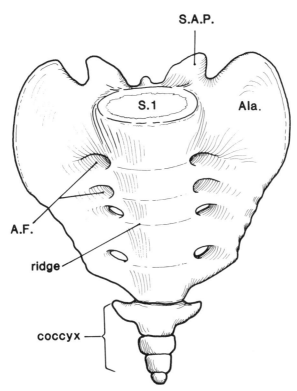

**Fig. 1-7.**  Anterior and superior surfaces of a female sacrum. The superior articular process *(SAP)* of S1 and the anterior sacral foramina *(AF)*, which transmit the ventral rami of sacral spinal nerves, are designated. The ridges mark the positions of fusion between the five centra forming the central part of the sacrum. The ala, or upper end of the sacral lateral mass, is crossed by the lumbosacral trunk as it descends to form the sciatic nerve with S1, S2, and S3.

directed downward and backward. The superior surface of the S1 vertebral body of the sacrum bears the weight of the head, trunk, and upper limbs, transmitted through the lumbar vertebral column. This axial force would tend to rotate the sacrum forward, but this tendency is resisted by the sacrotuberous and sacrospinous accessory ligaments (Fig. 1-8), which bind the lower parts of the sacrum and coccyx down to the lower parts of the hip bones. Equally important in preventing or reducing sacroiliac movement are the reciprocal irregularities of the adult articular surfaces, together with the great strength of the posterior and interosseous sacroiliac ligaments (Fig. 1-9). The cartilage-covered articular surfaces are smooth and flat in the child, where rotary movement in the sagittal plane is possible. They become irregular in the mature adult due to the growth of a ridge or ridges on the iliac surfaces. This makes movement almost impossible in most adults.[26,27] In young females, 8° of movement is said to be possible,[28] and during pregnancy there is a degree of ligamentous laxity, probably due to the effect of the hormone relaxin on fibrous tissues.

The sacroiliac joints should not be considered in isolation because they are part of a three-joint complex in the pelvis. A sacroiliac joint cannot rotate without some corresponding movement at the symphysis pubis. Bilateral differ-

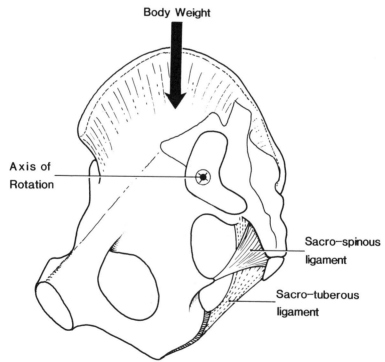

**Fig. 1-8.** Body weight, acting through the lumbar vertebral column, would tend to rotate the sacrum forward if its lower end were not "anchored" by the sacrospinous and sacrotuberous ligaments. The ligaments resist the anterior rotational effect of body weight.

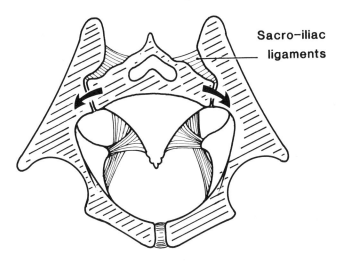

**Fig. 1-9.** The sacrum is "suspended" between the two ilia by very strong posterior sacroiliac ligaments. Body weight tends to compress the ilia against the sacrum at the sacroiliac joints.

ences in sacroiliac joint posture are sometimes seen on radiographs of adolescents who have a leg length discrepancy. Pelvic torsion occurs when one sacroiliac joint is rotated more than the other and a "step" is apparent between the right and left pubic bones on the anteroposterior radiograph.[29,30] The sacroiliac joint is deeply situated, medial to the posterior iliac spines, which are readily palpable, but the joint itself is difficult to palpate because it is covered by muscles.

## Joint: Mobility with Stability

The multisegmental construction of the spine combines strength with stability. The lumbar vertebral column is required to provide stability in loadbearing and a wide range of mobility. Mobility and stability are usually in inverse proportion to each other, but these two apparently contradictory requirements are achieved in the lumbar vertebral column by virtue of its multisegmental construction. Each mobile segment, consisting of one intervertebral disc and two zygapophyseal joints, has only a limited range of movement and therefore remains stable. However, the five lumbar mobile segments together provide large ranges of sagittal and coronal plane movement. There is a limited range of axial rotation, which is partly dependent on coupling with coronal and sagittal plane movement.

### Articular Triad

The intervertebral disc and its two associated synovial joints combine in a unique way to give strength and stability to the mobile segment, but at the same time provide it with adequate mobility.

The intervertebral disc provides the main strength and stiffness of the motion segment, but its slight compliance and its considerable thickness ensure a useful movement range. It is a structure of unique simplicity in concept, but with a complexity of fine structure in its parts. Though generally described as formed by the annulus fibrosus and the nucleus pulposus, it should be regarded as including the cartilage plates, which bind and unite it to the vertebral bodies above and below.[31] The cartilage plates and the inner annulus fibrosus form a continuous envelope enclosing the nucleus pulposus (see Fig. 1-2).

**Annulus Fibrosus.** The annulus fibrosus consists of 12 to 16 concentric lamellae, with two distinguishable parts. The outer fibrous annulus contains relatively little proteoglycan and attaches to the vertebral rim. The inner fibrocartilaginous annulus is rich in proteoglycan and is continuous with the cartilage plates. The annular lamellae have an outwardly convex arrangement and are arranged in spiralling sheets around the circumference of the nucleus. The parallel fibers of each successive sheet of collagen bundles cross the fibers of the next sheet at an interstriation angle of about 57°.[32] The arrangement is not unlike that of the layering of an onion and is similar to the architecture of collagen in the osteons of compact bone. In the intervertebral disc the arrangement gives the annulus great strength. The outer fibrous lamellae of the annulus are firmly embedded in the bony vertebral rim. The inner fibrocartilaginous lamellae of the annulus are shown by polarized light stidues[31] to be directly continuous with the horizontal lamellae of the ''hyaline'' cartilage plates above and below the nucleus. The inextensible but deformable envelope formed by the annulus and the cartilage plates encloses the elliptical sphere, which is the nucleus pulposus.

The cartilage plates not only form an essential part of the envelope containing the nucleus, they are also firmly bound to the end surface of the vertebral body; they were developmentally parts of the cartilage model of the vertebral body, and are sometimes described as its unossified epiphyses. In the growing individual, growth plates at the junction of the bony vertebral body and the cartilage plate ensure growth in vertebral height. The cartilage plates are best regarded as those parts where the vertebra and disc interlock. Observations of injuries suggest that they are more firmly attached to the disc than to the vertebra, particularly in children where injury may result in a cleft at the cartilage plate vertebral end-plate junction.[22]

**Nucleus Pulposus.** The infant nucleus pulposus is a viscous-fluid structure with a clear, watery matrix.[3] Its appearance and consistency are quite different in the adult, where the nucleus contains many collagen bundles, has a reduced water content, and is difficult to dissect clear of its envelope. However, the healthy young adult nucleus behaves hydrostatically as a viscous fluid, which is incompressible and changes shape freely.[33] By changing shape the disc acts as a joint. The nucleus receives axial loads and redistributes them centripetally to the surrounding envelope, dissipating vertical forces in horizontal directions and acting as a shock absorber. The elliptical envelope around the nucleus, formed by the inner annulus and cartilage plates with a high proteoglycan content, deforms under axial loading. The proteoglycan molecules resist this deformation, reinforcing the shock-absorbing function of the nucleus.

The outer six layers of the lumbar annulus are innervated, but nerves do not usually penetrate beyond its outer third; no nerves have been demonstrated in the nucleus or the cartilage plates.[34-36] The outer annulus and cartilage plates are vascular in the fetus and infant, but their vascularity is progressively reduced with maturation.[3,37] In the adult a few vessels penetrate the calcified cartilage layer binding the cartilage plate to the bony centrum and a few small blood vessels persist in the surface layers of the annulus.[38-40] The avascular nucleus contains a sparse cell population in a watery matrix rich in proteoglycans (PGs). The sparse cell population of the adult nucleus receives its nutrition by diffusion from the few vessels in the outer annulus and from the few vascular buds that penetrate the cartilage plates for a short distance from the vertebral marrow spaces.[40]

The nucleus is held under tension within the envelope formed by the annulus and cartilage plates. This tension (or turgor) is dependent on the inextensibility of the envelope, and is produced by the chemical force resulting from the water-attracting capacity of the PG macromolecules. These macromolecules make space for, or "imbibe," water. In recumbent posture, at night, the disc tends to swell, and during the course of each day when the disc is compressed by axial loading it "creeps" by squeezing out water, to become slightly thinner. All individuals lose about 17 mm of height due to axial weightbearing during the day, and regain it when recumbent at night.[3] At autopsy, discs that are cut open swell quite soon by absorbing water from the atmosphere. At discography, healthy discs actively resist the injection of contrast, while degenerate discs allow the contrast to enter with relatively little resistance.

## Zygapophyseal (Facet) Joints

Zygapophyseal joints are the principal guiding and restraining mechanism of the mobile segment. Although the disc is the strongest part of the motion segment, the zygapophyseal joints are essential to protect the lumbar discs from the rotational and translational strains that would damage the disc. Without the zygapophyseal joints the mobile segment would become unstable. The two zygapophyseal joints permit movement to occur in the sagittal and coronal planes, but they restrain axial rotation, and bring flexion to a halt at the end of the physiologic range.[12,41,42] They also widen the axial load-bearing base. In normal erect posture they bear 15 to 20 percent of axial loading.[33] This load-bearing function is larger in the flexed spine, particularly when lifting loads. The zygapophyseal joints can also be sources of back pain when their fibrous capsules or synovial folds are irritated.

**Joint Anatomy.** The zygapophyseal joints[6,43] are formed between the medially facing superior articular processes and the laterally facing inferior articular processes of the vertebra above. They are described as having plane or flat articular surfaces, but flat facets are relatively uncommon. The superior articular facets are usually concave in the horizontal plane, enclosing the smaller convex inferior articular facets, and resemble segments of the surface of a cylinder. Both articular surfaces are approximately vertically oriented, parallel to the long axis of the spine, although they may show a slight forward slope.

From the functional point of view, it is best to consider the facets as biplanar (see Fig. 1-3). The anterior third of each superior articular process is oriented close to the coronal plane and may be called the coronal component. This part prevents or severely limits forward translation of the upper vertebra in flexion and helps to control flexion. The posterior third is oriented close to the sagittal plane and may be called the sagittal component; it restrains or prevents axial rotation (Fig. 1-10). The articular surfaces of the superior articular process may be curved in a regular concavity, but not infrequently the coronal and sagittal components are distinct and meet at an angle greater than 90°; in transverse sections, the joints resemble a boomerang. The lumbar zygapophyseal joints show a gradual change in orientation from L1 down to L5: the sagittal component is largest in L1–L2 and the coronal component is largest in L5–S1. The upper lumbar and midlumbar joints are more consistently biplanar, while the lower joints are often truly planar (Fig. 1-11).

The joint is enclosed by a fibrous capsule posteriorly, and the elastic ligamentum flavum forms its anteromedial capsule (see Fig. 1-3). The posterior

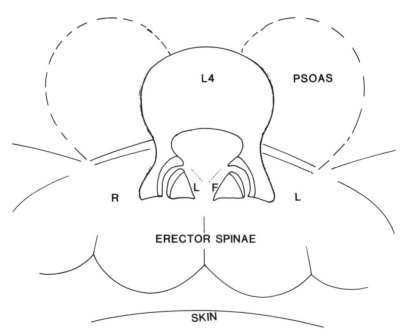

**Fig. 1-10.**   This tracing from a CT scan shows soft-tissue outlines of psoas, lateral and medial parts of erector spinae, and the outlines of the L3–L4 zygapophyseal joints. The "joint space" (articular cartilage) and the compact bone of the subchondral bone plate with its coronal and sagittal components are distinguished. *LF,* ligamentum flavum.

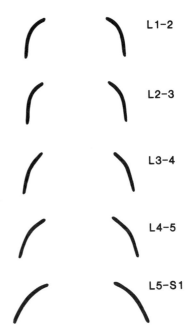

**Fig. 1-11.**    The segmental variation in the orientation of lumbar zygapophyseal joint planes is shown based on tracings from CT scans. It should be noted that there is a good deal of variation in structure between individuals. (From Taylor and Twomey,[6] with permission.)

capsule is frequently directly continuous with the posterior margin of the articular cartilage lining the superior articular facet. This capsular attachment gives the appearance of extending the concave socket for the convex inferior facet. The capsule is not as tight posteriorly as it is anteriorly, and depends on multifidus for "tensioning" (Fig. 1-12); it is quite loose above and below at the superior and inferior joint recesses.[6,43,44] A neurovascular bundle lies close to, and may be seen entering, each joint recess, where a large, vascular, fat-filled synovial fold extends from the inside of the fibrous capsule, projecting for a short distance between the articular surfaces. In young healthy joints, these vascular fat-pads adapt easily to the changing shape of the joint cavity in movement, but with aging, or after injury, they become fibrous, especially at the tips where they have been repeatedly compressed between the articular surfaces.[45] A variety of synovial, fibrofatty, or fibrous fringes extend around each joint as space fillers, from a base on the articular capsule to an apex projecting between the articular surfaces. The vascular fat-pads in the articular recesses of the lower lumbar and lumbosacral joints are particularly large,[44] and contrary to popular belief,[46] they are innervated by small nerves, which contain vasomotor fibers and also fibers that are separate from blood vessels, may contain substance P, and are probably both sensory and nociceptive.[47]

Small vertical ridges or tubercles, close to the posterior articular margin of each superior articular process, are termed the *mamillary tubercles*. These are formed by the attachments of the lumbar fascicles of multifidus. A lumbar fascicle of multifidus descends obliquely from the base of a spinous process two segments above, to the lateral margin of each joint (see Fig. 1-12). It uses

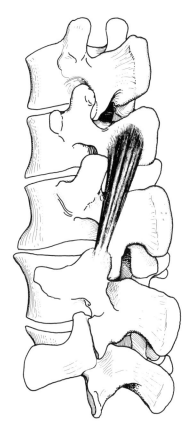

**Fig. 1-12.** Based on dissection studies, a single fascicle of the lumbar multifidus is shown descending obliquely from the spinous process of L2 to the mamillary tubercle on the superior articular process of L4, with some capsular insertion at the superior part of the L3–L4 joint.[25] This is one unit of a larger, more complex muscle. This obliquity of this deep fascicle would allow it both to extend the joints and to exert a small rotary force at the two mobile segments it crosses, but its principal function is probably as a fixator or stabilizer at the L3–L4 zygapophyseal joint. This view contrasts with most textbook descriptions. (From Taylor and Twomey,[6] with permission.)

this attachment to control joint posture and maintain congruity in the posterior sagittal component of the zygapophyseal joint.[6] This action is somewhat analogous to the rotator cuff function at the shoulder joint. Like the rotator cuff muscles, multifidus is partly inserted into the joint capsule. Observations on postmortem lumbar spines suggest that it helps to maintain joint congruity, because the posterior capsule is slack and the posterior joint surfaces separate slightly when the muscle is removed.[6,41]

The sagittal component of the joints appears well designed to block axial rotation around the usual axis of rotation near the posterior surface of the intervertebral disc, but some axial twisting is possible, as measurement studies show.[48] This movement is severely limited when individual mobile segments are tested in rigid experimental conditions, but when torque is applied to the whole lumbar spine, the resultant movement is a combination of true axial rotation with some coupled sagittal and coronal plane movements.

The function of the coronal components of the joints in limiting flexion is less well known. Posterior-release studies show that loading of these joints, by the forward translational force that accompanies flexion, is the single most important restraint to flexion at end range, and is more important than tension in the posterior ligaments in bringing flexion to a halt.[4] The chondromalacia that selectively occurs in the coronal components of the joints confirms that these are subject to greater compressive loads than the sagittal components.[6]

## Lumbosacral Joints

The anterior surface of the sacrum is normally inclined at an angle of about 60° to the vertical plane, giving a sharp change in direction from the approximately vertically oriented lumbar spine. This angulation involves a division of the vertical weight-bearing force through the lumbar spine into two vectors: one obliquely downward and backward through the sacrum, and the other obliquely downward and forward parallel to the upper surface of S1. The anteriorly directed vector of the weight-bearing force exerts a shearing force on the lumbosacral joints.[9] This shearing force is resisted by (1) the two lumbosacral zygapophyseal joints; (2) the lumbosacral intervertebral disc; and (3) the iliolumbar ligaments. The lumbosacral facets are the most rigid structures of the motion segment and bear most of the shearing stress.

The loading from each lumbosacral zygapophyseal joint is transmitted upward through the inferior articular process of L5 and through the pars interarticularis of L5, a narrow isthmus of bone between its superior and inferior articular facets. This narrow bridge of bone is the weakest link in the chain, and it is the part most likely to fail under loading.[49] A fracture of the pars interarticularis is quite common and is called spondylolysis. Deprived of this bony support, the lumbar column is now supported by ligamentous structures only, principally the lumbosacral disc. The L5 vertebral body may separate from its arch and slip forward (olisthesis) due to creep, stretch, and fissuring in the tissues of the disc. This anterior displacement is termed *spondylolisthesis*. Spondylolysis is seen frequently in sports involving repetitive and sudden loading of the lumbosacral joints in extension. It is found in L5 most often, from childhood and adolescence onward, but it is not found in fetuses and infants. It may be either painful or asymptomatic. There may be a developmental component in its etiology (e.g., a developmentally narrow isthmus in the pars interarticularis), but it is fundamentally a stress fracture and is painful in those cases where it occurs as a result of an identifiable sporting injury; in these individuals it remains painful when stressed.

Spondylolisthesis is more likely to follow spondylolysis in young people (under 25 years of age) with compliant discs than in older people with stiff discs. Spondylolysis is not the only possible result of the particular stresses at the lumbosacral joints and in the lower lumbar spine. Degenerative changes in the lumbosacral articular triad and in the L4–L5 articular triad are also common. Intervertebral disc rupture with nuclear extrusion is most common in the lowest two intervertebral discs,[50] and zygapophyseal joint arthritis is also most common in the lumbosacral joints.[51]

Retrolisthesis of L4 on L5 is also quite common in a lumbar spine with degenerative changes of the mobile segment.

## DEVELOPMENT AND GROWTH OF THE LUMBAR SPINE AND RELATED PATHOLOGY

### General Principles

The processes of development and growth influence structure, function, and pathology of the lumbar vertebral column in a number of important areas. Malformations result from abnormal genetic, chemical, or mechanical influences on growth. By growth we mean measurable increase in size. This involves increase in cell numbers and cell size, increased production of matrix and fibers, or any combination of these. Prenatal growth is characterized by cell multiplication and postnatal growth principally, but not entirely by increases in cell size and cell products. Development also involves differentiation of cells (i.e., cells become more specialized and less versatile in their function as they multiply). Connective tissue cells have a self-differentiating capacity depending on their genetic program, position in the developing embryo, and contact and interaction with other cells or tissues and on local and systemic hormonal influences. Some cells produce diffusible chemical substances, which influence the development of neighboring tissues. Other tissues influence the development of neighboring tissues by mechanical pressure, but the control mechanisms for many aspects of growth are still not completely understood.[52]

### Summary of Early Development

Before there is any vertebral column, in the third week of embryonic life the axis of the flat embryonic disc is determined by the appearance and growth of the notochord between the ectoderm and the endoderm. The appearance and growth of the notochord defines the axis of the flat embryonic disc, and it can now be described as having head and tail ends. At about the same time, mesoderm, the third primary layer of the embryo, develops on each side of the notochord, between the ectoderm and the endoderm.

The notochord is a long, thin rod of primitive cells, which have the potential to influence the development of other cells around them. The notochord induces thickening of the adjacent dorsal ectoderm to form the neural plate, which grows rapidly, folding to form the neural tube. The notochord and neural tube extend from the head to the tail of the embryo and together they attract the migration and condensation of mesodermal cells around them in order to form the original blastemal vertebral column. The paraxial mesoderm alongside the notochord and neural tube is originally in the form of two continuous columns but before the blastemal vertebral column is formed the paraxial mesoderm segments into a large number of somites or blocks of mesoderm. The medial parts of these blocks of mesoderm (somites) on either side the notochord and neural tube are used as building material to form the blastemal column.

The notochord, the neural tube, and the columns of paraxial mesoderm on each side of them are the essential elements for the formation of the vertebral

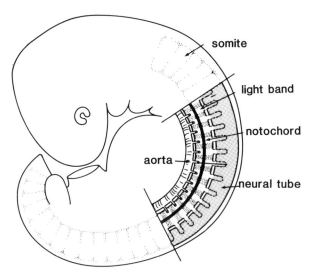

**Fig. 1-13.** A 7-mm crown-rump length (CRL) human embryo shows somites on the external surface. The center section shows median plane axial structures at the blastemal stage of vertebral development. The intersegmental branches of the aorta pass around the light bands, which are the promordia of the vertebral bodies. Neural processes grow around the neural tube to form the vertebral arches. The cylindrical notochord (black) passes through the centers of the light bands (primitive vertebrae) and dark bands (primitive intervertebral discs). (From Taylor and Twomey,[54] with permission.)

column. As the embryo grows, it folds and bends; the transverse folding of the flat disc encloses the endoderm to form a primitive gut tube and the longitudinal bending forms a ventral concavity with the primitive axial structures curved in a bow around the gut tube. Anterior to these structures, the primitive aorta runs down in the midline with blood already circulating to the area where the blastemal vertebral column will be formed (Fig. 1-13).

## Developmental Stages

The vertebral column will pass through three developmental stages: blastemal, cartilaginous, and osseous.

### Blastemal

The blastemal or mesenchymal column is formed around the notochord by the mesoderm from the ventromedial portions of the somites.[53–56] Although formed from segmented mesoderm, this original mesodermal condensation around the notochord is continuous and unsegmented. It resegments into alternate light and dark bands all the way along its length. Neural processes grow around the neural tube from each light band. The aorta, which lies immediately in front of the blastemal column, sends intersegmental branches around the middle of each light band. The light bands grow in height four times more rapidly than the adjacent dark bands.

## Cartilaginous

Each light band with its associated neural processes differentiates into a cartilaginous vertebra at the beginning of the fetal stage of development (2 months' gestation). This differentiation takes place throughout all the tissue of the light band at about the same time.[55] There is no evidence that there are two centers of chondrification as described by Schmorl and Junghanns.[57] The rapid differentiation and growth of the fetal cartilage models of vertebral bodies is accompanied by notochordal segmentation (Fig. 1-14). Each notochordal

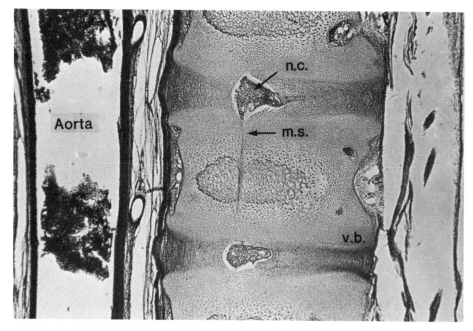

**Fig. 1-14.**   A median sagittal section of the thoracic spine of a 75-mm CRL (11th week) human fetus shows the cartilaginous stage of vertebral column development. At the center of each cartilage model of a vertebral body (*v.b.*), calcified zones with hypertrophied chondrocytes herald the formation of centers of ossification *(centra)*. The dark anterior rim around the calcified zone represents the first bone formation within the vertebral body. Vascular buds are seen within the posterior parts of the cartilaginous vertebrae. The notochord has segmented into notochordal aggregations *(n.c.)*, which will each form a nucleus pulposus. All that remains of the notochordal track through the vertebra is the mucoid streak *(m.s.)*.

segment will form a nucleus pulposus at the center of a dark band.[3] At the periphery of this primitive intervertebral disc, fibroblasts and collagen bundles appear in lamellar form. The cartilaginous stage of vertebral development is a short one. Soon, blood vessels grow into the cartilaginous vertebra, as centers of ossification appear.

### Osseous

Three primary centers of ossification are formed in each vertebra. Bilateral centers for the vertebral arch appear first, one for each half arch. The earliest vertebral-arch centers are in the cervicothoracic region, but the process rapidly extends up and down the column. The appearance of arch centers is generally sequential, with the most caudal appearing last, except that the appearance of midthoracic centers is delayed until all lumbar centers have appeared.[58] A single primary center for each vertebral body forms the centrum. There is no evidence that double centers appear in normal development of the centra, but a bilobed appearance is common in vertical sections through the plane of the notochord, due to a temporary inhibition of ossification in the immediate vicinity of the notochord.[3,59] The centra appear earliest near the thoracolumbar junction and then appear in sequence up and down the column.

The process of ossification extends through the cartilage model of each vertebra except for the growth plates, which persist to ensure continuing growth, and the cartilage plates on the upper and lower vertebral surfaces, which remain cartilaginous throughout life.

**Dorsal-Midline Growth Plate.** A single growth plate in the midline of the vertebral arch, dorsally (Fig. 1-15), which persists till about 1 year postnatally.

**Neurocentral Growth Plates.** Neurocentral growth plates persist on each side, between the arch and the centrum, until 3 to 7 years, ensuring growth of the spinal canal to accommodate growth of the spinal cord and cauda equina.

**Cartilage-Plate Growth Plates.** Growth plates at the upper and lower vertebral end-plates ensure growth in height of the vertebra. These growth plates are parts of the cartilage plates capping the cephalic and caudal surfaces of the vertebral body (Fig. 1-16). A rim of bone appears in the periphery of each cartilage plate between 9 and 12 years. This "ring apophysis" fuses with the vertebral body at 18 to 20 years in males,[60] and 2 years earlier in females (Fig. 1-17). An apophysis is comparable to an epiphysis, except that it does not itself contribute to growth.[53]

## Growth in Length of the Vertebral Column as a Whole

Growth is most rapid prenatally, and the rate of growth decreases progressively throughout infancy and childhood with a final increase in growth rate during the adolescent growth spurt. Measurements of sitting height at different ages can be used to chart postnatal growth in length of the spine.[41] The spine

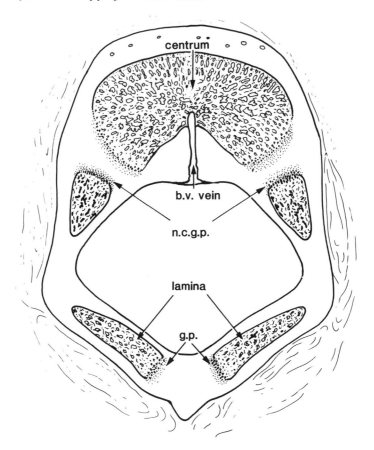

**Fig. 1-15.**    This tracing of a horizontal section of a human fetal lumbar vertebra (28.5-cm CRL, 32nd week) shows the centrum, the vertebral arches, the neurocentral growth plates *(ncgp),* and the vertebral arch growth plate *(gp).* There is only one center of ossification for each side of the vertebral arch, but the plane of the section has missed the bone of the middle part of each half arch, which appears as cartilage.

contributes 60 percent of sitting height. Sitting-height growth rate declines from 5 cm per year in the second year of life, to 2.5 cm per year at 4 years. It remains steady at this rate until 7 years, then declines further to 1.5 cm per year just before adolescence. The adolescent growth spurt for the spine begins at 9 years in females, lasting until 14 years, and peaking at 12 years with a sitting-height growth velocity of 4 cm per year. In males the growth spurt lasts from 12 to 17 years with a peak growth velocity of 4 cm per year at 14 years.

The thoracolumbar spine grows and matures earlier than the cervical or sacral regions. The lumbar spine grows more rapidly than the thoracic spine before puberty, but the thoracic spine grows more rapidly after puberty. Growth in length of the thoracolumbar spine is 60 percent more rapid in the female than in the male between the ages of 9 and 13 years (Fig. 1-18). After 13 years the

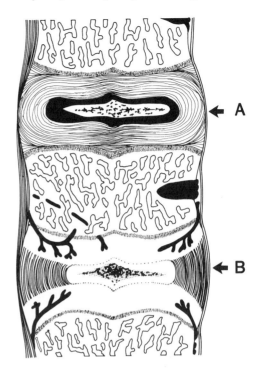

**Fig. 1-16.** (A) The intervertebral disc as it would appear in the median section of a full-term fetus when viewed by polarized light. There is direct continuity of the inner two-thirds of the annulus with the lamellar structure of the cartilage plates. (B) The lower disc as seen by normal transmitted light shows the outlines of the blood vessels supplying the disc. The angular indentations of the cartilage plates from the nucleus pulposus indicate where the notochordal track originally passed through the column. The growth plates of the vertebral end-plates are seen. The black area in the posterocentral vertebral body is the basivertebral vein. (From Taylor and Twomey,[54] with permission.)

male spine grows more rapidly. Sitting height and thoracolumbar spine length both reach 99 percent of their maximum by 15 years in girls and 17 years in boys. Risser's sign, involving the lateral appearance, medial excursion, and fusion of the iliac crest apophyses, is somewhat arbitrarily used to judge individual completion of spinal growth, which takes about 2 years from first appearance to fusion of the apophysis.[41] At completion of growth, the spine usually forms a greater proportion of the total stature in females than in males.

## Control Mechanisms in Normal and Abnormal Development

### Notochordal, Neural, Vascular, and Mechanical Influences

A summary of normal and abnormal aspects of development follows.

1. The notochord and neural tube induce formation of the blastemal vertebral column around them from the mesenchyme of the adjacent somites.[3]
2. Segmentation of the blastemal column is probably determined by the regular arrangement of intersegmental arteries within it.[61]
3. The notochord forms the original nucleus pulposus; after rapid growth

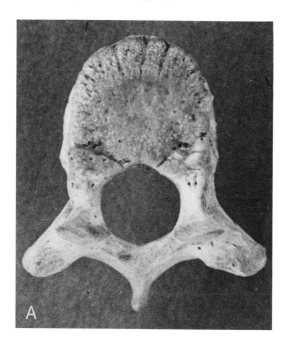

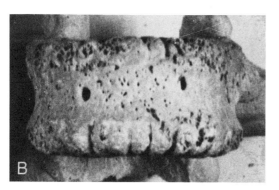

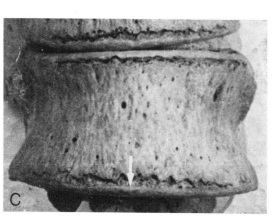

**Fig. 1-17.** **(A&B)** The superior and anterior surfaces of a juvenile thoracic vertebrae show the radial grooves due to the vascular canals entering the cartilage plates (Fig. **B**). **(C)** The lines of neurocentral fusion can also be seen. A fully grown vertebra shows the ring apophysis fusing with the centrum. Small vascular foramina pass between the apophysis and the centrum. (From Taylor and Twomey,[54] with permission.)

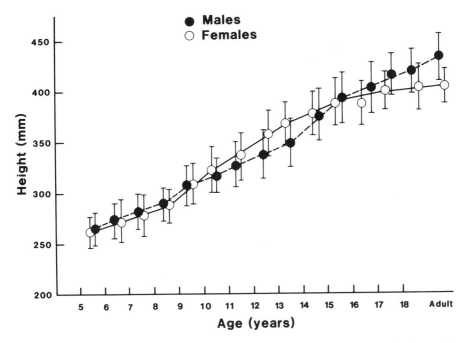

**Fig. 1-18.** Cross-sectional data for male and female growth in thoracolumbar spine length based on measurements in 1500 subjects.

of a notochordal nucleus pulposus in fetuses and infants, notochordal tissue atrophies and disappears during childhood.[3]

4. Persistence of live notochord cells in vertebrae may lead to the formation of chordomas in adults.[3] These rare, malignant tumors are usually seen in a high retropharyngeal or sacrococcygeal situation.

5. Anomalous vertebral development, such as block vertebrae, butterfly vertebra, or hemivertebra, may result from abnormal development of the notochord or the segmental blood vessels.[41]

6. When the notochordal track and vascular canals disappear from the cartilage plates of developing vertebrae, they leave weak areas, which are the sites of potential prolapse of disc material[54] into vertebral bodies (Schmorl's nodes).

7. Growth of the spinal cord and cauda equina influences growth of the vertebral arches and canal, just as brain growth influences skull-vault growth. An enlarged spinal cord results in an enlarged canal.[62] Spina bifida is a developmental anomaly, which varies from simple splitting of the skeletal elements of the vertebral arch (spina bifida occulta), which is common and innocuous, to complete splitting of skin, vertebral arch, and underlying neural tube (rachischisis) with associated neurologic deficits. In spinal bifida, abnormal development of the neural tube is probably the primary event and the skeletal defects are secondary.[62]

8. Asymmetric growth of right and left halves of the vertebral arches is very common in normal individuals. It produces slight rotation of the anterior elements to the left side in infancy and to the right side in adolescence. This probably determines the laterality (direction of curvature) of scoliosis in both its physiologic and progressive forms.[58]

9. Lumbar zygapophyseal joint facets grow backward from their lateral margins, and change from planar coronally oriented facets in infants, to biplanar facets with coronal and sagittal components in older children and adults. The coronal and sagittal components of the joint facets have different functions in controlling movements.[6,41]

10. When infants assume erect posture, there is an increase in the lumbosacral angle, increased lordosis, changes in the shape of intervertebral discs and the position of the nucleus pulposus. The vertebral bodies increase their anteroposterior growth rate, and the vertebral end-plates change their shape. These vertebral end-plates are convex in infants, but they become concave in children and adults. The end-plate concavity is opposite the maximum bulge of the nucleus.[1,63] Leg-length discrepancy and pelvic obliquity are associated with asymmetric concavities in the vertebral end-plates.

11. Sexual dimorphism in vertebral-body shape and spinal posture develops in childhood and adolescence in association with different hormonal influences and differences in muscle development.[64] These differences contribute to the greater prevalence of progressive scoliosis in females than in males.

12. Scheuermann's disease, with irregularity of the vertebral end-plates in adolescence, is associated with the development of multiple Schmorl's nodes.[41,65]

### Segmentation, Segmental, and Other Vertebral Anomalies

**Normal Segmentation.** A condensation of mesenchyme is formed around the notochord by the medial migration of cells from the sclerotomes, or ventromedial portions of the somites. Although the perichordal blastemal column is formed from segmented blocks of mesoderm, it is itself continuous and unsegmented. It resegments into alternate light and dark bands in such a way that the light bands, forming cartilaginous vertebrae, are at the level of the intersegmental branches of the aorta (see Fig. 1-13). The muscles, derived from the myotomes of the somites, bridge over the dark bands that form the discs, and are attached to upper and lower vertebral borders. The alternation of muscle and bone is essential to the proper function of the locomotor system.[55]

The intersegmental branches of the dorsal aorta have an important influence in vertebral-column resegmentation by virtue of their placement around the centers of the light bands, where they provide nutrition for the more rapid growth of the primitive vertebrae.[41] They are the only constant and regularly recurring structures in the blastemal vertebral column, and vascular anomalies may result in anomalies of segmentation.[61]

**Segmental Anomalies.** A unilateral hemivertebra results if one side of the vertebral body fails to develop. Normally there is only one primary center of ossification for the centrum, and it is likely that the anomaly originates during a preosseous stage of development. Absence of an intersegmental vessel on one side may give rise to a unilateral hemivertebra, which will be associated with a sharply angled congenital scoliosis after assumption of an erect posture. Absence of the anterior part of a vertebral body is also termed hemivertebra. The origin of this anomaly is difficult to explain. It gives rise to a congenital kyphosis (Fig. 1-19).

As the light bands grow rapidly, they appear to expel notochordal tissue into the more slowly growing intervertebral discs. Each notochordal segment forms a nucleus pulposus. Notochordal tissue grows rapidly by cell multiplication and production of mucoid matrix at the center of the fetal disc. Absence of a notochordal segment may cause the centra to fuse, forming congenital block vertebrae, because no nucleus pulposus forms to separate them.

**Later Notochordal Development, Chordoma, and Butterfly Vertebra.** The invasive nature of notochordal cells assists the rapid growth of the notochordal nucleus pulposus in the fetus and infant.[3] The notochordal cells produce substances that loosen and digest the inner margins of the surrounding envelope, incorporating these tissues into the expanding nucleus. The tissues of the envelope (annulus and cartilage plates) must grow rapidly just to keep pace with the "erosion" of their inner margins by the rapidly expanding nucleus. Notochordal

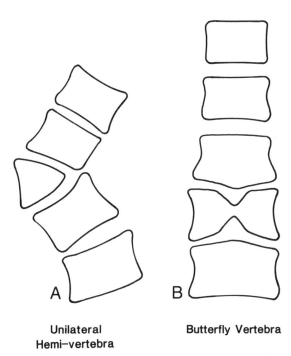

A    Unilateral
Hemi-vertebra

B    Butterfly Vertebra

**Fig. 1-19.** (A) A tracing of vertebral outlines from an anteroposterior radiograph shows the appearance of a unilateral hemivertebra, with consequent angled scoliosis. (B) A tracing from an anteroposterior radiograph shows a butterfly vertebra. Soft tissues are continuous through the vertebral body from one intervertebral disc to the next.

cells do not normally survive beyond early childhood—except perhaps deeply buried in the developing sacrum or possibly in Schmorl's nodes. Their fortunate demise during childhood is associated with the progressive decrease in vascularity of the surrounding tissues. If notochordal cells do survive, they may be "released" by trauma to the containing tissues, and begin to multiply again. The cells of malignant chordomas strongly resemble embryonic notochordal cells.[3]

The mucoid streak persists for a while in the cartilage models of the vertebrae as an acellular notochordal track, but when ossification of the centrum commences, it is usually obliterated. The mucoid streak has a temporary inhibiting effect on ossification of the centrum, which may have a bilobed appearance in vertical sections through the plane of the notochord. Persistence of parts of the notochordal track through the centrum is quite common in infancy,[3] but is probably rare after infancy. If a complete notochordal track persists, a butterfly vertebra is the result (see Fig. 1-19). Persistence of the notochordal track in infancy produces a misshapen vertebra with a nipple-shaped deformity (Fig. 1-20) of the vertebral end-plates. This may be responsible for the "Cupid's bow" appearance frequently seen in lower lumbar vertebral bodies in adults.[59,66]

### Other Vascular and Notochordal Influences

**Disappearance of Notochordal Cells from the Nucleus Pulposus.** The cartilage plates of infants have an excellent blood supply from the adjacent vertebral periosteum. This brings nutrition to the rapidly growing intervertebral disc.[31] The capillary plexuses of the vascular arcades approach close to the growing notochordal nucleus pulposus (see Fig. 1-16B). When the disc mass grows and its vessels disappear during childhood, the notochordal cells die off and are replaced by chondrocytes, cells better adapted to an avascular environment.

**Schmorl's Nodes.** The vascular canals are plugged by loose connective tissue, leaving channels of reduced resistance from near the nucleus to the peripheral vertebral spongiosa.[54] These channels, arching around the advancing ossification front of the centrum, inhibit ossification locally, causing a toothed or grooved surface on the vertebral end surfaces of adolescents (see Fig. 1-17 A & B).

The cartilage plates also have a consistently situated funnel-shaped defect on their nuclear aspect, where the notochordal track formerly penetrated the column, just behind the center of each vertebral end-plate (see Fig. 1-16). These notochordal weak points are the sites of central Schmorl's nodes and the vascular channels are probably the sites of peripheral Schmorl's nodes, either in the anterior spongiosa or forming a limbus vertebra (Fig. 1-21). They occur almost as frequently in adolescents and young adults as in older adults,[57] indicating their association with developmental factors.

Schmorl's nodes occur in thoracic and lumbar vertebrae of 38 percent of adult spines. The central nodes are an incidental finding, and may not cause

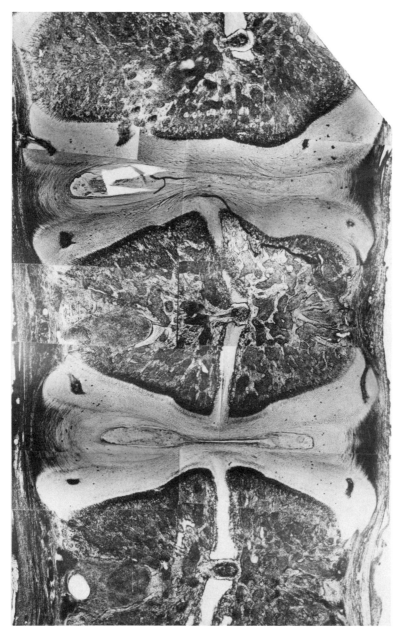

**Fig. 1-20.**  A montage of a median sagittal section of three thoracic vertebrae and two discs in a 1-month-old infant demonstrates continuity of the notochord track through the thoracic vertebral bodies. The notochordal track normally disappears from the vertebrae at about 20 weeks' gestation. The track may temporarily inhibit ossification, but in this case the deformities of the vertebral end-plates appear to result from attempts by the bone to "grow around" it. The nucleus pulposus is bilocular because of the bony deformity. (From Taylor,[59] with permission.)

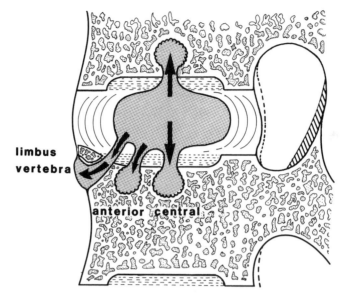

**Fig. 1-21.** Varieties of Schmorl's nodes (intraspongious disc prolapse). Central nodes are very common and occur through weaknesses in the cartilage plates left by the notochordal track (see Fig. 1-16). Peripheral nodes are less frequent and occur along the lines of vascular canals. Blood vessels atrophy during maturation and the vascular canals are plugged by loose connective tissue (see Figs. 1-16 and 1-17). Disc prolapse between the centrum and the ring apophysis is termed a *limbus vertebra*. Vascular canals are more plentiful anteriorly, and peripheral prolapses are usually anterior. Note: Central nodes are slightly posterior of center. (Modified from Taylor and Twomey,[54] with permission.)

any symptoms, but the anterior nodes may be associated with a traumatic incident, and the patient may complain of localized somatic back pain.[41]

**Scheuermann's Disease.** Multiple Schmorl's nodes, both large and small, are seen in Scheuermann's juvenile kyphosis, with a radiologic appearance of irregularity of the vertebral end-plates. Large anterior nodes are frequently seen, and are sometimes associated with anterior vertebral body collapse and wedging. The cause of the multiple Schmorl's nodes is uncertain, but one suggestion is that there may be an associated osteoporosis predisposing to vertebral end-plate weakness.[67] Alternatively, an "abnormally" vascular end-plate would have a correspondingly large number of "weak points" on attrition of the vessels, predisposing to a larger number of Schmorl's nodes than usual. We have noted an increased vascularity of vertebral end-plates containing Schmorl's nodes.[65]

## Scoliosis and Growth

When ossification centers appear in the fetal thoracic vertebral arches, those on the right commonly appear before the corresponding left centers. Taylor[68] advanced the hypothesis that in the fetal circulation, the better oxygenated blood from the left ventricle supplied the right midthoracic vertebral arches, and the less well oxygenated blood from the right ventricle, through the ductus arteriosus, supplied the left vertebral arches. This would occur through slow mixing of the two streams of blood from the proximal aorta and the ductus arteriosus.

This could explain why right arch centers often appear before corresponding left arch centers in midthoracic vertebrae.[58,68] This asynchrony in appearance of paired ossification centers correlates with measured asymmetry in infant vertebral arches (right greater than left), and with the observation that infantile thoracic scoliosis tends to be convex to the left (Fig. 1-22).

There is evidence of asynchronous maturation and growth of vertebral arches (right greater than left) in fetuses and infants persisting until closure of the neurocentral growth plates at 6 to 7 years, and of a reversal of this asynchrony and asymmetry in thoracic vertebral arches in older children (left greater than right) after closure of the neurocentral growth plates.

In older children and adolescents the left arches are larger than the corresponding right arches.[58] The consequent reversal of the twist of the midthoracic anterior elements from 7 years onward changes the direction of any spinal curvature so that it becomes convex to the right in the midthoracic spine. This change is related to asynchrony of closure of the neurocentral growth plates. At the same time, left-sided flattening of the anterior surfaces of midthoracic vertebrae begins to appear in older children, where the vertebral bodies are in contact with the aorta. The aortic pressure that flattens the anterior left surfaces of thoracic vertebral bodies also supplies the force that twists these vertebral bodies to the right.[41,58,68] The different position of the lumbar aorta on the anterior surfaces of L2 to L4 and the different shape of the lumbar vertebral bodies may be related to the observation that slight twisting of vertebral bodies

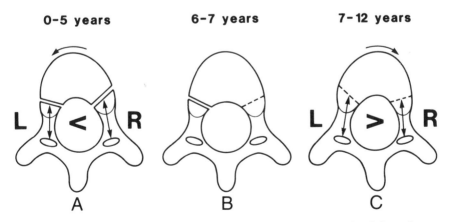

**0-5 years**        **6-7 years**        **7-12 years**

A                    B                    C

**Fig. 1-22.** Diagram representing the normal asynchrony in growth of thoracic vertebrae. **(A)** In later fetal and infant life, the right neural arch generally matures earlier than the corresponding left arch and therefore is slightly larger. **(B&C)** At neurocentral closure this symmetry is "reversed" by earlier closure on the right (see text). (From Taylor and Twomey,[41] with permission.)

to the left is more common here.[68,69] The asymmetries described are minor in nature. They accompany normal growth and probably determine the side of scoliosis, whether it be physiologic or progressive, but they are not by themselves the cause of progressive scoliosis. Other causes also operate in the multifactorial etiology of structural scolioses.

## Growth of Lumbar Zygapophyseal Joints

Lumbar zygapophyseal joints, like thoracic facets, are oriented in a coronal plane in fetuses and infants, but from late infancy onward, the lumbar articular facets grow in a posterior direction from their lateral margins, changing their shape and orientation. The original coronally oriented part remains, but a sagittal component is added to the joint by posterior growth from its lateral margins (Fig. 1-23). In the adult joints, from L1 to L2 to L3 to L4, the posterior two-thirds of the joint is approximately sagittal and the anterior third is approximately coronal (see Fig. 1-11). Remodeling at the junction of the two components usually makes the joints surfaces curved. In transverse sections or computed tomography (CT) scans the concave superior articular facet is seen to "embrace" the smaller convex inferior facet (see Fig. 1-10). Both curved articular surfaces are inclined approximately parallel to the long axis of the lumbar spine so that they resemble segments of cylinders. The lower lumbar joints are more nearly coronal in their overall orientation than the upper joints and tend to be flatter or less curved than the upper joints.[6,43,70]

The coronal and sagittal components of the articular surfaces relate to two different functions: restraint of flexion and restraint of axial rotation, respectively. The subchondral bone plate (SCP) of the superior articular facet becomes much thicker in its anterior coronal part than in the sagittal part, developing a wedge shape in transverse section, which reflects the greater physiologic compressive loading in the coronal part of the joint.[6] The SCP and articular cartilage reach their maximum thickness in young adult life. The adult hyaline cartilage is about 1 mm thick on each facet. It has a very smooth surface and the matrix and cells stain lightly and evenly in the healthy young adult joint. It is joined to the underlying SCP by a thin, regular calcified layer. In the growing joint the subchondral bone is very vascular, but with maturation this vascularity declines.

The articular cartilage is avascular and has no nerves, so that it is insensitive, except at its periphery, where it may be in continuity with the well-innervated joint capsule. It receives its nutrition from the synovial fluid that bathes it, the circulation of the fluid being aided by movements of the joint. From the fourth decade onward, there are changes in the staining characteristics of the articular cartilage of the coronal component of the joint, with hypertrophy of chondrocytes and increased intensity of staining of the matrix, especially in the mid-zone, suggesting a response to high compressive loading in these parts of the joints, probably in flexion.[6] The cellular changes eventually change the

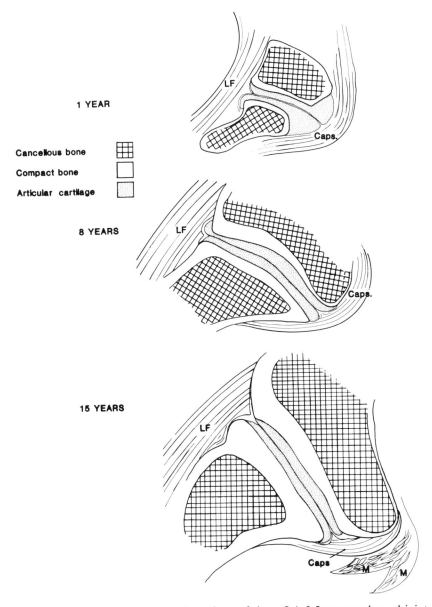

1 YEAR

Cancellous bone

Compact bone

Articular cartilage

8 YEARS

15 YEARS

**Fig. 1-23.** Tracings from horizontal sections of three L4–L5 zygopophyseal joints at 1, 8, and 15 years show the "rotation" of the joint plane from the coronal plane, toward the sagittal plane during growth. The concave anterior facet is on the superior articular process of the lower vertebra. The convex facet is on the inferior articular process of the upper vertebra. Note that the anteromedial capsule is formed by the ligamentum flavum *(LF)*, and that multifidus *(M)* partly insets into the posterior fibrous capsule *(Caps)*. Articular cartilage is seen *(stippled)*, and deep to it the subchondral bone plate *(white)* becomes thicker with growth and is generally wedge-shaped and thus thicker anteriorly in the concave facet.

nature of the matrix so that splitting of the cartilage occurs, along lines parallel to the collagen framework. This is characteristic of chondromalacia.

## Growth of Vertebral Bodies and Intervertebral Discs

### Shape Changes on Assumption of Erect Posture

There are marked changes in the shape of lumbar vertebral bodies after infancy. These are due to the changed mechanical forces on the spine with erect posture and are closely related to a change in the position of the growing nucleus pulposus as lordosis is established.[71] Fetal and infant lumbar vertebral bodies have convex upper and lower surfaces, so that the intervertebral discs are biconcave. In the fetus and small infant, the primary spinal curve is maintained and each lumbar nucleus pulposus appears wedge shaped in sagittal section, with its main mass situated posteriorly. As the infant sits up, stands, and learns to walk, the secondary lumbar curvature appears, the disc changes its shape, and the nucleus pulposus moves forward to a central position. The weight-bearing vertebral end-plates gradually change their shape from convex to concave during childhood, the concavities appearing opposite the maximum bulge of the nucleus pulposus.[3,63]

Other important changes in lumbar spinal shape following assumption of the erect posture are the relative increases in the anteroposterior and transverse dimensions of vertebral bodies and discs. These changes in the predominant direction of growth give the lumbar spine more stability in the sagittal and coronal planes. We have studied the increased anteroposterior growth of the lumbar vertebral bodies and intervertebral discs. The changes in vertebral-body shape following weightbearing in the erect posture reflect the plasticity of vertebral bone and its ready response to mechanical forces at this age. In nonambulatory children, these normal growth changes of early childhood do not appear. Such children have very square vertebrae on lateral radiographs, without the normal concavities in the endplates and with relatively short anteroposterior dimensions (Fig. 1-24). This abnormal shape is due to decreased hori-

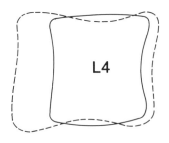

— **non-ambulant (14 year female)**

--- **ambulant (15 year female)**

**Fig. 1-24.** Tracings from lateral radiographs show the effect of weightbearing on growth. In the absence of normal weightbearing in erect posture, no endplate concavity appears and anteroposterior vertebral body growth is severely retarded. (From Taylor,[63] with permission.)

zontal growth rather than to any increase in vertical growth.[72] A similar square shape, but from a different cause, is seen when the posterior surfaces of vertebral bodies are scalloped by resorption in the presence of a tumor in the vertebral canal.

### Sexual Dimorphism in Vertebral Body Shape

From the age of 8 or 9 years onward, further interesting differences in shape appear in normal lumbar vertebrae in males and females.[64] Female vertebrae grow in height more rapidly than male vertebrae, giving a more slender vertebral column. Male vertebrae grow more in both transverse and anteroposterior dimensions than female vertebrae throughout the whole adolescent growth period, and appear on radiographs wider and more squat than female vertebrae (Fig. 1-25).[64] A measurement survey of a growing population showed that the thoracolumbar spine grows in height 1.7 times more rapidly in females than males between the ages of 9 and 13 years.[30] After the age of 14 years, the male spine grows in length more rapidly than the female spine, but the greater transverse growth of male vertebrae maintains the shape difference described. Accompanying these differences in vertebral growth patterns in males and females are differences in muscular support, since the effect of testosterone on muscle is to increase both its bulk and its strength-per-unit cross-sectional area. Thus the broader or thicker male vertebral column also has better muscular support than the average female column. When axially loaded, an average slender female column will buckle more easily than a wide male column, particularly if it already has a slight physiologic scoliosis. This may explain the greater tendency to progression of scoliosis in females than in males.[64]

The increased anteroposterior vertebral growth we have observed in both sexes in early childhood, and the greater increase in transverse vertebral growth in males than in females around puberty, relate to mechanical influences on bone growth. In the first case, the horizontal growth is the result of the new

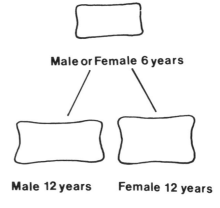

**Male or Female 6 years**

**Male 12 years**     **Female 12 years**

**Fig. 1-25.** The appearance of sex differences in vertebral-body shape is shown in tracings from anteroposterior radiographs of normal vertebrae. Male vertebral bodies grow more in width than female vertebrae, and female vertebral bodies tend to be relatively taller than male vertebrae. (From Taylor and Twomey,[54] with permission.)

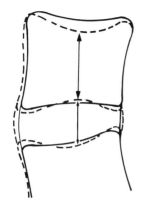

Fig. 1-26. Diagram based on tracings of vertebral bodies and on measurements of vertebral bodies and intervertebral discs shows the changes in their shapes with age. "Ballooning" of the central part of the disc is related to collapse of the vertebral end-plates, and there is some increase in anteroposterior dimension with aging. (From Twomey and Taylor,[80] with permission.)

———— Young adult outline

– – – – Elderly adult outline

forces of weightbearing in erect posture, and in the second case it is probably related to differences in muscle activity on growing vertebrae. There may also be hormonal influences independent of muscle activity. It is interesting to compare these growth changes in shape to the aging changes in shape in elderly adults, where there is "thickening of the waist" of vertebral bodies, and loss of the sex difference in shape.[4,73] This is associated with reduced mechanical loading (and reduced response of osteoblasts to mechanical loads), and reduced estrogen levels in postmenopausal women (Fig. 1-26).

## AGE CHANGES IN THE LUMBAR SPINE

### Anterior Elements

**Vertebral Bodies**

Measurement studies on large series of lumbar vertebral columns of all ages[4,5,73,74] demonstrated that the length of the column decreases with aging, as expected, but the reason for this is not usually loss in disc height, but gradual collapse of vertebral end-plates, associated with reduced bone density. The primary osseous change is loss of horizontal trabeculae in the vertebral bodies. These horizontal trabeculae form cross-ties, binding together and stiffening the vertical trabeculae, which act like weight-bearing "beams."

The loss of the cross-ties leads to buckling and fracturing of the unsupported vertical trabeculae or beams of bone, which hold up the vertebral end-plates. Measurements demonstrate a gradual increase in vertebral end-plate concavity with aging. This appears earlier in females than in males. In hemisected spines, the increased bowing of the vertebral end-plates is accompanied by "ballooning" of the center of each disc into the adjacent vertebral bodies. The traditional assumption that discs generally get thinner with aging is incorrect. Measurements of average disc thickness and mass in a large series of lumbar spines show increases in central disc thickness and disc mass in the majority of old lumbar spines.[74]

There are also age changes in the horizontal dimensions of the vertebral bodies, characterized as a "thickening of the waist" (see Fig. 1-26). These late changes in vertebral shape gradually eliminate the sex differences in vertebral-body shape that are present from adolescence to middle age. Female vertebrae are relatively taller and more slender during this child-bearing period. The effects of testosterone on muscle may provide a mechanism for the development of broader vertebrae in adult males, as the pull of muscle attachments affects bone shape. Other hormonal influences, such as the fairly dramatic estrogen loss at the female menopause, lead to the earlier loss in bone density in aging females. However, it is unwise to regard bone loss with aging as inevitable. Some of it may be difficult to avoid, but as noted in Chapter 2, regular exercise, adequate calcium intake, and possibly hormone replacement therapy, can reduce or prevent some of the bone loss associated with aging.[75]

**Intervertebral Discs**

Contrary to popular belief, aging lumbar discs do not, in the majority of people, become thinner and bulge like underinflated car tires. A minority of the population shows disc thinning and degeneration in one or more lumbar discs with aging, but the majority of discs, in a majority of individuals, maintain or even increase their average thickness, due to their central expansion, in an osteoporotic spine. When thinning and degeneration are found, they are seen most often in the L4–L5 and L5–S1 discs. In subjects over 60 years of age, 30 percent of the L4–L5 and L5–S1 discs are classified as Rolander grade 3.[4,74] Aging of intervertebral discs is generally associated with a reduction in water content, particularly in the nucleus pulposus, but the greater part of this loss occurs during maturation rather than in old age. The nucleus becomes less well differentiated from the annulus both in its water content and its histologic structure.[3] There are increases in the absolute amounts of collagen in the nucleus pulposus and changes in the types of collagen present. There is also an increase in the ratio of keratin sulfate (KS) to chondroitin sulfate (CS) in the disc during childhood growth and maturation, in parallel with the decreased water-binding capacity of the disc. The progressive substitution of KS for CS takes place in childhood when growth of the disc is accompanied by a disappearance of its blood vessels, and not in old age. In conditions of oxygen lack, KS acts as a functional substitute for CS in maintaining the turgor and water content of the disc.[37] The degenerative changes observed in lumbar discs with aging include the appearance of fissures in the annulus, first circumferential and later radial fissures. The nucleus has usually, by this stage, lost some of its fluidity, so that it does not "flow" into the fissures. However, if fissures or tears occur in relatively young discs, with a high turgor, the nucleus may be forced out through the fissure, most often in a posterolateral direction. Disc rupture with extrusion of its nucleus is less frequent than was once supposed. Disc aging is generally accompanied by increased disc stiffness and decreased ranges of movement, which is fully discussed in Chapter 2.

## Kissing Spines

With the collapse of vertebral end-plates allowing the discs to "sink into" shortened vertebral bodies, there is shortening of the column, and spinous processes, which were formerly well spaced, may come into contact with each other. Histologic studies on four lumbar spines from elderly cadavers showing radiologic evidence of "kissing spines" revealed adventitious joints with a fibrocartilaginous covering on the bone and a bursalike cavity, surrounded by fat and lined by synovial membrane, between the "kissing spines" (Taylor 1984, unpublished data). In the view of Sartoris et al,[76] "kissing spines" are attributable to increased lordosis with aging.

# Zygapophyseal Joints

## Articular Surfaces and Subchondral Bone Plate

The geometry of these biplanar joints at different lumbar levels has already been described. Age changes in young and middle-aged adults are described first.[6,43]

**Coronal Component (Anteromedial Third of Joint).** The loading stress imposed on the coronal components of the joints, by the tendency to forward translational during flexion, is reflected by changes in the articular cartilage and its supporting SCP. In normal adolescents and young adults a thicker SCP develops in the coronal component of the concave superior articular facet. Later, in middle life, this subchondral bone in the coronal component of the concave facet shows further thickening and an intense hematoxylin staining suggestive of sclerosis. In young adults between 30 and 40 years old, the articular cartilage lining this thicker part of the SCP in the anteromedial third of the joint generally shows cell hypertrophy and increased staining of chondrocytes and their pericellular matrix, which begin in the mid-zone of the articular cartilage of the concave facet. These articular cartilage changes occur in the concave facet first, anteriorly and at the deepest part of its concavity. They occur in the coronal component of the convex facet soon afterward. Generally, they do not affect the sagittal component of either facet. They appear in the fourth decade of life and often progress to swelling and vertical splitting (chondroma-lacia) of the cartilage (Fig. 1-27).

These changes in bone and cartilage appear to be reactions to compressive loading of the coronal components of the joint. This would occur in flexion, as the convex inferior articular process (IAP) glides upward in the concavity of the superior articular process (SAP). The resistance offered by the SAP to forward translation by the IAP, which hooks down behind it from the vertebra above, would create this compressive loading. In many respects the changes described are analogous to those of patellofemoral chondromalacia, where the stress also involves gliding movement accompanied by compression of the con-vex patella against the concave trochlea of the femur.

**Sagittal Component (Posterior Two-Thirds of Joint).** The age changes in the posterior, sagittally oriented two-thirds of the zygapophyseal joints are quite different in character, and tend to occur at a later stage than the changes de-scribed in the coronal component of the articular facets. The sagittally oriented parts of the SCPs are relatively thin, suggesting less compressive loading. How-ever, in middle-aged or elderly adults, the sagittal components of a number of joints show splitting of the articular cartilage near the posterior joint margin, parallel to the articular cartilage–SCP interface. The direction of the tear is related to the force producing it. This is conditioned by the peculiar anatomy at the posterior joint margin, where we have frequently observed a direct attach-ment of the posterior fibrous capsule to the posterior margin of the articular cartilage. This capsule–cartilage continuity is seen most often at the posterior margin of the superior articular facet. The potential for biomechanical mischief is accentuated by the partial insertion of multifidus through the posterior cap-sule (see Fig. 1-27). Tension transmitted to the cartilage from the capsule, and frequently repeated, may shear the articular cartilage from the subchondral bone. Even movement without muscle activity could exert this tension. The activity of axial rotation around an axis in the posterior disc would exert tension in the posterior capsule on one side and compression of the articular cartilage on the other side, particularly in a motion segment that had lost its tightness and its original mechanical efficiency. Some slight forward or backward sliding of one facet on the other may accompany axial rotation in loose joints. This would produce complex forces on the articular cartilage, including tension at the capsular margin and compression and shearing deeper in the sagittal compo-nent of the joint.

## Meniscoid Inclusions, Back Pain, and "Locked Back"

In a previous section we described the different varieties of synovial-lined, vascular, fibrofatty pads, which project up to 3 mm between the articular sur-faces from the polar joint recesses of a normal joint. Smaller folds from the anterior and posterior capsules fill the small triangular gaps between the rounded joint margins. A survey of 80 adult joints found that there are larger fat-pads in older joints, which show the wear and tear changes of osteoarthrosis,

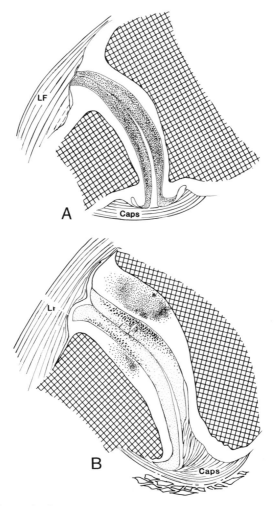

**Fig. 1-27.** Drawings of mid-joint horizontal sections of L3–L4 zygapophyseal joints, which were stained by hematoxylin and light green. **(A)** A normal joint from a 20-year-old woman shows smooth articular cartilage with regularly distributed chondrocytes and even staining of the matrix. The subchondral bone plate *(white)* is thicker anteriorly than posteriorly in the concave facet. The elastic ligamentum flavum *(LF)* forms the anterior capsule, which maintains close apposition of the anterior articular surfaces, but, in the absence of multifidus, the posterior fibrous capsule *(Caps)* is lax and the posterior part of the joint is open. **(B)** A joint of a 37-year-old man shows chrondrocyte hypertrophy in the articular cartilages of the coronal component. This is most evident in the concave facet of the superior articular process of L4, where two small splits in the articular cartilage are seen. There is thickening of the SCP, particularly in the coronal component, compared to the joint in **(A)**. Increased staining of the thickened SCP suggests hypercalcification or "sclerosis." The posterior fibrous capsule is covered by some fibers of multifidus. Note the continuity of the capsule with the posterior margin of the articular cartilage of the concave facet. Splitting of this cartilage away from the SCP is apparent. *LF,* ligamentum flavum; *Caps,* posterior fibrous capsule. *(Figure continues).*

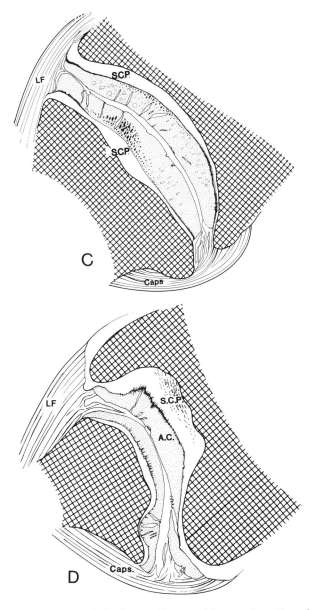

**Fig. 1-27.** *(Continued).* **(C)** A joint from a 62-year-old man where there is some atrophy of chondrocytes and loss of staining in the concave facet, and some cell hypertrophy in the convex facet. Fibrillation of both articular cartilages, most marked in the coronal parts of the joint, may be seen. The SCP has lost thickness compared to the SCP in Fig. **B.** There are osteophytes at the posterior joint margin. **(D)** A joint from a 61-year-old man showing advanced arthritic changes with widespread fibrillation of articular cartilage *(AC)*. There are infractions and irregularity of the SCP. The coronal component of the SCP appears to have collapsed into the spongy bone of the concave facet. The SCP at this point shows local thickening and increased staining suggestive of "sclerosis."

than in younger adult joints. They appear to act as cushions in lateral or medial joint recesses adjacent to osteophytes, and to extend further between articular surfaces where cartilage loss has occurred (Taylor and Connell, unpublished data). These vascular structures are innervated, and also directly connected to the joint capsule, which has many pain-sensitive nerve fibers. They are particularly large in the inferior joint recess of the lowest two lumbar mobile segments.[44,45,47] They are capable of causing back pain if entrapped between articular surfaces, either due to direct stimulation of the innervated inclusions or due to traction on the innervated capsule. Their potential importance in this latter regard has been questioned by Engel and Bogduk[77] on the grounds that they are too friable to exercise tension on the capsule if caught between the articular surfaces.

In our study,[6] we have found a number of instances of fibrocartilaginous inclusions projecting into the posterior aspect of zygapophyseal joints, which

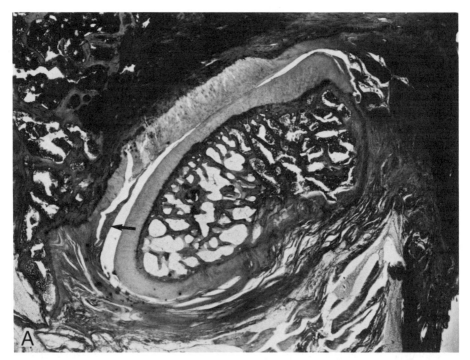

**Fig. 1-28.** **(A)** Horizontal section from the lower third of a left L3–L4 joint in a 37-year-old man that shows a joint inclusion, which may be a torn-off portion of the damaged articular cartilage of the concave facet, attached at its base to the posterior fibrous capsule. There is continuity of the capsule with the posterior margin of the cartilage on the concave facet, and also metaplastic formation of articular cartilage around the posterior margin of the convex facet under the capsule in the form of a "wrap-around bumper" (×4). *(Figure continues.)*

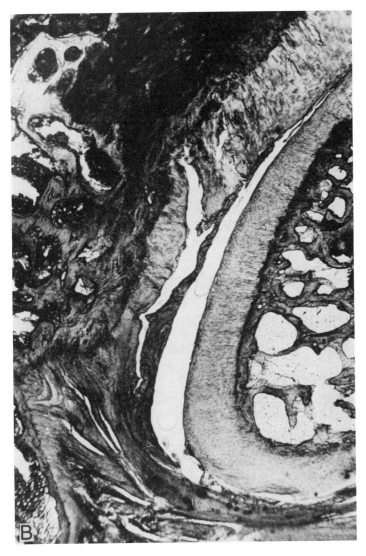

**Fig. 1-28.**   *(Continued).* **(B)** A higher-power view of the joint inclusion in Fig. **A** shows the templatelike fit of the inclusion on the underlying damaged cartilage, which shows signs of repair (× 10). (Fig. **B** from Taylor and Twomey,[81] with permission.)

appeared to be torn-off portions of articular cartilage that remained attached to the fibrous capsule. Their origin in the articular cartilage is attested by their templatelike fit on the underlying damaged cartilage, which is repairing (Fig. 1-28). They appear to be analogous to torn menisci in the knee joint. Like torn knee joint menisci, they could be displaced in certain circumstances, and being firmer and more strongly attached to the capsule than other fibrofatty inclusions, their entrapment could cause a reduction in the normal range of spinal movement or even "locked back." It is highly likely that this would be painful because of traction on the joint capsule. In this regard, the action of multifidus in controlling accurate apposition of the joint surfaces would be important. If joint congruity is not maintained by tone in multifidus there would be an opportunity for the torn portions of cartilage to be displaced, particularly if the joint surfaces separate in sudden rotary movements. Manipulative techniques would be appropriate in "freeing" such entrapped torn pieces of articular cartilage. On the other hand, manipulative techniques that "gap" the joints too forcefully could also damage joints with capsule–cartilage continuity by "shearing off" articular cartilage.

In comparative anatomic and radiologic studies, Taylor and McCormick[44] showed that loose joints may contain enlarged fat-pads that extend from a polar recess down to mid-joint levels. These may represent an attempt to fill the potential space in unstable joints with a loose capsule.

### Age Changes in Middle-Aged and Elderly Zygapophyseal Joints

Age changes in middle-aged and elderly zygapophyseal joints include those already described: the chondromalacia and subchondral sclerosis in the coronal components of the facets, which probably result from repetitive compressive loading, and also the loosening or "shearing off" of articular cartilage flaps at the posterior joint margins from wear and tear associated with capsule–cartilage continuity. They also include the more general age changes of osteoarthrosis (e.g., surface fibrillation and irregularity), with thinning of articular cartilage, osteophytic lipping, facet enlargement, and irregularity at the articular margins, and sclerotic thickening of the subchondral bone. Subchondral bone cysts are also found, but less often than in the hip and knee joints. Constant rubbing of enlarged posterior joint margins against an overlying thickened capsule leads to the extension of metaplastic cartilage around the posterior joint margins under the posterior fibrous capsule. These rounded "wrap-around bumpers" can be recognized on CT scans of the joints.

Measurements of articular cartilage thickness suggest that an increase in central thickness may occur in middle age. Histologic examination shows chondrocyte hypertrophy with swelling of the matrix. This swelling may disrupt the matrix, splits occurring normal to the subchondral bone, parallel to the collagen fibers in the mid-zone. The underlying SCP may show thickening, or infractions and collapse of its anterocentral portion. Measurements of concavity indexes of the zygapophyseal joints at L1–L2, L3–L4, and L4–L5, from 70 lumbar spines of all ages, show increased concavity of the superior articular facets in old age. This index measures the degree of concavity at the bone–cartilage interface in the superior articular facet. The concurrent increase in central cartilage thickness may simply represent an attempt to maintain joint congruity. Some osteoporotic joints with very thin SCPs show a marked increase in concavity. Other joints show infractions or local collapse of central parts of the

SCP. This phenomenon is similar to the osteoporotic collapse of the vertebral body end-plate, which has reduced bony trabecular support.

### Changes at Joint Margins: Tension Effects

**Articular Cartilage.** While the initial and more dramatic age changes in articular cartilage take place in the coronal and central parts of the joints as described, in the long term, the more destructive effects are at the joint margins, particularly at the polar regions and at the posterior margins of the joints. Actual loss of cartilage is most common in these regions, probably due to the "shearing off" of cartilage by tension from capsular attachments.[6] This is often accompanied by the intrusion of enlarged fat-pads into the defect.

**Bone Changes.** In middle-aged joints, osteophytes appear at the joint margins in addition to the subchondral bony sclerosis previously described in the coronal components of the superior articular facets. They are another manifestation of response to tension, both by extension of ossification from the laminae into the ligamenta flava, and at the posterior articular margins with associated enlargement of the mamillary processes.

**Radiologic Diagnosis.** The assumption that subchondral bone thickening and sclerosis are reliable indicators of wear and tear changes may be valid in the joints of middle-aged active patients, but in elderly osteoporotic joints there may be arthritic changes without subchondral bony sclerosis. Our studies show that many elderly subjects with advanced fibrillation and cartilage loss have extremely thin SCP due to concomitant osteoporosis.

## Relation of Age Changes in Discs and Facet Joints

It is commonly stated[78] that disc degeneration (as a primary change) leads to secondary zygapophyseal joint degeneration. The coexistence of disc and facet changes in advanced degeneration of the motion segment is often observed, but it cannot be assumed that facet changes are always secondary to disc degenerations. The facets are vitally important in protecting the discs from damage, and in fulfilling this function they endure repetitive loadbearing. In spondylolysis, when the protective influence of the zygapophyseal joint is removed, damage to the intervertebral disc will ensue. The anterior, coronally oriented parts of lumbar zygapophyseal joints protect intervertebral discs from translational shearing forces and bear high loads when they bring flexion to a halt at the end of the physiologic range or when the spine is loaded in a flexed position. The facets also limit the range of extension when the tips of the inferior articular processes abut on the subjacent laminae. The observation of a build-up of sclerotic compact bone in the laminae at the inferior joint recesses in adults of all ages is witness to this effect. The important protective effects of the zygapophyseal joints on the intervertebral discs are largely substantiated by the evidence we have presented.[6,12,41,43] The increased ranges of movement amounting to instability that result from experimental sectioning of pedicles would place additional stress on the intervertebral discs. It is apparent from our studies of discs and zygapophyseal joints from the same individuals that in some cases the zygapophyseal joints show more advanced degeneration than is apparent in the intervertebral discs. However, the mobile segments interact in a mutually dependent way and it is likely that any defect in one joint of the articular triad would adversely influence the other joints of the triad. This is recognized by spinal surgeons who fuse the lumbar spine to avoid instability, when a wide laminectomy is required for spinal stenosis (see Ch. 11).

## SUMMARY

1. The strong construction of lumbar vertebrae and motion segments reflects the need for regional stability in weightbearing and movement.

2. The thick young discs, rich in proteoglycans, are designed to allow useful ranges of movements and bear high compressive loads.

3. The biplanar facets restrain torsion and translation, protecting the annular fibers of the discs from the stresses to which they are most vulnerable.

4. In resisting translation in flexion, the coronal components of the facets may develop chondromalacia and thickening of the SCP in young adults.

5. In protecting the discs in deceleration injuries, the facets show infractions of their articular surfaces. In flexion compression injuries, the motion segment hinges on the facets and the vertebral bodies are compressed with endplate fractures or vertebral wedging.

6. Spondylolysis in young athletes implies failure of the facet function, with consequent exposure of the disc to shearing forces, which may lead to spondylolisthesis.

7. Degenerative spondylolisthesis in the elderly implies slow failure of the facets' protective function with segmental instability.

8. In the "dysfunctional" phase of early loosening of the motion segment, with disc fissuring, tension at the posterior facet margins, where the capsule and articular cartilage are continuous, may "shear off" a flap of articular cartilage forming a loose cartilaginous inclusion in the joint, with the possibility of locking of the joint.

9. In elderly spines, osteoporosis leads to vertebral end-plate collapse with "ballooning" of discs into the concave vertebral end-plates and shortening of the spine; this reduces the vertical dimensions of the nerve-root canals.

10. Loosening of the motion segment may allow vertebral retrolisthesis with reduction in the horizontal dimensions of the nerve-root canals.

## REFERENCES

1. Giles LGF, Taylor JR: Lumbar spine structural changes associated with leg length inequality. Spine 7:159, 1982
2. Giles LGF, Taylor JR: The effect of postural scoliosis on lumbar apophyseal joints. Scand J Rheumatol 13:209, 1984

3. Taylor JR: Growth and development of the human intervertebral disc. Ph.D. Thesis, University of Edinburgh, 1973

4. Twomey LT: Age changes in the human lumbar vertebral column. Ph.D. Thesis, University of Western Australia, 1981

5. Twomey LT, Taylor JR: Age-related changes in the lumbar spine and spinal rehabilitation. CRC critical review. Phys Rehab Med 2:153, 1991

6. Taylor JR, Twomey LT: Age changes in lumbar zygapophyseal joints: observations on structure and function. Spine 11:739, 1986

7. Taylor JR, Twomey LT, Corker M: Bone and soft tissue injuries in postmortem lumbar spines. Paraplegia, 28:119, 1990

8. Hutton W, Adams MA: The forces acting on the neural arch and their relevance to low back pain. p. 49. In: Engineering Aspects of the Spine. Mechanical Engineering, London, 1980

9. Davis PR: Human lower lumbar vertebrae: some mechanical and osteological considerations. J Anat 95:337, 1961

10. Ramsey RH: Anatomy of ligamentum flava. Clin Orthop 44:129, 1966

11. Yong-Hing MD, Reilly J, Kirkaldy-Willis WH: The ligamentum flavum. Spine 1: 226, 1976

12. Twomey LT, Taylor JR: Sagittal movements of the human lumbar vertebral column: a quantitative study of the role of the posterior vertebral elements. Arch Phys Med Rehab 64:322, 1983

13. Heylings D: Supraspinous and interspinous ligaments of the human lumbar spine. J Anat 125:127, 1978

14. Twomey L, Taylor JR: Age changes in the lumbar spine and intervertebral canals. Paraplegia 26:238, 1988

15. Knutsson F: Growth and differentiation of postnatal vertebrae. Acta Radiol 55:401, 1961

16. Eisenstein S: The morphometry and pathological anatomy of the lumbar spine in South African negroes and caucasoids with specific reference to spinal stenosis. J Bone Joint Surg 59B:173, 1977

17. Parkin IG, Harrison GR: The topographical anatomy of the lumbar epidural space. J Anat 141:211, 1985

18. Crock HV, Yoshizawa H: Blood supply of lumbar vertebral column. Clin Orthop 155:6, 1976

19. Romanes GJR: The arterial blood supply of the spinal cord. Paraplegia 2:199, 1965

20. Dommisse GF: Blood supply of spinal cord. J Bone Joint Surg 56B:225, 1974

21. Sunderland S: Meningeal-neural relationships in the intervertebral space. J Neurosurg 40:756, 1974

22. Kakulas BA, Taylor JR: Pathology of injuries of the vertebral column and spinal cord. p. 21. In Frankel HL (ed.): Handbook of Clinical Neurology. Elsevier, New York, 1992

23. Twomey LT, Taylor JR, Oliver M: Sustained flexion loading, rapid extension loading of the lumbar spine and the physiotherapy of related injuries. Physiother Pract 4:129, 1988

24. Taylor JR: Age changes in lumbar zygapophyseal joints. p. 121. In: Archives of Biology VIIth Symposium Internationale des Sciences Morphologiques. Louvain-en-Wolue, 1986

25. Taylor JR, Twomey LT: Lumbar multifidi: rotator-cuff muscles of zygapophyseal joints. J Anat 149:266, 1986

26. Bowen V, Cassidy JD: Macroscopic and microscopic anatomy of the sacro-iliac joint from embryonic life until the 8th decade. Spine 6:620, 1981

27. Palfrey AJ: The shape of sacroiliac joint surfaces. J Anat 132:457, 1981
28. Clayson SJ: Evaluation of mobility of hip and lumbar vertebrae of normal young women. Arch Phys Med 43:1, 1962
29. Bourdillon JF: Spinal Manipulation. 2nd Ed. Heinemann, London, 1973
30. Taylor JR, Slinger BA: Scoliosis screening and growth in Western Australian students. Med J Aust 1:475, 1980
31. Taylor JR, Twomey LT: Development of the human intervertebral disc. p. 39. In Ghosh P (ed): Biology of the Intervertebral Disc. CRC Press, Boca Raton, FL, 1988
32. Horton WG: Further observations on the elastic mechanism of the intervertebral disc. J Bone Joint Surg 40B:552, 1958
33. Nachemson A, Elfstrom G: Intravital dynamic pressure measurements in lumbar discs. Scand J Rehabil Med 1:1, 1970
34. Taylor JR, Twomey LT: Innervation of lumbar intervertebral discs. Med J Aust 2: 701, 1979
35. Taylor JR, Twomey LT: Innervation of lumbar intervertebral discs. N Z J Physiol 8:36, 1980
36. Bogduk N: The innervation of the lumbar spine. Spine 8:286, 1983
37. Taylor JR, Scott JE, Cribb AM, Bosworth TR: Human intervertebral disc acid glycosaminoglycans. J Anat 180:137, 1992
38. Hirsch C, Schazowicz F: Studies on structural changes in the lumbar annulus fibrosus. Acta Orthop Scand 22:184, 1953
39. Walmsley R: The human intervertebral disc: development and growth. Edin Med J 60:341, 1953
40. Maroudas A, Nachemson A, Stockwell RA: Factors involved in the nutrition of the human lumbar intervertebral disc: cellularity and diffusion of glucose in vitro. J Anat 120:113, 1975
41. Taylor JR, Twomey, LT: Vertebral column development and its relation to adult pathology. Aust J Physiother 31:83, 1985
42. Twomey L, Taylor J: Age changes in the lumbar articular triad. Aust J Physiother 31:106, 1985
43. Taylor JR, Twomey LT: Structure and function of lumbar zygapophyseal (facet) joints. Ch. 8. In Boyling JD, Palastanga N (eds): Grieve's Modern Manual Therapy of the Vertebral Column. Churchill Livingstone, Edinburgh, 1993
44. Taylor JR, McCormick CC: Lumbar facet joint fat pads. Neuroradiology 33:38, 1991
45. Giles LGF, Taylor J: Intra-articular synovial protrusions in the lower lumbar apophyseal joints. Bull Hosp Joint Dis 42:248, 1982
46. Wyke B: The neurology of joints: a review of general principles. Clin Rheum Dis 7:223, 1981
47. Giles LG, Taylor JR, Cockson A: Human zygapophyseal joint synovial folds. Acta Anat 126:110, 1986
48. Taylor JR, Twomey L: Sagittal and horizontal plane movement of the lumbar vertebral column in cadavers and in the living. Rheum Rehabil 19:223, 1980
49. McCormick CC, Taylor JR, Twomey LT: Facet joint arthrography in lumbar spondylolysis: anatomic basis for spread of contrast. Radiology 171:193, 1989
50. Spangfort EV: The lumbar disc herniation. Acta Orthop Scand suppl 142: 1972
51. McRae DL: Radiology of the lumbar spinal canal. p. 92. In Weinstein PR, Ehni G, Wilson CB (eds): Lumbar Spondylosis: Diagnosis, Management and Surgical Treatment. Year Book Medical Publishers, Chicago, 1977
52. Wolpert L: The cellular basis of skeletal growth during development. Br Med Bull 37:152, 1981

53. Taylor JR, Twomey LT: Factors influencing growth of the vertebral column. p. 30. In Grieve GP (ed): Modern Manual Therapy. Churchill Livingstone, Edinburgh, 1986

54. Taylor JR, Twomey LT: The role of the notochord and blood vessels in development of the vertebral column and in the aetiology of Schmorl's nodes. p. 21. In Grieve, GP (ed): Modern Manual Therapy of the Vertebral Column. Churchill Livingstone, Edinburgh, 1986

55. Verbout AJ: The development of the vertebral column. p. 1. In: Beck F, Hild W, Ortmann R (eds): The Development of the Vertebral Column. Advances in Anatomy, Embryology and Cell Biology. Vol. 90. Springer Verlag, Berlin, 1985

56. O'Rahilly R, Meyer DB: The timing and sequence of events in the development of the human vertebral column during the embryonic period proper. Anat Embryol 157:167, 1979

57. Schmorl G, Junghanns H: p. 68. The Human Spine in Health and Disease. 2nd Ed. (Translated by Besemann EF.) Grune & Stratton, New York, 1971

58. Taylor JR: Scoliosis and growth: patterns of asymmetry in normal growth. Acta Orthop Scand 54:596, 1983

59. Taylor JR: Persistence of the notochordal canal in vertebrae. J Anat 111:211, 1972

60. Dale Stewart TD, Kerley ER: Essentials of Forensic Anthropology. p. 136. Charles C. Thomas, Springfield, IL, 1979

61. Tanaka T, Uhthoff HK: The pathogenesis of congenital vertebral malformations. Acta Orthop Scand 52:413, 1981

62. Watterson RL, Fowler I, Fowler BJ: The role of the neural tube and notochord in development of the axial skeleton of the chick. Am J Anat 95:337, 1954

63. Taylor JR: Growth of human intervertebral discs and vertebral bodies. J Anat 120: 49, 1975

64. Taylor JR, Twomey LT: Sexual dimorphism in human vertebral growth. J Anat 138:281, 1984

65. McFadden KD, Taylor JR: End-plate lesions of the lumbar spine. Spine 14:867, 1989

66. Dietz GW, Christensen EE: Normal ""'cupid's bow'"" contour of lower lumbar vertebrae. Radiology 121:577, 1976

67. Bradford DS, Moe JH: Scheuermann's juvenile kyphosis: a histological study. Clin Orthop 110:45, 1975

68. Taylor JR: Vascular causes of vertebral asymmetry and the laterality of scoliosis. Med J Aust 144:533, 1986

69. Dickson R, Lawton JO, Butt WP: Pathogenesis of idiopathic scoliosis. p. 16. In Dickson R, Bradford D (eds): Management of Spinal Deformities. Butterworths, London, 1984

70. Van Shaik JPJ, Verbiest H, Van Shaik FDJ: The orientation of laminae and facet joints in the lower lumbar spine. Spine 10:59, 1985

71. Taylor JR, Corker M: Age related responses to stress in the vertebral column: a review. In: The Growing Scope of Human Biology: Proceedings of the Australasian Society for Human Biology 2:213. Centre for Human Biology U W A, University of Western Australia, 1989

72. Taylor JR: Growth of lumbar vertebral bodies and IVDs in relation to weightbearing in the erect posture. J Anat 119:413, 1975

73. Twomey LT, Taylor JR, Furniss B: Age changes in the bone density and structure of the lumbar vertebral column. J Anat 136:15, 1983

74. Twomey L, Taylor J: Age changes in lumbar vertebrae and intervertebral discs. Clin Orthop 224:97, 1987

75. Twomey LT, Taylor JR: Old age and physical capacity: use it or lose it. Aust J Physiother 30:115, 1984
76. Sartoris DJ, Resnick D, Tyson R, Haghighi P: Age-related alterations in the vertebral spinous processes and intervening soft tissues: radiologic-pathologic correlation. Am J Roentgenol 145:1025, 1985
77. Engel R, Bogduk N: The menisci of the lumbar zygapophyseal joints. J Anat 135: 795, 1982
78. Vernon-Roberts B: The pathology and interrelation of intervertebral discs lesions, osteoarthrosis of the apophyseal joints, lumbar spondylosis and low back pain. p. 83. In Jayson MIV (ed): The Lumbar Spine and Back Pain. 2nd Ed. Pitman, London, 1985
79. Last S: Anatomy: Regional and Applied. 2nd Ed. Churchill Livingstone, Edinburgh, 1959.
80. Twomey LT, Taylor JR: Age changes in lumbar intervertebral discs. Acta Orthop Scand 56:496, 1986
81. Taylor JR, Twomey LT: Structure, function, and age changes in the lumbar zygaphophyseal joints. Spine 11:739, 1986.

# 2 | Lumbar Posture, Movement, and Mechanics

*Lance T. Twomey*
*James R. Taylor*

The adult vertebral column is a segmented, jointed, flexible rod that supports the loads of weightbearing in the erect posture, protects the spinal cord and emerging spinal nerves, allows a considerable range of movements in all directions, and serves as the axial support for the limbs. The vertebral column's capacity to fully subserve these functions alters through the different phases of the life cycle. The extremely malleable C-shaped column of the neonate remains almost as flexible and mobile in childhood as it grows and develops its finely balanced curves. Further growth and maturation are associated with progressive increases in the strength and "dynamic" stability of the adolescent and young-adult columns, and with a continuing small decline in its mobility. The middle years demonstrate an increasing incidence of minor traumatic and degenerative pathology, with a further decline in range of movement. In old age, with its osteoporotic decrease in bone strength, there is progressive increase in joint stiffness with a considerable decline in movement ranges, and a flattening of the lumbar spine. The lumbar spine is markedly lordotic in children, with a small decline in lordosis in adolescents and young adults, and a pronounced flattening of the region in middle life and old age.

*Posture* is a term that indicates the relative position of the body segments during rest or activity, while *stature* indicates the height of a subject. In most individuals their resting supine length exceeds their standing height (or stature) by about 2 cm.

## POSTURE

*Posture* refers to a composite of the positions of all of the joints of the body at any given moment.[1] A minimum of muscle work is required for the maintenance of good posture in any human static or dynamic situation. In good standing posture, the head is held tall and level, while the spine is nicely balanced so that its sagittal curves allow free movement of the chest and abdomen, and prevent the shoulders from sagging forward. The lower limbs serve as balanced support. In a side view of most individuals, a plumb line would intersect the mastoid process, the acromion process, and the greater trochanter. It would pass just anterior to the center of the knee joint and through the ankle joint.

The usual static posture for the lumbar spine is that of lordosis. Normal spinal posture is expressed as a balanced series of curves when viewed from the side (Fig. 2-1). The adult spine is supported on a symmetrical level pelvis by two equal-length lower limbs. In normal sitting posture, the level pelvis is supported with body weight distributed equally through both ischial tuberosities. There is no discernible lateral curvature or rotation of the spine when viewed from the front or behind.

**line of gravity**

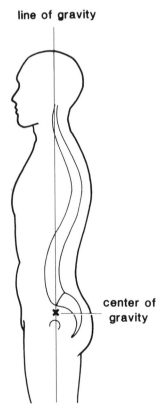

**center of gravity**

**Fig. 2-1.**   The relationship between the vertebral column and the line of gravity.

The cervical lordosis begins to appear at birth and develops as a permanent curve at about 3 months of age, while the permanent lumbar lordosis appears with the extension of the legs and weightbearing in the erect posture, usually between 12 and 18 months of age. These curves continue to change until the completion of spinal growth, usually between the ages of 13 and 18 years.[2-4]

## Sagittal Pelvic Tilt and Muscle Action

Pelvic tilt in the sagittal plane and lumbar lordosis are inextricably linked together, because the lumbar spine and the sacrum are united at the strong, relatively immobile sacroiliac joints. Thus, when the pelvis is tilted further forward, it brings about an increase in lordosis, and when tilted backward, the lumbar spine flattens. The muscles responsible for pelvic posture include erector spinae (sacrospinalis), abdominals (rectus abdominus and oblique muscles), psoas major and iliacus, gluteus maximus, and hamstrings (Fig. 2-2).

It is the interaction between these muscles that is the major factor determining pelvic tilt and lumbar lordosis at any point in time. Thus, while the back extensor muscles primarily increase lumbar lordosis, the abdominal muscles,

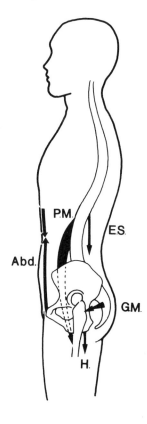

**Fig. 2-2.** The muscles responsible for the maintenance of pelvic tilt. *Abd*, abdominal muscles; *ES*, erector spinae; *GM*, gluteus maximus; *H*, hamstrings; *PM*, psoas major.

gluteals, and hamstrings act together to flatten lumbar lordosis by their action about the lever of the pelvis. The psoas muscles, which attach to the lateral margins of the lumbar vertebrae, can also increase lumbar lordosis when the lower limbs are extended by pulling the lumbar vertebrae forward around the "pulley" of the hip joint (see Fig. 2-2). In this way they pull the pelvis and lumbar vertebrae ventrally. In the course of everyday activity we are constantly adjusting our posture to allow for comfort, ergonomic advantage, and in response to our environment. Muscle tightness affecting any of the muscle groups listed can change both habitual resting posture and the total range of dynamic postures available. Tightness of psoas major and hamstring muscles is associated with increased lordosis in some individuals. Shortened hamstrings should pull down on the pelvis and flatten the lumbar spine. For this reason, it is possible that tight hamstrings are the *result* of lordotic posture rather than its cause.

## Analysis of the Lumbar Curve

The lumbosacral lordosis is a compound curve (Fig. 2-3) with the degree of curvature greatest at the L5–S1 level, and least at the L1–L2 level. In general, at all ages the intervertebral discs contribute to a greater proportion of the

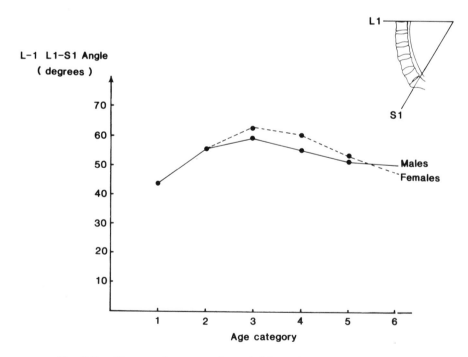

**Fig. 2-3.** Changes that occur through life to the lumbosacral angle.

lordosis in both sexes than do the vertebrae. However, at the lumbosacral junction, the L5 vertebral body makes a significant contribution. The L5–S1 disc is also more wedge-shaped than any of the higher discs.

## Sexual Dimorphism

During the childbearing years (i.e., between adolescence and middle age) the L1–S1 angle of lumbar lordosis is greater in women than in men.[5] This sexual dimorphism is not apparent in childhood and disappears again in old age. Although the reasons for this difference remain obscure, its place in the life cycle suggests that it has a hormonal basis. One of the hormones that may be involved consists of three closely related polypeptides collectively called relaxin. It is secreted by the ovary and has been shown to relax the symphysis pubis, sacroiliac joints, and spinal ligaments.[6] These hormones, which are secreted in relatively large amounts by the corpus luteum of pregnancy, are also found in small amounts in the circulating blood of nonpregnant women of childbearing age. It is suggested that the effects of relaxin in "loosening" pelvic and lumbar ligaments may coincidentally allow an increase in the lumbar curve during that period in the female life cycle (adolescence and early adult life) when the hormones are present in relatively large amounts.

Another suggestion advanced to explain the gender differences in lordosis relates to Treanor's demonstration[7] that the wearing of high-heel shoes tips the body's center of gravity forward and brings about an associated increase in pelvic tilt and an increase in lumbar lordosis, because lumbar lordosis is dependent on pelvic posture (Fig. 2-4). The habitual wearing of high heels (predominantly a female fashion) in the "developed" countries may eventually contribute to a difference in lordosis between men and women in Western societies. This is less likely to be a feature in societies where outdoor activity in bare feet or soft-heel shoes is possible for most of the year.[8]

Recent studies[8,9] show that an increase in pelvic tilt due to high heels does not always bring about an increase in lumbar lordosis in nonpregnant young women. An equal number of women demonstrated a flattening of their lumbar curve as showed an increase. However, pregnant women showed a significant increase in lordosis when wearing 2-inch-high heels. The response of the lumbar spine to changes in pelvic posture would appear to relate to the location of the center of gravity. In pregnancy, the center of gravity is displaced ventrally and is balanced by an increase in lumbar lordosis.

An analysis of the components of the L1–S1 angle in a major cadaveric study[5] showed that the principal difference between the lumbar posture of females and males occurs at the lumbosacral junction, because the composite L1–L5 angles are similar throughout life in both sexes (Fig. 2-5). Thus, it is the increased sacral and pelvic tilt of females that is primarily responsible for the difference in lordosis during adolescence and early adult life. In this regard, it is interesting to note that anatomists such as Romanes[10] consider that in normal erect posture, the anterosuperior iliac spines and the symphysis pubis

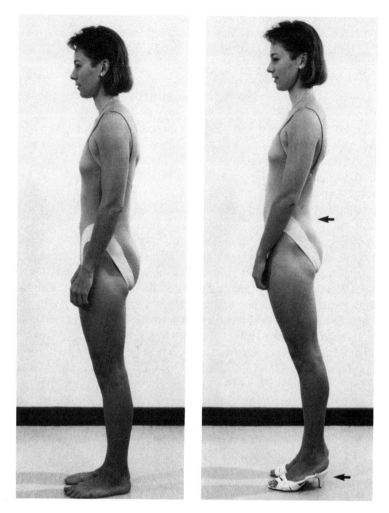

**Fig. 2-4.**   The increase in lumbar lordosis due to wearing high-heel shoes.

lie in the same plane. This was confirmed in a measurement study by Taylor and Alexander[11] of 39 nonpregnant females. Obstetric experience suggests that the symphysis pubis lies in a more anterior plane than do the iliac spines.[12] The greater L5–S1 angle in females may well be related to a greater degree of pelvic tilt during the childbearing years.

## Variations in Lumbar Lordosis

Lumbar lordosis is maintained by intrinsic features such as the shape of the vertebrae, discs, and the sacrum, and by extrinsic factors such as position of center of gravity, body weight and its distribution, muscle strength, and

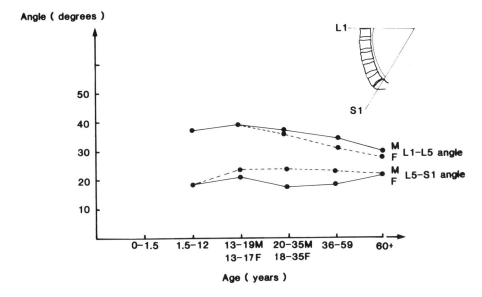

**Fig. 2-5.**   An analysis of the change in L1 to L5 and L5–S1 angles with increasing age.

sociocultural preferences. In regard to sociocultural preferences, it is commonly observed that an individual's lumbar lordosis and thus habitual posture is based on factors such as fashion (e.g., wearing high heels), repetitive daily activity (e.g., a schoolchild carrying a heavy schoolbag), life-style (e.g., the "typical" military posture), affect and attitude (e.g., depression or elation), and aesthetics or training (e.g., model's swayback posture).

### Prolonged Maintenance of the Static Erect Posture

Standing in the upright position for long periods of time tends to produce an increase in lumbar lordosis as muscles begin to fatigue and as the slow creep of the soft tissues often emphasizes the natural tendency toward extension of the region. This occurs because the center of gravity is usually ventral to the sacral promontory in most adults.[13] The effect of gravity acting through this center pulls the lumbar spine into a more lordotic posture in those individuals. This postural change accompanies the diurnal decline in height (see Diurnal Variation in Stature, below). Vertebral column posture is ideally dynamic rather than static, as the tissues adapt to prolonged static loading by further creep of the column.

### The Effects of Age on Lumbar Lordosis

The lumbar spinal lordosis flattens considerably in old age in both sexes (see Fig. 2-5),[2,5] although a few individuals do show small increases in lordosis. Increases are usually associated with increased abdominal girth and weight and declines in abdominal-muscle strength, so that their physique approximates that of a pregnant female. Thus, the explanation for an increase in lordosis is the same as that for pregnant women (see above). However, Twomey's large study[5] of a typical Australian society clearly shows a significant decrease in lumbar lordosis with increasing age after adolescence of 32 percent in females and 20 percent in males.

### Lumbar Lordosis in Association with Back Pain

Clinicians often report a flattening of the lumbar lordosis during episodes of back pain. However, a study of 600 men between the ages of 23 and 60 years has shown that the distribution and range of lordosis (as viewed on radiographs) do not vary in acute or chronic low-back pain more than they do in men without back pain.[14]

## Leg-Length Inequality and Pelvic Obliquity

Whereas pelvic tilt in the sagittal plane is inextricably linked with lumbar lordosis, coronal-plane obliquity of the pelvis is associated with lumbar scoliosis. The most common cause of this functional situation is leg-length inequality.[15] Functional scoliosis must be distinguished from idiopathic structural scoliosis. Structural scoliosis progresses during the growth period, is seen most frequently in girls,[16] and is usually convex to the left in the lumbar spine. Leg-length inequality and postural scoliosis have been associated with low back pain, degenerative changes in the intervertebral discs and zygapophyseal joints, and with a higher incidence of osteoarthritic changes in hip and knee joints. Interestingly, it is most often the left leg that tends to be longest, particularly in men,[17] since most right-handed people put more weight on their left foot.[18]

Unequal leg length may be associated with pathologic conditions (e.g., Perthes disease, previous fracture), but in the vast majority of situations, it accompanies normal growth. In most of this latter group, the degree of asymmetric growth of the lower limbs is very common. It is associated with "out of phase" growth, where one of a pair of bones is more advanced than the other at maturity.[17] A leg-length difference of 1 cm or greater is twice as common at the peak of the adolescent growth spurt (13 percent) than at maturity (7 percent).[19] Indeed, it is very rare to find exactly equal leg lengths in normal communities.

Giles and Taylor[20,21] showed that unequal leg length and the associated "postural" scoliosis are linked with minor structural changes in lumbar discs and vertebral end-plates, and with asymmetric changes to the articular cartilage and subchondral bone of the lumbar zygapophyseal joints. The joints on the convex side of the scoliotic curve show thicker subchondral bone plates and thinner articular cartilage than those from the concave side, suggesting greater loading on the convex side of the curve. This may be related to the greater postural muscle forces necessary on the convex side to prevent buckling of the scoliotic column under axial loading. A number of surveys have shown a statistical association between leg-length inequality and low back pain.[15,22,23] Leg-length inequality is twice as common in low back pain patients (13 to 22 percent) than in control populations (4 to 8 percent). Giles and Taylor[15] also suggested that the response to manipulative therapy in low back pain associated with leg-length inequality is much improved when a foot-raise shoe insert is provided as part of the treatment.

## STATURE

The topics of stature and posture are closely related. Stature is affected by posture in a number of ways.

## Postural Fatigue

Laxity in posture causes "creep" of soft tissues (see Prolonged Maintenance of the Static Erect Posture, above).

## Diurnal Variation in Stature

In 1777, Buffon noted that a young man was considerably shorter after spending the night at a ball but he regained his previous height after a rest in bed. Merkel (1881) measured his own daily loss in height (2 cm standing, 1.6 cm sitting) by measuring the height of his "visual plane" from the floor. He found that half his loss in statute occurred in the first hour after rising, and that a greater loss occurred after vigorous exercise.

De Puky[24] measured diurnal variation in stature and found the daily loss in height to average 15.7 mm. Diurnal variation as a percentage of total body height decreases steadily with increasing age. Blackman[25] showed a decrease in stature of 0.76 cm 1 hour after rising and 1.77 cm 4 hours after rising; this order of decrease was confirmed by Stone and Taylor,[26] who showed that loss in sitting height was equivalent to 80 percent of the loss in standing height.

In an interesting study, Tyrrell et al[27] showed that average daily variation in stature was about 1 percent of normal stature, and that the greatest loss occurred in the first hour after rising in the morning. Approximately 70 percent of this lost stature was gained during the first half of the night. The carrying of heavy loads increased the rate of shrinkage loss (i.e., by creep). Interestingly, rest with the lumbar spine in full flexion produced more rapid gains in stature than in other positions. This also suggests that the diurnal loss involves creep into extension (see Prolonged Maintenance of the Static Erect Posture, above). Adams and Hutton[28] have recently demonstrated that the flexed position induces the transport of metabolites and fluids into the intervertebral discs. If most of the diurnal loss in stature is a loss of trunk length due to small diurnal reductions in disc height,[26] then the use of flexion as a tool to maintain disc height and to preserve normal erect posture without excessive lordosis becomes of clinical interest for physical therapists.

The mechanism involved in diurnal variation in stature is discussed further under later sections on creep of vertebral structures.

## The Influence of Changes in Posture on Stature

When parents measure their child's stature as a record of their growth rate, the usual instructions given are to "stand tall, like a soldier." This implies a general understanding that stature is dependent in part on a person's posture. When "standing tall," the child flattens the spine as much as possible, tucks the chin in, and attempts to push the top of the head as far upward as possible. Similarly, after surgical correction of moderate to severe scoliosis, when the spine is surgically "straightened," children can gain up to 8 cm in height.

The thoracic spine makes the largest contribution to spine length. The lumbar spine constitutes one-third, the cervical spine one-fifth, and the thoracic spine the remainder of the total length of the presacral spine in the adult.[29]

## The Effect of Growth and Aging on Stature

The rates of growth and decline in stature are described in Chapter 1. The spinal component in the decline in stature that occurs in old age is much more a result of a decrease in vertebral height than it is a decrease in intervertebral disc height.[30,31] An increasing thoracic kyphosis (particularly in women) also contributes significantly to the loss of stature in old age.

## MOVEMENTS OF THE LUMBAR VERTEBRAL COLUMN

At each level in the vertebral column there are three interacting joints allowing and controlling movement. This unique combination is known as the *articular triad* or as the *mobile segment* (see Ch. 1). Each articular triad allows only a few degrees of movement. However, lumbar movement usually involves a complex interaction of mobile segments at multiple levels. The thickness of each intervertebral disc, the compliance of its fibrocartilage, and the dimensions and shape of its adjacent vertebral end-plates are of primary importance in governing the extent of movement possible. The shape and orientation of the vertebral-arch articular facets, with the ligaments and muscles of the arch and its processes, guide the types of movement possible and provide restraints against excessive movement.

## Ranges of Disc Movement

The anterior elements (vertebrae and discs) of the articular triads are capable of certain ranges in movement depending on disc dimensions (thickness and horizontal dimensions) and disc stiffness.

### Disc Dimensions

A large range of movement would occur when disc height was relatively great and vertebral end-plate horizontal dimensions relatively short (Fig. 2-6). Adolescent and young adult females have shorter vertebral end-plates *(a)* than males, whereas disc height *(b1, b2, and b3)* and disc stiffness are substantially the same. Thus, females possess the necessary combination of dimensions for a larger range of movements than is possible in males.[5,32] In old age, when male and female vertebrae and disc shapes become very similar and hormonal differences are reduced, the range of movement of men and women becomes almost identical (Fig. 2-7).

### Disc Stiffness

The general reduction in movement ranges in both sexes is attributable to increased disc stiffness. This has been demonstrated by the posterior release experiment of Twomey and Taylor,[33] which demonstrated a 40 percent increase in disc stiffness in the elderly.

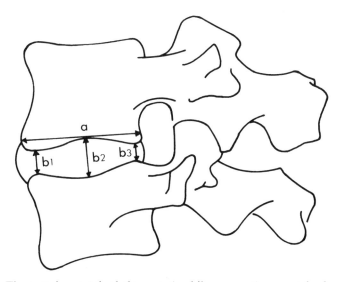

**Fig. 2-6.** The anterior vertebral elements (mobile segment): *a,* vertebral end-plate, and *b,* disc thickness.

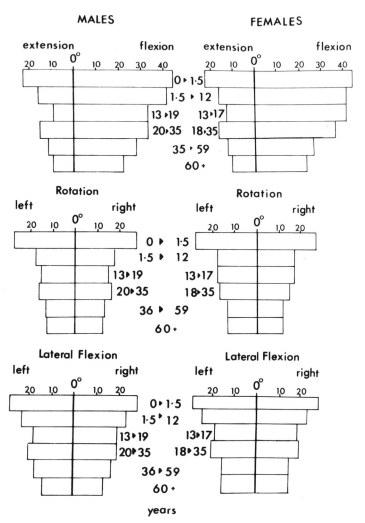

**Fig. 2-7.**   Age changes in the range of lumbar movements in both sexes. (From Taylor and Twomey,[32] with permission.)

## Planes of Movement

The movements possible at each lumbar-motion segment are traditionally described as being in the sagittal (flexion–extension), coronal (lateral flexion), and horizontal (axial rotation) planes. Each movement occurs along one of three coordinate axes x, y, and z (Fig. 2-8). Thus, all mobile segments of the lumbar spine possess 6° of freedom and each movement consists of an angular or rotary displacement together with translation of a vertebra on its subjacent vertebra. It is rare for movement to occur exclusively in a single plane. Move-

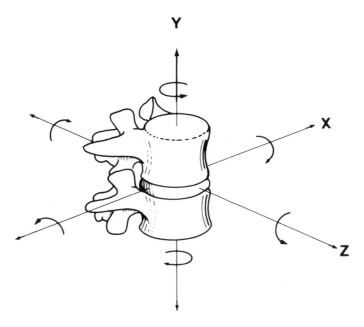

**Fig. 2-8.**   Planes and axes of movement. Sagittal plane movements occur along the x axis; rotational plane movements occur along the y axis; and coronal plane movement occurs along the z axis.

ments are generally "coupled" in habitual movement,[34] and occur across the standard descriptive planes of motion.

## Ranges of Lumbar Movement

Despite the availability of simple, reliable methods for measuring spinal mobility, these have not been applied to studies of normal lumbar spine movement until recently. The literature records considerable variation in the values given for the ranges of movements of the lumbar spine. This variation stems largely from the different measurement methods used and the differences in age, sex, race, and numbers of subjects studied. The clinical measurements most frequently used include indirect estimates of spinal mobility from measurement of (1) the distance from the fingertips to the floor when the patient bends forward, and (2) the use of a tape measure to measure the increase in distance between two skin landmarks, often the S1 and L1 spinous processes. These methods are most inaccurate, and give no direct measure of the range (angular deflection) of spinal movement. The former is dependent on hamstring muscle length and the latter fails to show a reasonable level of consistency between repeated measures. Published studies of lumbar spinal movement have mostly concentrated on sagittal and coronal plane movements, and include direct measurement in living subjects, using a wide variety of equipment,[32,35-43] radiographic studies,[44-51] cadaveric studies that have mostly involved a single mobile segment in a small number of specimens,[3,49,52-64] photographic techniques,[65,66] and theoretical studies based on mathematical models.[67-72]

Estimates of the range of sagittal motion of the lumbar region vary widely from 121° in a young male acrobat,[44] to 21.8° in elderly women.[47] However, Begg and Falconer[73] considered 70° to be the "normal" average total range of lumbar flexion–extension. Few studies have attempted to measure axial rotation in the lumbar spine, largely because of methodologic problems. It has proven difficult to measure lumbar rotation in the living either directly or radiographically with any degree of accuracy, and cadaveric studies have mostly been confined to motion segments rather than to the whole lumbar column. Some authorities maintain that rotary movement does not exist as a separate entity in the lumbar region,[74-76] or that if rotation does occur, it is in spite of the fact that the facets are designed to prevent it.[77] Other sources have assessed the total range of rotation as between 5° and 36° of movement.[3,38,40,78-80]

## Clinical Measurement

In an effort to provide instrumentation that would be relatively easily applied in the clinical situation and provide reasonably accurate objective data, two instruments have been devised to measure lumbar sagittal and horizontal plane movement, and have been tested in clinical trials.[32,64,81] The lumbar spondylometer is noninvasive, has good interperson and intertest reliability, and measures lumbar sagittal motion (Fig. 2-9). Since its base rests on the sacrum, the measurement is not confounded and invalidated by the inclusion of hip motion. Tests of its accuracy made by comparing living subjects with fresh, cadaveric specimens suggest that it underestimates the range of movement by an average of 1°.[32] Inter- and intraoperator repeatability trials show high correlations.[82] The lumbar spondylometer is comparable in accuracy and in some respects in principle to an inclinometer, but with a more complex geometry.[35] It is also easier to use in a clinical situation where separate readings from two inclinometers would be required. Its use requires a thorough knowledge of the surface anatomy of the lumbar region, with consistently accurate placement of the cushions, and the precise location of the L1 spinous process.

The cushions of the lumbar spondylometer rest on the dorsal surface of the sacrum, with the top cushion at the level of S1. The distal end of the instrument rests on the spinous process of L1 (Fig. 2-9). The physical therapist reads off the initial starting position in degrees, asks the subject to fully extend, and reads off the new position in degrees. The subject returns to the starting position (checked by the operator), and then moves into full-range flexion, with the operator recording the result. Thus, flexion, extension, and full-range sagittal motion are recorded. This entire process takes an experienced physical therapist less than 2 minutes to administer and record, and is a useful objective

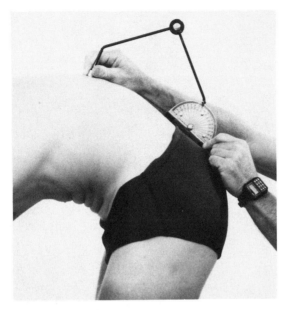

**Fig. 2-9.**   The lumbar spondylometer.

clinical measurement in the assessment of the progress of treatment for back conditions.[81]

The external measurement of rotation in the clinical situation has been made possible by the development of a lumbar rotameter.[32,64] The apparatus consists of a large protractor strapped at right angles to the subject's sacrum, and a belt with a pointer strapped around the trunk at L1. The tip of the pointer rests just above the protractor (Fig. 2-10). The subject is asked to rotate fully to the right and the left, and angular deflections of the pointer are read off on the protractor. Intertrial and interoperator reliability tests show a maximum variation of 5° in a range of 56°, and these measurements correlate well with cadaveric motion.[32] The rotameter is relatively cumbersome, and it takes about 3 minutes for an experienced physical therapist to use it in a clinical setting. For these reasons, it has proven less useful as a clinical tool. It has the additional disadvantage that its reading may be influenced to a minor degree by lower rib cage movements.

Ranges of lumbar movements, for both sexes in six age-group categories using the spondylometer and the rotameter, and the gravity inclinometer[37] for side flexion, are listed in Table 2-1.

## Age Changes in Ranges of Movements

Table 2-1 clearly demonstrates a decline in the ranges of all lumbar movements in the living with increasing age. This decline parallels the reductions observed in cadaveric studies by other authors.[5,33,47,48,83]

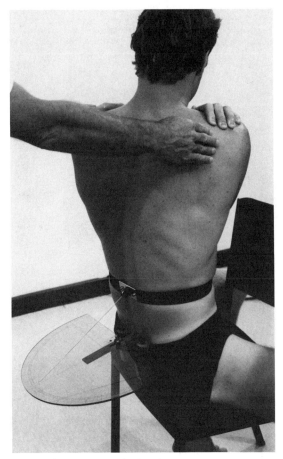

**Fig. 2-10.**    The lumbar rotameter.

**Table 2-1.** The Mean and Standard Deviation for the Total Ranges of Sagittal, Horizontal, and Coronal Plane Movements in Living Subjects (Population 960 Persons)

| | Ranges of Movements | | | | | |
|---|---|---|---|---|---|---|
| | Sagittal Range (Flexion–Extension) | | Horizontal Range (Rotation to Both Sides) | | Coronal Range (Side Flexion) | |
| Age (yr) | Male | Female | Male | Female | Male | Female |
| 5–12 | 58° ± 9° | 58° ± 9° | 34° ± 6° | 34° ± 6° | 47° ± 6° | 47° ± 6° |
| 13–19 | 45° ± 10° | 57° ± 8° | 30° ± 4° | 34° ± 4° | 38° ± 5° | 37° ± 4° |
| 19–35 | 42° ± 6° | 42° ± 7° | 33° ± 6° | 33° ± 6° | 40° ± 5° | 40° ± 5° |
| 35–59 | 38° ± 7° | 38° ± 7° | 26° ± 6° | 27° ± 6° | 32° ± 4° | 30° ± 3° |
| 60+ | 30° ± 7° | 28° ± 6° | 22° ± 5° | 20° ± 4° | 28° ± 4° | 30° ± 5° |

In old age the ranges of lumbar movement in men and women become almost identical. It would appear that when hormonal differences are reduced, sexual differentiations in vertebral shape, posture, and spinal-movement ranges disappear. The general reduction in ranges in both sexes occurs as a result of increased "stiffening" of the intervertebral disc in association with disc-shape changes involving increases in the anteroposterior length and concavity of the vertebral end-plate.[33] A reason often provided for the decline in average ranges of movements in aging populations (i.e., a general tendency to thinning of inter-vertebral discs in old age) has recently been shown to be false.[30,31] In old age most discs increase in volume and become thicker and more convex at the disc–vertebral interface. Only about 30 percent of discs become thinner. The principal reason for decreased range of movement is increased disc stiffness.[33]

The 40 percent increase in disc stiffness with age is associated with well documented histologic and biochemical changes. These include an increase in the total number of collagen fibers and in the ratio of type I to type II collagen, a decrease in water content and a change in the proteoglycan ratios where the proportion of keratan sulfate; chondroitin sulfate increases.[84] There is also an associated increase in "fatigue failure" of collagen in older cartilage. It is uncer-tain whether it is collagen fibers that undergo "fatigue" or splitting or whether it is the bonds between adjacent collagen fibers that separate. Collectively, these changes and the associated decrease in compliance render the disc fibro-cartilage less capable of acting efficiently as a shock absorber or joint, and of transmitting loads along the vertebral column.[33,85,86]

## Lumbar Intersegmental Motion

It is an essential part of a physical therapist's examination to determine ranges of movement of the whole lumbar spine. In addition to measurement of these physiologic ranges of movements, the manipulative physical therapist always conducts a manual assessment of lumbar intersegmental motion. This involves the displacement of a lumbar motion segment by the application of an external, manual force applied directly through the spinous processes, or indirectly via the ligaments and joints of the adjacent vertebrae. Small rotations and translations about and along the axes of movement can be achieved in this way (see Fig. 2-8). No techniques are currently available for objective clinical local anomalies (increases or decreases in movement) to be confidently diag-nosed. While these techniques involve subjective evaluation of vertebral mo-tion, it is interesting to note its current excellent correlation with other diagnos-tic studies.[38]

Many clinical reports have associated either hypo- or hypermobility with a variety of lumbar disorders and low back pain.[34] At this point in time, there is very little real evidence linking ranges of motion and back pain,[87] although anecdotal and clinical stories abound. However, Farrell and Twomey,[81,82] in a study of acute low back pain and manipulative therapy, did show an improve-ment in lumbar sagittal motion (measured manually) associated with improvement in back pain symptoms. Giles and Taylor[15] also showed increased lumbar range of movement following recovery from episodes of low back pain, but this increase was only in patients under the age of 50 years. Similarly, Jull[88] has shown an increase in intersegmental motion associated with remission of symptoms in patients with low back pain. It is likely that current research will throw further light on this question over the next few years.

## BIOMECHANICS

The orientation of the lumbar articular processes facilitates sagittal movement and allows for a considerable range of motion in this plane. From the "normal" erect standing posture, flexion usually comprises about 80 percent and extension 20 percent of the total range of sagittal movement. Flexion ceases due to apposition of lumbar zygapophyseal joint surfaces and tightening of posterior ligaments and muscles, whereas extension is blocked by bone contact when the inferior joint facets come into contact with the laminae of the vertebra below or the spinous processes meet.[33]

## Control of Flexion

### Muscular Control

The lumbar back muscles exert considerable control over active ranges of lumbar movement (see Ch. 4). Erector spinae and multifidis are principally responsible for all movements[72] by exerting an eccentric control (i.e., by paying out) on movements that are gravity assisted. Thus trunk flexion in standing or sitting is controlled by an eccentric contraction of these muscle groups. In exerting this control, the muscles tend to restrict the total range of movements possible, particularly in the sagittal plane.[32,64,79] This helps explain why cadavaric studies show a slightly greater range of lumbar sagittal movement than is usually recorded in the living.[5]

It has been shown that after suitable warm-up exercises, ranges of lumbar flexion increase by a few degrees,[32] and that a change in posture from the upright to the side-lying position brings about an additional increase, which equates with the ranges observed in the cadaveric studies. It would appear that warm-up exercises achieve their effect by relaxation or stretching of the sacrospinalis muscle group and it is not unreasonable to assume that the slightly larger increase obtained in side lying is due to the elimination of antigravity activity in the long back muscles. Research has shown[64] an "electrically silent" phase in the back muscles at the limit of lumbar flexion. Although they conclude that the spine is supported passively by tension in postvertebral connective tissue structures at this point, it may also be due in part to passive elastic tension of the posterior muscles themselves. Indeed, the apposed zygapophyseal facets play the greater restraining role.[33]

Each lumbar multifidus muscle attaches strongly to a mamillary process on a superior articular process and also into the capsule of zygapophyseal joint. It acts as a rotator cuff muscle and maintains the approximation and congruity of the zygapophyseal facets on the posterolateral aspect of the joint (the ligamentum flavum maintains the articular surfaces in close apposition on the anteromedial side of the joint). The close relation of this muscle to the joint capsule and its similar innervation would readily explain how with other postvertebral muscles it would severely limit flexion and rotation in any painful condition of the joints.

### Other Factors Controlling Lumbar Flexion

In addition to the postvertebral muscles, the posterior elements of the lumbar spine consist of a complex ligamentous system and the articulating bony arches. Over the years there have been a number of conflicting views on the relative roles played by these posterior elements in limiting and controlling the range of lumbar flexion. In general, it has been considered that the interspinous and supraspinous ligaments and the strong elastic ligamentum flavum served principally to act as a "brake" to flexion.[89] In this regard, the elasticity of the ligamentum flavum was seen as important because tension increased as the movement continued, while the dense, strong, and inelastic inter- and supraspinous ligaments acted as a physical barrier to the movement.

Adams et al,[90] in a sequential posterior release experiment, quantitated the relative parts played by the supraspinous–infraspinous ligaments, the ligamentum flavum, the zygapophyseal joint fibrous capsule, and the intervertebral disc in resisting flexion of individual motion segments. They showed that the joint fibrous capsule and intervertebral disc play the more important roles, with the ligamentum flavum and spinous ligaments making lesser contributions. They found it most surprising that the relatively unimpressive fibrous capsule should exert such large restraining forces, and noted that technical problems in sectioning all capsular fibers made it difficult to distinguish the role of capsular forces from articular facet forces exerted through the articular processes.

In our study[33] of the role of the posterior elements, each of the posterior ligaments was sectioned in turn (supraspinous and interspinous, ligamentum flavum and capsule), as was the bony arch to assess the influence of each on the range of lumbar flexion. The range of flexion was measured before and after sectioning of each of the elements and the results are listed in Table 2-2.

**Table 2-2.** Average Increases (Degrees) in Sagittal Range Following Section

| Section | Flexion Increase | Extension Increase | Sagittal Range Increase |
|---|---|---|---|
| Supraspinous and interspinous ligaments | 2.0 | 1.5 | 3.5 |
| Ligamenta flava | 2.5 | 1.0 | 3.5 |
| Joint capsules | 3.0 | 2.0 | 5.0 |
| Pedicles | 14.0 | 3.0 | 17.0 |

Analysis demonstrated small regular increases in sagittal range on each successive ligamentous release and a large abrupt increase in range following section of the vertebral arches. Young and middle-aged subjects showed almost a 100 percent increase in lumbar sagittal range after removal of all posterior elements, whereas elderly subjects showed a 60 percent increase (Fig. 2-11).

This study confirms that all the ligamentous elements offer some resistance to lumbar flexion, with the joint capsules having the greatest influence, as suggested by Adams, et al.[90] However, by far the greatest restraining influence on flexion is the pressure between the apposed articular facets of the zygapophyseal joints. Radiographic analysis of flexion in a young cadaveric lumbar spine showed that the movement includes both forward rotation of a vertebra on the vertebra beneath along an axis in the posterior part of the intervertebral disc, and an associated forward translation or slide of the superior vertebrae on the inferior vertebra (Fig. 2-12). The zygapophyseal joints guide the plane of rotation and resist the forward slide. The coronally oriented anterior component of each articular facet bears the resultant stress. When the pedicles are cut, a greater degree of forward slide permits further rotation.

Joint loading in axial weightbearing has been described by Nachemson[91] and by Shah et al.[92] It seems clear from our studies that flexion involves progressive joint loading to the point where the horizontal moment prevents further rotation from occurring. The lumbar vertebral arches through the zygapophyseal joints thus provide an essential restraint limiting or preventing the transmission of shearing forces to the intervertebral discs. This could lead to instability (as in spondylolisthesis) with danger to the cauda equina and to the nerve roots in the intervertebral canals.

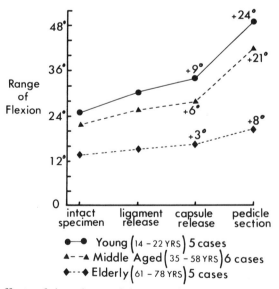

**Fig. 2-11.** The effects of the release of the posterior vertebral elements on the range of lumbar flexion. (From Twomey and Taylor,[33] with permission.)

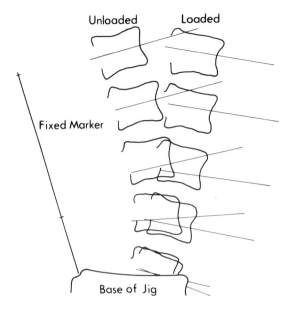

Unloaded    Loaded

Fixed Marker

Base of Jig

**Fig. 2-12.** Tracings of superimposed radiographic plates showing the range of flexion produced and indicating the types of movement involved. (From Twomey and Taylor,[33] with permission.)

Age differences in response to the posterior sectioning procedure cited above throw light on the effect of increased stiffness with aging in the intervertebral discs. Following ligamentous release and also more dramatically following pedicle section, the available increase in movement range is much reduced in elderly subjects compared to young subjects. This demonstrates that the increased stiffness or the reduction in disc compliance with aging is the principal reason for the observed decrease in lumbar range of movement. The important conclusions drawn from the studies described above are summarized below:

1. Lumbar sagittal movement involves both forward rotation and slide of one vertebra on the vertebra beneath around a coronal axis located in the posterior annulus of the intervertebral disc.
2. Sagittal movement of the vertebral column is restricted more by progressive increase in loading of apposed facetal joint surfaces in flexion than by tension or compression in posterior ligaments.
3. The decline in sagittal range of movement in old age is principally due to increasing stiffness in the intervertebral disc.

## Creep in the Lumbar Spine

We have argued (above) that the stiffness in intervertebral discs and the progressive loading of the zygapophyseal joints are the factors bringing the normal range of flexion to a halt. However, prolonged loading in flexion (10 minutes or more) *does* produce further flexion of the spine. This movement is due to creep, which is the progressive deformation of a structure under constant load when the forces are not large enough to cause permanent damage to the vertebral structures.

## Axial Creep

In the normal erect posture, approximately 16 to 20 percent of axial compressive load on the lumbar spine is borne by zygapophyseal joints, while the rest is carried by the intervertebral discs,[91,93] which are well suited to this purpose. When axial loads to intervertebral discs are maintained, the discs progressively lose height until the chemical forces developed within them equal those mechanical forces applied externally.[94] Provided that the forces used are below the levels that would cause permanent damage, the greater the external force then the greater the loss of height that occurs.[94,95]

During the day, a person's body weight acts as an axial compression force through the vertebral column, and the subsequent creep brings about a reduction in stature. When body weight is relieved (e.g., at night in bed) and axial loads reduced, the intervertebral discs and other soft tissues are able to rehydrate and stature increases.[96] It has recently been demonstrated that a period of rest in full flexion brings about a more rapid increase in stature than does rest in the fully extended position.[27] This presumably occurs because flexion acts as a distracting force on the lumbar region, causing the discs to "suck in" water at a greater rate.

## Creep in Flexion

When full-range lumbar flexion is maintained under load for a period of time, the articular triad is distorted so that the anterior disc region is "squeezed" while the posterior region is stretched; the zygapophyseal joint surfaces are compressed tightly together as the coronal part of the articular surfaces bear most of the load; the soft tissues adjust by creep.[91,94,95,97]

Creep in flexion is observed as progressive ventral movement into further flexion, so that the endpoint of flexion is increased (i.e., range increases). The amount of creep in the elderly is greater than in the young and both the creep and the recovery from creep take place over a longer period of time. During the process fluid is extruded from the soft tissues and they become relatively deprived of their nutrition.[98] Repetitive loading causes cartilage degeneration and bone hypertrophy in the various elements of the articular triad.[99]

If the amount of creep involved after prolonged loadbearing in flexion is considerable, then recovery back to the original starting posture (hysteresis) is extremely slow. It takes considerable time for the soft tissues to imbibe fluid after it has been expressed during prolonged flexion loading. Many occupational groups (e.g., stonemasons, bricklayers, roofing carpenters) regularly submit their lumbar spines to this category of insult. They work with their lumbar column fully flexed and under load for considerable periods of time. There is often little movement away from the fully flexed position once it has been reached and little opportunity for recovery between episodes of work in this position. It is therefore not at all surprising to find so many bricklayers, for instance, with chronic back pain and with occasional episodes of acute pain. These occupational groups need considerable ergonomic advice and require alterations to their working conditions if this situation is to be rectified.[95]

## Control of Extension

### The Role of Muscles

The control of lumbar extension has not been investigated and analyzed to the same extent as flexion. In the erect standing or sitting postures, the movement is initiated by contraction of the long back-extensor muscles, and then controlled by the eccentric contraction of the abdominal muscle group once the movement has begun. The range of extension from the neutral erect standing position is much less than the range of flexion, but the muscular control mechanisms are very similar.

### Other Contributing Factors

It seems probable that the range of extension is not controlled by ligamentous tension, but that it ceases when the two inferior articular processes at any level are forced against the laminae of the vertebrae below or perhaps when the spinous processes "kiss." This is witnessed by the build-up in compact bone, which is evident in the lamina beneath the inferior process. Extension occurs along an axis in the posterior part of the intervertebral disc at that level. This position probably does not place the soft tissues under the same constant strain as flexion does except at the limits of lordosis after prolonged standing, when zygapophyseal joints probably take a larger amount of the load of body weight. When hyperextension occurs, it is likely that the axis of movement shifts even further posteriorly and is located where the tips of the inferior facets articulate with the laminae. This would cause stretching of the anterior soft tissues, notably the anterior longitudinal ligament and the anterior annulus fibrosus, which are extremely strong and capable of withstanding such forces. It is apparent from our investigations that considerable osteoarthritic change takes place in the articular cartilage and subchondral bone. This change occurs at the polar region of the inferior recesses of the zygapophyseal joints corresponding to the areas of extension impact and compression.[99]

**Creep in Extension**

Prolonged maintenance of an extended posture or of loading in extension are rare, and few if any occupational groups have such a working situation. The position of the line of gravity is described as passing anterior to the thoracic vertebrae and through the lumbar vertebrae.[100] Theoretically, prolonged standing (i.e., axial loading with body weight) would tend to increase thoracic kyphosis (by creep), but not alter lumbar lordosis. However, present evidence indicates that in prolonged standing there is a tendency for the axial load of body weight to increase lumbar lordosis. In this way, the zygapophyseal joints will take an increasing proportion of the load of body weight. Although long, continued lordotic posture and loading are rare, a number of sports activities involve full extension movements of an explosive nature. These may be repetitive movements and may involve high peaks of loading in full extension. Thus, fast bowlers in cricket, gymnasts, and high jumpers are three groups that place tremendous impact forces through this posterior arch complex. At heel strike during these sports, the chisel-like inferior articular processes are forced down suddenly into the laminae of the vertebrae below. The forces involved are very considerable, as the load borne by the facets increases dramatically with the amount of extension of the region.[101] Repetition over long periods of time results in soft-tissue inflammation and bone sclerosis that may become obvious on radiographic examination, but which may later result in fracture and perhaps displacement. The bone area that absorbs this force is the isthmus between the zygapophyseal facets (i.e., the pars interarticularis). As is well known, this is the site at which spondylolysis occurs. It is even more likely that the repetitive combination of alternative explosive full extension followed suddenly by full flexion places enormous strain on the pars interarticularis region. This extension/flexion repetition moment at the pars may cause fatigue fracture in a similar way to that of fatigue in metal caused by successive opposite movements.

Considerable research on the mechanics of this region has taken place in recent years.[93]

## VULNERABILITY OF THE DISC TO LOADING: INTRADISCAL PRESSURE

The nucleus of the intervertebral disc is contained under pressure within its protective fibrous and cartilaginous envelope. Intradiscal pressure is a useful index of disc function and has been shown to vary according to posture, movement, external loading, and age. Nachemson's comprehensive study[91] on lumbar intradiscal pressure in 128 discs from 38 cadavers of both sexes from 6 to 82 years of age concluded the following:

1. The loaded disc behaves hydrostatically in that the nucleus acts as a fluid, distributing external pressures equally in all outward directions to the annulus.

2. Axial loading produces lower pressure readings in children under the age of 16 years than in adults.

3. The level of the lumbar spine does not influence the pressures recorded in "loaded" or resting discs (the L5–S1 disc was not included in the study).

4. The posterior vertebral structures (pedicles and articular processes) absorb 16 to 20 percent of the axial loading forces.

5. "Moderately degenerated" discs (as suggested by disc "thinning") show similar pressure behavior to "intact" discs, and the mechanical behavior of a lumbar disc does not change appreciably if "degeneration" is not advanced.

Since Nachemson's original study,[91] it has been shown in living subjects that intradiscal pressures are higher in the sitting than the standing posture[102,103]; they are less in the physiologic lordotic posture than in the straight or kyphotic posture[103]; pressures are increased with passive lumbar flexion of 20°[104]; they are further increased during active trunk flexion exercises[105]; and the largest increases accompany heavy lifting, particularly when the Valsalva maneuver is performed.[106] Nachemson et al[30] and Merriam et al[107] showed that abnormal degenerated discs did not behave in a consistent way, as they showed patterns of pressure changes in different postures that were often dissimilar from that shown by normal discs. Similarly, other studies have shown that the ability of the disc to withstand compressive forces depends on both the integrity of the disc envelope and the turgor of the contained nucleus pulposus.[55,108,109] This contrasts with the claim of Belytschko et al[110] that in a theoretical model annular tears would reduce intradiscal pressures more than degenerative nuclear lesions.

## Clinical Considerations

The effects of different postures, exercises, and loading conditions on intradiscal pressure are of interest to the physical therapist as an indicator of how the disc responds to these variables and of the possible abnormal response in disc degeneration. However, intradiscal pressure alone does not appear to be able to indicate which activities are likely to be either safe or dangerous for a patient's back. Although it is probably important to take the environmental condition of the disc into account when prescribing exercise, as yet there are no clear indications that any particular exercises are contraindicated on the grounds that a rise in intradiscal pressure would be prejudicial to the disc or risk injury to the vertebral end-plates.

It is quite clear that movements such as lumbar flexion and lateral bending and tasks such as the lifting of heavy weights increase intradiscal pressure. For this reason, many clinicians approach these activities with considerable care and watch their patients very carefully when they begin such activities. Similarly, patients need to be aware of the effect of these activities on their lumbar spine and approach tasks that involve rises in intradiscal pressure with reasonable care. In the same way, because it is known that intradiscal pressure is lowest in supine and prone lying, is lower in standing than in sitting, and remains quite low in activities involving lumbar extension and rotation, then some clinicians may wish to use this information in the exercise programs they prescribe. While this may be useful, no direct link has yet been established between a rise in intradiscal pressure and the production of a disc lesion. Similarly, ergonomic advice as to lifting technique, seat design (including car seat design), working posture, and activities of daily living that emphasizes the maintenance of a lordosis is often given on the basis of the effects of these tasks on intradiscal pressure. It still remains uncertain just what role raised intradiscal pressure may play in the production of disc lesions and low back pain or whether reduced pressure may prevent disc lesions. Therefore, it remains an interesting observation that may ultimately prove to be of practical use, but at present its relevance is uncertain.

## THE INFLUENCE OF INTRATRUNKAL PRESSURE

Until quite recent times, intrathoracic and intraabdominal pressure have been considered to be important in relieving the spine of a large part of the axial compression and shear loads by converting the trunk into a more solid cylinder and transmitting part of the load over the wider area. It was considered highly likely that intraabdominal pressure exerted a major force in this regard by the simultaneous contraction of abdominal muscles, the diaphragm, and the muscles of the pelvic diaphragm. These are mostly transverse and obliquely oriented muscles, all capable of exerting considerable torque and compressive force on the cavity they enclose.

The thoracic spine bears less weight than the lumbar spine and is supported ventrally and laterally by the physical presence of the ribs and to a lesser extent, when the glottis is closed, by a rise in intrathoracic pressure. The role of intraabdominal pressure in reducing forces acting on the spine and protecting vulnerable vertebral bodies and intervertebral discs from excessive loading was initially investigated by Bartelink,[111] and since then has excited the imagination of other researchers.[106,112–116]

Contraction of the muscles of the trunk cavity to raise intraabdominal pressure probably functions as a protective reflex mechanism, both to protect abdominal viscera from damage by a blow and to assist in protecting the vertebral column from excessive loading. Thus, when loads are placed on the vertebral column, the muscles are involuntarily called into action to fix the rib cage and to restrain and compress the contents of the abdominal cavity so that it becomes like a "balloon."[115] The positions of the trunk and the load influence the extent of any rise in intraabdominal pressure. The greater the spine is flexed and the further the load is away from the body, the greater is the increase in intraabdominal pressure required to balance the load and help distribute the compression forces.

The mechanism may be compared to an inflated balloon, which acts on an anterior moment arm two or three times the length of the posterior moment arm of the back extensor muscles. Pressures generated in the abdominal cavity will produce a net positive moment, and tend to restore the lordotic curvature of the lumbar spine. This will counteract the flexion moments produced by the upper body and the anterior load carried. Eie[114] described the relieving force of intraabdominal pressure as reducing by about 40 percent the required compressive effect of the contraction force of the erector spinae muscles. However, recent studies have clearly shown that the effect is nowhere near as substantial.[30] They have shown a much smaller relieving net effect due to intratrunkal pressure and have also clearly demonstrated that there is not a linear relationship between the increase in intratrunkal pressure and the strength of contraction of the abdominal musculature.[30,117]

Intraabdominal pressure thus plays a small role in stabilizing the spine and pelvis at the onset of the lift by resisting trunk flexion, although it probably does little to reduce intervertebral compression forces. This helps allow the pelvis to be rotated backward and the lumbar curve to be flattened by the powerful gluteal and hamstring muscles, which have a longer moment arm and a greater cross-sectional area (and thus power) than do the spinal extensors. Thus they are the most suitable and capable muscles to be recruited in initiating the task of heavy lifting,[118] and help to reduce the moment of the load, allowing the erector spinae muscles to take over and extend the spine on a stable pelvis.[119]

While the suggested ability of intratrunkal pressure to relieve loads acting on the lumbar spine received significant support in the 30 years since Bartelink,[111] there are currently many questions raised about its validity. These have arisen since studies of lifting have not demonstrated sufficiently large rises in intraabdominal pressure that correlate with either the size of the load being lifted, or the stresses measured on the vertebral column.[30,106,117,120] Similarly, increasing intraabdominal pressure by using the Valsalva maneuver may actually increase the load on the lumbar spine, whereas strengthening abdominal muscles in normal people or in those with back pain does not appear to increase the capacity to raise intraabdominal pressure as measured during lifting.[30,106,117,120] It should also be taken into account that it has been clearly shown that to raise intraabdominal pressure high enough to generate a sufficient antiflexor moment, the pressure would be so high as to obstruct blood flow in the vena cava and abdominal aorta,[121] a point that Bartelink[111] noted in his early study.

The lowest intraabdominal pressures have been recorded in the smallest people, whereas largest pressures are evident in taller, heavier subjects.[122] Strong atheletes are able to produce enormous rises in intraabdominal pressure.[120] Gait shows phasic changes in this pressure, with increases as the speed of the activity increases. Jumping in place or from a height raises the pressure, as do pushing and pulling activities. It is uncertain whether or not the Valsalva maneuver or the use of a lumbosacral corset does any more than produce marginal increases in intraabdominal pressure.

## Clinical Considerations

In the past, intraabdominal pressure was considered to be a potent influence for reducing the loads applied to the spine. This rationale was used to explain the need for the development of strong abdominal musculature surrounding the abdominopelvic cavity. However, more recent research has demonstrated that intraabdominal pressure does not dramatically reduce loads on the spine. The previous estimates of the loads generated at the L5–S1 junction during maximal lifting were an overestimate and the back musculature has been shown to be stronger and able to generate a considerably greater power than was first estimated.[117] These observations, together with a greater understanding of the role of the thoracolumbar fascia in assisting in distributing a small percentage of the load and in "tying" the long back muscles down (see Ch. 4) has meant that the inherent strength of the back mechanism as a whole is better recognized. Similarly, Waddell[123] has demonstrated that those with back pain respond very favorably to programs of intensive exercise, including a strong trunk-strengthening program. This adds weight to the argument that musculoskeletal fitness is a major factor in the management of back pain and lifting disorders. The role of intraabdominal pressure in this equation is now under serious debate and would benefit from further research. It may be that improvements in abdominal muscle strength achieve an effect through the better control of pelvic and spinal posture rather than by a greater capacity to raise intraabdominal pressure.

## ZYGAPOPHYSEAL JOINT INTRACAPSULAR PRESSURE

In 1983, physical therapists Giovanelli, Thompson, and Elvey[124] conducted a pilot trial investigating lumbar zygapophyseal intracapsular joint pressures in living subjects. They placed two needles within the joint under radiographic control, one needle to inject saline and the other to record pressure changes. They showed that there is no intracapsular pressure at rest. Once fluid was injected into the joint, most active and passive movements caused a drop in the pressure produced by the injection, the pressure rising again on return to the starting position. The greatest drops in pressure occurred when passive techniques were directed specifically to the joint concerned. This highlighted a possible mechanism of pain relief by the use of localized manipulative and mobilizing techniques because raised intracapsular pressure with outpouring of fluid may result from some forms of joint pathology. This pilot trial needs to be extended considerably before much regard can be placed on its conclusions, but it does provide interesting information useful to the manipulative physical therapist on the ways in which manipulative techniques directly influence the joints moved. The anatomic studies of the fat-pads of the lumbar facet polar recesses show that in movement, the fat moves in and out of the joint in response to any changes in pressure.

## SKELETAL HEALTH AND EXERCISE

As described in Chapter 1, the internal architecture of lumbar vertebrae consists of vertical bony trabeculae (beams or struts of bone) supported by horizontal trabeculae, which are aligned parallel to the lines of stress. Thus the vertical trabeculae absorb the axial loads of weightbearing, and transmit the load downward and outward to the vertebral shell via the transverse trabeculae, which resist buckling of the vertical weight-bearing beams. It is likely that the horizontal trabeculae are also important in absorbing and transmitting the lateral forces applied through the body as a consequence of muscular activity. Old age is associated with a significant selective decline in the numbers of horizontal trabeculae. The compressive load of body weight, which is usually maintained in old age, brings about fractures of the now less-well-supported vertical trabeculae, and collapse of the vertebral end-plate. Lumbar vertebrae become shorter and wider in old age, and more concave at the disc–vertebral junction.[125]

This pattern of selective bone loss and associated changes in vertebral body shape is part of the general picture of osteopenia and osteoporosis seen in the elderly. In Western society, at age 65 radiographic comparison with a "standard" suggests that 66 percent of women and 22 percent of men have osteoporosis. In women the incidence increases by about 8 percent for each additional decade, whereas a large increase does not occur until after the age of 76 in men.[126] The principal sites of fracture and pain due to osteoporosis are the vertebral column, the distal radius, and the neck of the femur. It causes over 200,000 hip fractures annually in the United States. Pain and shortened stature accompanied by "dowager's hump" or hunchback in elderly women are major symptoms of advanced osteoporosis, which often leads to vertebral collapse and functional disability.[127]

The prevention of osteoporosis at present focuses on the need for relatively high levels of dietary calcium (1000 to 1200 mg/day), particularly in women, and for estrogen replacement therapy in some women.[128,129] Recently, considerable attention has also been paid to the important role of exercise in prevention. Important studies by Aloia et al[130] and Smith et al[131] have shown bone gain to follow exercise even in very elderly subjects. Physical therapists dealing with the prevention and treatment of back pain and disability need to stress these factors with their middle-aged and elderly patients. There is no doubt that bone loss occurs in the absence of physical activity, and that bone hypertrophy follows increased exercise activity.[132] It is likely that the incidence of osteoporotic bone fractures in the elderly could be reduced if regular exercise was generally maintained into old age. This reduced risk of fracture may relate as much to the maintenance of muscle strength and neuromuscular coordination as to the associated maintenance of bone mass.

## REFERENCES

1. Kendall FP, McCreary EK: Muscles, Testing and Function. 3rd Ed. Williams & Wilkins, Baltimore, 1983
2. Schmorl G, Junghanns H: The Human Spine in Health and Disease. 2nd Ed. Grune & Stratton, New York, 1971

 3. Horak FB: Clinical measurement of postural control in adults. Phys Ther 67:1881, 1987
 4. Taylor JR: Growth of human I/V discs and vertebral bodies. J Anat 120:49, 1975
 5. Twomey LT: Age changes in the human lumbar spine. PhD Thesis, University of Western Australia, 1981
 6. Landau BR: Essential Human Anatomy and Physiology. 2nd Ed. Scott Foresman, Glenview, IL, 1980
 7. Treanor WJ: Motions of the hand and foot. In Licht SH (ed): Therapeutic Exercise. Waverly Press, Baltimore, 1965
 8. Opila KA, Wagner SS, Schiowit Z, Chen J: Postural alignment in barefoot and high heel stance. Spine 13:542, 1988
 9. Youngman A, Elliott M: The effect of high heel shoes on lumbar lordosis. BAppSc project, Western Australian Institute of Technology, 1985
10. Romanes CJ: Cunningham's Textbook of Anatomy. 11th Ed. Oxford University Press, Oxford, 1972
11. Taylor JR, Alexander R: BSc project, University of Western Australia, 1983
12. Ostgaard HC, Andersson GBJ, Karlsson K: Prevalence of back pain in pregnancy. Spine 16:549, 1991
13. Day JW, Smidt GL, Lehmann T: Effect of pelvic tilt on standing posture. Phys Ther 64:510, 1984
14. Hansson T, Sandstrom J, Roos B et al: The bone mineral content of the lumbar spine in patients with chronic low back pain. Spine 10:158, 1985
15. Giles LGF, Taylor JR: Low back pain associated with leg length inequality. Spine 6:510, 1981
16. Willner S: A study of height, weight and menarche in girls with idiopathic structural scoliosis. Acta Orthop Scand 46:71, 1975
17. Taylor JR, Halliday M: Limb length asymmetry and growth. J Anat 126:634, 1978
18. Ingelmark BE, Lindstrom J: Asymmetries of the lower extremities and pelvis and their relationship to lumbar scoliosis. Acute Morphol Neerl Scand 5/6:227, 1963
19. Taylor JR, Slinger BS: Scoliosis screening and growth in Western Australian students. Med J Aust 17:475, 1980
20. Giles LGF, Taylor JR: Intra-articular synovial protrusions. Bull Hosp J Dis Orthop Inst 42:248, 1982
21. Giles LGF, Taylor JR: The effect of postural scoliosis on lumbar apophyseal joints. Scand J Rheumatol 13:209, 1984
22. Terjesen T, Benum P, Rossvoll I et al: Leg length discrepancy measured by ultrasonography. Acta Orthop Scand 62:121, 1991
23. Sicuranza BJ, Richards J, Tisdall LH: The short leg syndrome in obstetrics and gynaecology. Am J Obstet Gynecol 107:217, 1970
24. De Puky MD: Diurnal variation in stature. Acta Orthop Scand 6:338, 1935
25. Blackman J: Experimental error inherent in measuring the growing human being. p. 389. In Boyd E (ed): Am J Phys Anthropol 13, 1924
26. Stone M, Taylor JR: Factors influencing stature. BSc anatomy dissertation, University of Western Australia, 1977
27. Tyrrell AP, Reilly T, Troup JDG: Circadian variation in stature and the effects of spinal loading. Spine 10:161, 1985
28. Adams MA, Hutton WC: The effect of posture on the lumbar spine. Bone Joint Surg 67B:625, 1985
29. Sullivan WE, Miles M: The lumbar segment of the vertebral column. Anat Rec 133:619, 1959

30. Nachemson AL, Schultz AB, Berkson MH: Mechanical properties of human lumbar spine motion segments. Spine 4:1, 1979
31. Twomey LT, Taylor JR: Age changes in the lumbar intervertebral discs. Acta Orthop Scand 56:496, 1985
32. Taylor JR, Twomey LT: Sagittal and horizontal plane movement of the human lumbar vertebral column in cadavers and in the living. Rheumatol Rehabil 19:223, 1980
33. Twomey LT, Taylor JR: Sagittal movements of the human lumbar vertebral column: a quantitative study of the role of the posterior vertebral elements. Arch Phys Med Rehabil 64:322, 1983
34. White AA, Panjabi MM: The Clinical Biomechanics of the Spine. JB Lippincott, Philadelphia, 1978
35. Dunham WF: Ankylosing spondylitis: measurement of hip and spine movements. Br J Phys Med 12:126, 1949
36. Lindahl O: Determination of the sagittal mobility of the lumbar spine: a clinical method. Acta Orthop Scand 37:241, 1966
37. Leighton JR: The Leighton flexometer and flexibility test. J Assoc Phys Ment Rehabil 20:86, 1966
38. Gregersen G, Lucas DB: An in vivo study of the axial rotation of the human thoracolumbar spine. J Bone Joint Surg 49A:247, 1967
39. Loebl WY: Measurement of spinal posture and range of spinal movement. Ann Phys Med 9:103, 1967
40. Loebl WY: Regional rotation of the spine. Rheumatol Rehabil 12:223, 1973
41. Macrae IF, Wright V: Measurement of back movement. Ann Rheum Dis 28:584, 1969
42. Moll JMH, Liyanage SP, Wright V: An objective clinical method to measure spinal extension. Rheum Phys Med 11:293, 1972
43. Moll J, Wright V: Measurement of spinal movement. p. 93. In Jayson M (ed): The Lumbar Spine and Back Pain, Pitman Medical, Kent, England, 1976
44. Wiles P: Movements of the lumbar vertebra during flexion and extension. Proc R Soc Med 28:647, 1935
45. Gianturco C: A roentgen analysis of the motion of the lower lumbar vertebrae. Am J Roentgenol 52:261, 1944
46. Hasner E, Schalintzek M, Snorrason E: Roentgenological examination of the function of the lumbar spine. Acta Radiol 37:141, 1952
47. Tanz SS: Motion of the lumbar spine. A roentgenologic study. Am J Roentgenol 69:399, 1953
48. Allbrook D: Movements of the lumbar spinal column. J Bone Joint Surg 39B:339, 1957
49. Rolander SD: Motion of the lumbar spine with special reference to the stabilising effect of posterior fusion. Acta Orthop Scand, suppl. 90, 1966
50. Troup JDG, Hood CA, Chapman AE: Measurements of the sagittal mobility of the lumbar spine and hips. Ann Phys Med 9:308, 1967
51. Froning EC, Frohman B: Motion of the lumbosacral spine after laminectomy and spine fusion. J Bone Joint Surg 50A:897, 1968
52. Virgin WJ: Experimental investigations into the physical properties of the intervertebral disc. J Bone Joint Surg 33B:607, 1951
53. Hirsch K: The reaction of the intervertebral discs to compression forces. J Bone Joint Surg 37A:1188, 1955
54. Hirsch K, Nachemson A: A new observation on the mechanical behavior of lumbar discs. Acta Orthop Scand 23:254, 1954

55. Brown T, Hansen RJ, Yorra AJ: Some mechanical tests on the lumbosacral spine with particular reference to the intervertebral discs. J Bone Joint Surg 39A:1135, 1957

56. Evans FG, Lissner HR: Biomechanical studies on the lumbar spine and pelvis. J Bone Joint Surg 41A:278, 1959

57. Roaf R: Vertebral growth and its mechanical control. J Bone Joint Surg 42B:40, 1960

58. Galante JO: Tensile properties of the human lumbar annulus fibrosis. Acta Orthop Scand, suppl. 100:1, 1967

59. White AA: Analysis of the mechanics of the thoracic spine in man. Acta Orthop Scand, suppl. 127, 1969

60. Farfan HF, Cossette JW, Robertson GH et al: The effects of torsion on the lumbar intervertebral joints: the role of torsion in the production of disc degeneration. J Bone Joint Surg 52A:468, 1970

61. King AL, Vulcan AP: Elastic deformation characteristics of the spine. J Biomech 4:413, 1971

62. Kazarian L: Dynamic response characteristics of the human lumbar vertebral column. Acta Orthop Scand, suppl. 146:1, 1972

63. Panjabi MM: Experimental determination of spinal motion segment behavior. Orthop Clin North Am 8:169, 1977

64. Twomey LT, Taylor JR: Physical Therapy of the Low Back. Churchill Livingstone, New York, 1987

65. Keegan JJ: Alterations of the lumbar curve related to posture and seating. J Bone Joint Surg 35A:589, 1953

66. Davis PR, Troup JDG, Burnard JH: Movements of the thoracic and lumbar spine when lifting: a chrono-cyclophotographic study. J Anat 99:13, 1965

67. Schultz AB, Belytschko TP, Andriacchi TP et al: Analog studies of forces in the human spine: mechanical properties and motion segment behaviour. J Biomech 6:373, 1973

68. Panjabi MM: Three-dimensional mathematical model of the human spine structure. J Biomech 6:671, 1973

69. Belytschko TB, Andriacchi TP, Schultz AB et al: Analog studies of forces in the human spine: computational techniques. J Biomech 6:361, 1973

70. Panjabi MM, Brand RA, White AA: Mechanical properties of the human thoracic spine. J Bone Joint Surg 58A:642, 1976

71. Panjabi MM, Krag MH, White AA: Effects of preload on load displacement curves of the lumbar spine. Orthop Clin North Am 8:181, 1977

72. Bogduk N, Macintosh JE, Pearcy MJ: A universal model of the lumbar back muscles in the upright position. Spine 17:897, 1992

73. Begg AG, Falconer MA: Plain radiographs in intraspinal protrusion of lumbar intervertebral discs: a correlation with operative findings. Br J Surg 36:225, 1949

74. Lovett RW: A contribution to the study of the mechanics of the spine. Am J Anat 2:457, 1902

75. Tondury G: Functional anatomy of the small joints of the spine. Ann Med Phys 15:2, 1971

76. Kapandji IA: The Physiology of the Joints. 2nd Ed. Vol. 3. Trunk and Vertebral Column. Churchill Livingstone, London, 1974

77. Lewin T, Moffett B, Viidik A: The morphology of lumbar synovial intervertebral joints. Acta Morphol Neerl Scand 4:229, 1961

78. Rissanen PM: The surgical anatomy and pathology of the supraspinous and interspinous ligaments of the lumbar spine with special reference to ligament ruptures. Acta Orthop Scand, suppl. 46, 1960
79. Bogduk N, Twomey LT: Clinical Anatomy of the Lumbar Spine. 2nd Ed. Churchill Livingstone, Melbourne, Australia, 1991
80. Lumsden RM, Morris JM: An in vivo study of axial rotation and immobilisation at the lumbosacral joint. J Bone Joint Surg 50A:1591, 1968
81. Farrell JP, Twomey LT: Acute low back pain: comparison of two conservative treatment approaches. Med J Aust 1:160, 1982
82. Farrell J: A comparison of two conservative treatment approaches to acute low back pain. MAppSc Thesis, Western Australian Institute of Technology, 1982
83. Nachemson A: Lumbar spine instability: a critical update and symposium summary. Spine 10:290, 1985
84. Adams P, Eyre DR, Muir H: Biomechanical aspects of development and ageing of human lumbar intervertebral discs. Rheum Rehabil 16:22, 1977
85. Bushell GR, Ghosh P, Taylor TFK et al: Proteoglycan chemistry of the intervertebral disc. Clin Orthop 129:115, 1977
86. Nachemson AL: The lumbar spine: an orthopaedic challenge. Spine 1:59, 1976
87. Hilton RC, Ball J, Benn RT: In-vitro mobility of the lumbar spine. Ann Rheum Dis 38:378, 1979
88. Jull G: The changes with age in lumbar segmental motion as assessed by manual examination. Master's Thesis, University of Queensland, 1985
89. Ramsey RH: The anatomy of the ligamenta flava. Clin Orthop 44:129, 1966
90. Adams MA, Hutton WC, Stott MA: The resistance of flexion of the lumbar intervertebral joint. Spine 5:245, 1980
91. Nachemson A: Lumbar intradiscal pressure. Acta Orthop Scand, suppl. 43, 1960
92. Shah JS, Hampson WGJ, Jayson MIV: The distribution of surface strain in the cadaveric lumbar spine. J Bone Joint Surg 60B:246, 1978
93. Miller JAA, Haderspeck KA, Schultz AB: Posterior element loads in lumbar motion segments. Spine 8:331, 1983
94. Kazarian LE: Creep characteristics of the human spinal column. Orthop Clin North Am 6:3, 1975
95. Twomey LT, Taylor JR, Oilver MJ: Sustained flexion loading, rapid extension loading of the lumbar spine and the physical therapy of related injuries. Physiother Pract 4:129, 1988
96. Shirazi-Adl A: Finite element simulation of changes in the fluid content of intervertebral discs. Spine 17:206, 1992
97. Twomey LT, Taylor JR: Flexion creep deformation and hysteresis in the lumbar vertebral column. Spine 7:116, 1982
98. Adams MA, Hutton WC: The effect of posture on the fluid content of lumbar intervertebral discs. Spine 8:665, 1983
99. Twomey LT, Taylor JR: Age changes in the lumbar articular triad. Aust J Physiother 31:106, 1985
100. Pearsall DJ, Reid JG: Line of gravity relative to upright vertebral posture. Clin Biomech 7:80, 1992
101. Yang KH, King AI: Mechanism of facet load transmission as a hypothesis for low back pain. Spine 9:557, 1984
102. Nachemson A, Morris JM: In vivo measurements of intradiscal pressure. J Bone Joint Surg 46A:1077, 1964

103. Andersson BJG, Ortengren R, Nachemson A et al: Lumbar disc pressure and myoelectric back muscle activity during sitting. Scand J Rehabil Med 6:104, 1974
104. Nachemson A: The effect of forward bearing on lumbar intradiscal pressure. Acta Orthop Scand 35:314, 1965
105. Nachemson A, Elfstrom G: Intravital dynamic pressure measurements in lumbar discs. Scand J Rehabil Med, suppl. 1:1, 1970
106. Andersson BJG, Ortengren R, Nachemson A: Quantitative studies of back loads in lifting. Spine 1:178, 1976
107. Merriam WF, Quinnell RC, Stockdale HR et al: The effect of postural changes on the inferred pressures within the nucleus pulposus during lumbar discography. Spine 9:406, 1984
108. Virgin WJ: Anatomical and pathological aspects of the intervertebral disc. Indian J Surg 20:113, 1958
109. Panjabi MM, Krag MH, Chung TQ: Effects of disc injury on mechanical behavior of the human spine. Spine 9:707, 1984
110. Belytschko T, Kulak RF, Schultz AB et al: Finite element stress analysis of an intervertebral disc. J Biomech 4:277, 1974
111. Bartelink DL: The role of abdominal pressure in relieving the pressure on the lumbar intervertebral discs. J Bone Joint Surg 39B:718, 1957
112. Morris JM, Lucas DB, Bresler B: Role of the trunk in stability of the spine. J Bone Joint Surg 43A:328, 1961
113. Davis PR, Troup JDG: Pressures in the trunk cavities when pulling, pushing and lifting. Ergonomics 7:465, 1964
114. Eie N: Load capacity of the low back. J Oslo City Hosp 16:73, 1966
115. Kumar S, Davis PR: Lumbar vertebral innervation and intra-abdominal pressure. J Anat 114:47, 1973
116. Grillner S, Nilsson J, Thorstensson A: Intra-abdominal pressure changes during natural movements in man. Acta Physiol Scand 103:275, 1978
117. McGill SM, Norman RW: Portioning of the L4–L5 dynamic movement into disc, ligamentous and muscular components during lifting. Spine 11:666, 1986
118. Farfan HF: Muscular mechanism of the lumbar spine and the position of power and efficiency. Orthop Clin North Am 6:135, 1975
119. Ortengren R, Andersson GBJ: Electromyographic studies of trunk muscles, with special reference to the functional anatomy of the lumbar spine. Spine 2:44, 1977
120. Ortengren R, Andersson GBJ, Nachemson AL: Studies of relationships between lumbar disc pressure, myoelectric back muscle activity and intra-abdominal pressure. Spine 6:98, 1981
121. Gracovetsky S, Farfan HF: The optimum spine. Spine 11:543, 1986
122. Davis PR, Stubbs DA, Ridd JE: Radio pills: their use in monitoring back stress. J Med Eng Technol 1:209, 1977
123. Waddell G: A new clinical model for the treatment of low back pain. Spine 12:632, 1987
124. Giovanelli B, Thompson E, Elvey R: Measurement of variations in lumbar zygapophyseal joint intracapsular pressure: a pilot study. Aust J Physiother 31:115, 1985
125. Twomey LT, Taylor JR, Furniss B: Age changes in the bone density and structure of the lumbar vertebral column. J Anat 136:15, 1983
126. Eisman JA: Osteoporosis: prevention, prevention and prevention. Cur Ther 33:25, 1992
127. Pardini A: Exercise, vitality and aging. Age Ageing 344:19, 1984
128. Dixon AStJ: Non hormonal treatment of osteoporosis. Br Med J 286:999, 1983

129. Spencer H, Kramer L, Lesniak M et al: Calcium requirements in humans. Clin Orthop 184:270, 1984
130. Aloia JF, Cohn SH, Ostuni JA et al: Prevention of involutional bone loss by exercise. J Clin Endocrinol Metab 43:992, 1978
131. Smith EL, Reddan W, Smith PE: Physical activity and calcium modalities for bone mineral increase in aged women. Med Sci Sports Exerc 13:60, 1981
132. Menard D, Stanish WD: The aging athlete. Am J Sports Med 17:187, 1991

# 3  Innervation, Pain Patterns, and Mechanisms of Pain Production

*Nikolai Bogduk*

Fundamental to the interpretation of lumbar pain syndromes is a knowledge of the mechanisms by which local and referred pain can be produced. If the mechanisms involved in a particular patient are properly understood, then treatment can be prescribed logically and appropriately. However, when interpretations are based on misconception or restricted knowledge, there is a risk of treatment being inappropriate and unsuccessful.

What has compromised the evolution of thought on lumbar pain syndromes has been a tendency simply to infer or deem that a particular mechanism or cause is responsible for a particular syndrome, without actually proving it to be so. Indeed, if reiterated often and strongly enough, such inferences, even if incorrect, seem to gain the respectability of a "rule" or "dogma," and sometimes become so "sacred" as to be exempt from challenge. Yet in some instances, new facts or correct logic expose the limitations or errors in concepts evolved in this way.

As far as possible, concepts should be based on scientific fact. This chapter presents those experimental observations that are relevant to the comprehension of the mechanisms of lumbar pain syndromes, to provide a rational basis for interpretation and challenging or dispelling certain common misconceptions that are no longer tenable.

## INNERVATION

For any structure to be a source of pain it must be connected to the nervous system; conversely, any structure that has a nerve supply is a potential source of pain. For this reason, the innervation of the lumbar spine has been the subject of several studies[1-4] and reviews[5,6]; only a summary is provided here.

The posterior elements of the lumbar vertebral column are those parts that lie dorsal to the intervertebral foramina, and they are all innervated by branches of the dorsal rami of the lumbar spinal nerves. The dorsal rami themselves are very short nerves directed backward and caudally through the intertransverse spaces (Fig. 3-1). As each dorsal ramus approaches the subjacent transverse process, it divides into two or three branches.[3] Lateral branches are distributed to the lateral column of the lumbar erector spinae—the iliocostalis muscle. The lateral branches of the L1 to L3 dorsi rami emerge from this muscle and cross the iliac crest to become cutaneous over the buttock.[3,7] Intermediate branches of the lumbar dorsal rami arise independently from each dorsal ramus or from

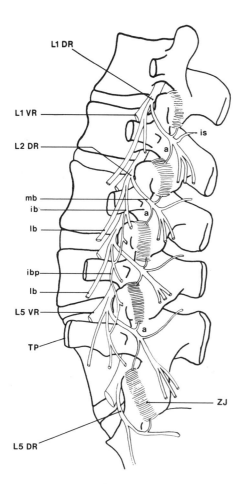

**Fig. 3-1.** Left posterolateral view of the lumbar dorsal rami showing the disposition of their branches. *VR*, ventral ramus; *DR*, dorsal ramus; *mb*, medial branch; *ib*, intermediate branch; *lb*, lateral branch; *ibp*, intermediate branch plexus; *is*, interspinous branch; *a*, articular branch; *ZJ*, zygapophyseal joint. (From Bogduk and Twomey,[52] with permission.)

its lateral branch[3] and are distributed to the medial column of the lumbar erector spinae—the longissimus thoracic muscle.[8]

The medial branches of the lumbar dorsal rami have been considered the most relevant clinically; in addition to innervating the multifidus muscle and the interspinous muscles and ligaments they supply the lumbar zygapophyseal joints.[3,9–12]

The anterior elements of the lumbar vertebral column are the vertebral bodies and the intervertebral discs and their related ligaments, but include also the anterior aspect of the lumbar dural sac, which not only lies anterior to the spinal nerves and their roots, but is innervated by branches of the same nerves that innervate the other anterior elements. No nerve endings occur in the posterior dura[4,13]; therefore, for present purposes, no controversy need be raised as to whether the posterior dura should be classified as an anterior or posterior element.

The anterior elements of the lumbar vertebral column are innervated by dense, microscopic plexuses of nerves stemming from the lumbar sympathetic trunk, the gray rami communicantes, and the ventral rami of the lumbar, spinal nerves. An anterior plexus accompanies the anterior longitudinal ligament along the front of the vertebral column and a posterior plexus accompanies the posterior longitudinal ligament[4] (Figs. 3-2 and 3-3). Within the posterior plexus certain larger nerves can be identified on microdissection, and in the past have been referred to as the sinuvertebral nerves[2,8,9,10,14] (see Fig. 3-3). They represent the main sources of the posterior plexus and stem from the gray rami communicantes and the lumbar ventral rami. They reach the plexus by passing through the intervertebral foramina.

From both the anterior and posterior plexuses many fine branches enter the vertebral bodies and intervertebral discs from their posterior, anterior, and lateral aspects (Fig. 3-4). Osseous branches accompany vessels into the vertebral bodies and penetrate deeply into the spongiosa. Branches to the discs penetrate only the outer third or so of the annulus fibrosus and do not extend further than the outer half of the annulus. Ligament branches innervate the posterior and anterior longitudinal ligaments. From the posterior plexus, branches innervate the anterior aspect of the dural sac and the dural sleeves of the lumbar nerve roots.[4,15]

Histologic studies have demonstrated nerve fibers and nerve endings not only in the superficial laminae of the annulus fibrosus,[16–18] but also as deeply as the outer third or outer half of the annulus.[1,2,4,19] More comprehensive reviews of this issue are available elsewhere.[5,6]

This summary of neurologic anatomy establishes that the possible sources of lumbar pain are the lumbar zygapophyseal joints, the various back muscles, the interspinous ligaments (all innervated by dorsal rami), the vertebral bodies, intervertebral discs, longitudinal ligaments, and the dura mater (all innervated by ventral rami). Anatomy alone, however, does not prove that a structure can be a source of pain. It shows only that the necessary nerve supply is present. Additional physiologic evidence is needed to show that stimulation of a structure can actually cause pain.

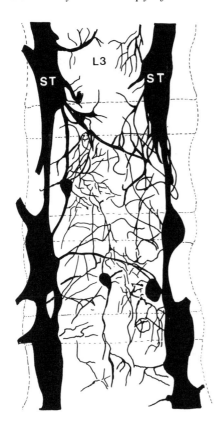

**Fig. 3-2.** The nerve plexus accompanying the anterior longitudinal ligament at the levels of the L3 and lower vertebrae, as seen in whole mounts of human fetuses. *ST*, lumbar sympathetic trunk. (Adapted from Groen et al,[4] as appeared in Bogduk and Twomey,[52] with permission.)

## Physiology

At one time or another, each of the structures listed above has been incriminated as source of low back pain. However, it has taken many years to collect the experimental evidence that proves these assertions. Thus, in 1938 and 1939, Kellgren[20,21] demonstrated that low back pain could be induced by noxious stimulation of the lumbar back muscles and interspinous ligaments, while, reciprocally, Steindler and Luck[22] showed that certain forms of low back pain syndromes could be relieved, at least temporarily, by anesthetizing these same structures. Although the term *facet syndrome* was introduced in 1933,[23] it was not shown until 1976 that experimental stimulation of lumbar zygapophyseal joints could cause low back pain in normal volunteers,[24,25] and that back pain stemming from these joints could be relieved by radiologically controlled blocks of the joints themselves[26–33] or their nerve supply.[34–37]

Two lines of evidence revealed that the intervertebral discs could be a source of back pain. Operating on patients under local anesthesia, Wiberg[38] showed that pressing on the posterior annulus fibrosus could evoke low back pain, as did Falconer et al.[39] Later, after the introduction of discography as a diagnostic procedure, it was recognized that back pain could be reproduced by

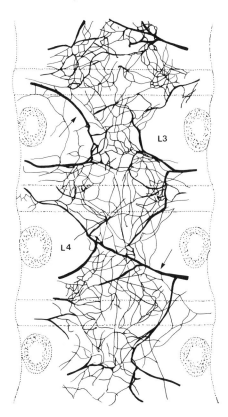

**Fig. 3-3.** The nerve plexus accompanying the posterior longitudinal ligament at the levels of the L3 and lower vertebrae, as seen in whole mounts of human fetuses. The large fibers *(arrows)* represent the sinuvertebral nerves. (Adapted from Groen et al,[4] as appeared in Bogduk and Twomey,[52] with permission.)

injections of contrast medium into lumbar intervertebral discs.[40] Subsequent experience with provocation discography has confirmed that the injection of contrast medium or even normal saline into intervertebral discs can evoke back pain, even if the disc is structurally intact and appears normal on myelography.[41–45]

The dura mater has been shown to be capable of causing back pain in two types of clinical experiments. First, it was shown that back pain could be evoked by traction on the dural sleeves of lumbar nerve roots by pulling on sutures threaded through the dura at operation for laminectomy.[46] More recently it has been shown that chemical irritation of the dura in the form of injections of hypertonic saline can evoke back pain.[47] Pain stemming from the dura mater of nerve root sleeves has been relieved by microsurgical transection of the nerves supplying them.[48,49]

There is, therefore, a wealth of clinical experimental data confirming that the ligaments, muscles, joints, discs, and dura mater of the lumbar spine are all capable of being a source of back pain. Of the innervated structures of the lumbar spine, only the epidural blood vessels and the vertebral bodies have not been subjected to experimental study to determine whether they too can be a source of pain. Circumstantial evidence is conducive to the notion that

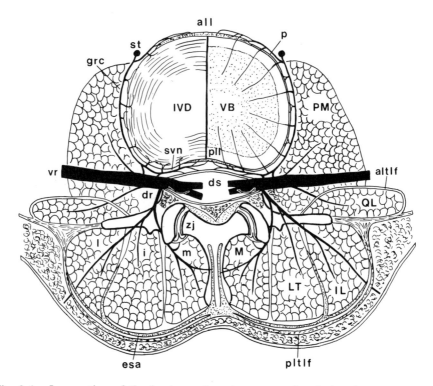

**Fig. 3-4.** Innervation of the lumbar spine. A cross-sectional view incorporating the level of the vertebral body *(VB)* and its periosteum *(p)* on the right and the intervertebral disc *(IVD)* on the left. *PM*, psoas major; *QL*, quadratus lumborum; *IL*, iliocostalis lumborum; *LT*, longissimus thoracis; *M*, multifidus; *altlf*, anterior layer of thoracolumbar fascia; *pltlf*, posterior layer of thoracolumbar fascia; *esa*, erector spinae aponeurosis; *ds*, dural sac; *zj*, zygapophyseal joint; *pll*, posterior longitudinal ligament; *all*, anterior longitudinal ligament; *vr*, ventral ramus; *dr*, dorsal ramus; *m*, medial branch; *i*, intermediate branch; *l*, lateral branch; *svn*, sinuvertebral nerve; *grc*, gray ramus communicans; *st*, sympathetic trunk. (From Bogduk and Twomey,[52] with permission.)

distension of epidural veins can cause pain[50]; however, although it is presumed that the pain of spinal osteoporosis arises from vertebral bodies, there have been no formal experimental studies of low back pain stemming from bone.

## Pathology

Given that various structures in the lumbar spine have been shown to be capable of producing low back pain, it is important to realize that in each case, the mechanism involved is the stimulation of nerve endings in the affected structure. Lumbar nerve-root compression is in no way involved. To relate this to pathology, the possible causes of low back pain would be any pathologic process that stimulates the nociceptive nerve endings in one or other of the pain-sensitive structures of the lumbar spine. In this respect, there are only two known mechanisms by which nerve endings can be stimulated: chemical or mechanical irritation.

Chemical irritation occurs in inflammatory diseases or follows tissue damage. Although it is very difficult to validate experimentally, the mechanism seems to involve the direct stimulation of nerve endings by chemicals. These may include hydrogen and potassium ions or enzymes that are liberated from inflammatory cells or damaged tissue cells. Mechanical irritation, on the other hand, involves the stretching of connective tissue without the involvement of any chemical mediators. Exactly how mechanical irritation causes pain remains unclear, but a plausible explanation is that when an array of collagen fibers in a ligament, joint capsule, or periosteum is placed under tension, it deforms and closes the available space between individual collagen fibers. Nerve endings or perhaps nerve fibers within the array would then be stimulated by being squeezed between the encroaching collagen fibers.

It is beyond the scope of this chapter to expand on the pathology of the lumbar spine, but other publications have explored the pathomechanics of pain arising from discs,[5,6,51] dural pain,[52] and pain mediated by the lumbar dorsal rami.[53,54] However, it is worth elaborating on the issue of primary disc pain.

## Primary Disc Pain

In contradistinction to pain caused by the compression of spinal nerves by herniated intervertebral discs, primary disc pain is pain that stems directly from the disc itself. It is caused by the stimulation of the nerve endings within the annulus fibrosus. Pathologic processes theoretically responsible for this stimulation include excessive mechanical strain of the annulus, chemical irritation as a result of inflammation following trauma to the annulus, and involvement of the annulus in the chemical degrading processes that occur in internal disc disruption.[51]

Logical deduction reveals that not every pathologic process affecting a disc will necessarily be painful, as only the peripheral annulus is innervated. Disc pain will occur only if a pain-producing process affects the innervated periphery of the disc. Processes such as disc degradation or degeneration that are restricted to the nucleus and central portions of the annulus do not have access to the nerve supply of the disc, and therefore cannot directly cause pain. Thus even severely degenerated discs may not be painful. However, should centrally located processes extend to the innervated periphery, as in a radial fissure[5,6,51] or if the peripheral annulus itself is primarily damaged, as in a torsional strain,[5,6,51] then nerve endings may be affected, and if enough are stimulated, then pain may ensue. On the other hand, an otherwise healthy and innervated portion of an annulus could become painful if it is called on to bear a greater mechanical load as a result of disease in other portions of the disc, and is thereby secondarily subjected to excessive strain.[5,6,51] Variations and permutations like these explain why discs apparently affected by similar disease processes may be inconsistently painful or painless.

## Referred Pain

Referred pain is pain perceived in a region topographically displaced from the area that is the source of the pain. In lumbar pain syndromes, referred pain is generated by lesions in the lumbar spine but is perceived in the buttocks and lower limbs or sometimes in the groin or abdominal wall.

There are two common types of referred pain from the lumbar spine. The mechanisms and their diagnostic and therapeutic implications are so different in each that the two must be recognized and distinguished. The first is somatic-referred pain and the other is radicular pain.

### Somatic-Referred Pain

The term *somatic-referred pain* is used to emphasize the skeletal or "somatic" origin for this form of pain, and to distinguish it from radicular pain and referred pain caused by visceral or vascular disease.

Virtually any source of local lumbar or lumbosacral pain is also capable of producing somatic-referred pain. The mechanism appears to be that afferent impulses from the lumbar spine activate neurons in the central nervous system, which also happen to receive afferents from the lower limbs, buttocks, or groin. Stimulation of such central nervous system neurons by impulses from the lumbar spine results in the perception of pain arising from all the tissues subtended by these neurons. Thus the patient complains of pain in the lower limbs as well as the back even though there is no signal actually emanating from the limbs.

The evidence for such a mechanism stems from several experimental and clinical studies. Kellgren[20,21] showed that low back pain experimentally induced by stimulating interspinous ligaments and back muscles could be accompanied by referred pain in the lower limbs. These observations were later corroborated by other investigators.[55,56]

Experimental noxious stimulation of lumbar zygapophyseal joints can cause referred pain in various regions of the lower limbs, buttocks, and groin.[24,25] Traction on the dura mater has been shown to produce buttock and thigh pain,[46] and in some patients, disc stimulation can reproduce not only their back pain but their referred pain as well.[17,42–44] Complementing these experimental studies are the reports that anesthetizing intervertebral discs,[44] and anesthetizing[24–27,29,32,33] or denervating[31,37,53] zygapophyseal joints in certain patients relieves not only their local pain but also their lower limb pain.

The critical feature of these various studies is that the stimuli used to evoke referred pain or the anesthetics used to relieve it were delivered directly to somatic elements of the lumbar spine. Nerve roots were not stimulated or anesthetized. The mechanisms for the referred pain, therefore, must lie beyond the nerve roots, and the only possible site is in the central nervous system.

An overemphasized aspect of somatic-referred pain is its apparent segmental distribution. Early investigators sought to establish charts of the segmental pattern of pain referral in the anticipation that the axial origin of referred pain could be diagnosed on the basis of its peripheral distribution, just as dermatomes are used to diagnose the segmental level of a root compression or spinal cord injury.[21,55,56] However, it is now evident that the fields of referred pain from individual segments overlap greatly within a given individual and the patterns exhibited by different individuals vary significantly.[25,53,54] These irregularities preclude the use of charts of so-called sclerotomes for any legitimate diagnostic purpose. Such charts serve only to illustrate that lumbar pain may be referred into the lower limbs, but do not pinpoint constant locations.

In this context, it is sometimes maintained that somatic-referred pain does not extend beyond the knee and that pain distal to the knee must be radicular in origin. However, while it is true that somatic-referred pain most commonly is distributed in the region of the buttock,[24,39,56] it nevertheless can extend as far as the foot.[21,24,55] Indeed, there is even some evidence that the distance of referral into the lower limb is proportional to the intensity of the stimulus to the spine.[24]

An important (although overlooked) legacy of the experimental studies on somatic-referred pain relates to its quality. All the studies showed that the referred pain was deep and aching in quality, and was hard to localize. This contrasts with the sharper, lancinating nature of radicular pain and putatively may be used to distinguish somatic-referred pain from radicular pain.

## Radicular Pain

The concept of *sciatica* stems from the coincidental similarity between the distribution of some forms of referred pain and the course of the sciatic nerve. Consequently, sciatica was originally ascribed to intrinsic disease of the sciatic nerve, then later to muscular compression, and eventually to compression of the lumbosacral nerve roots by disorders of the vertebral column (hence the term *radicular pain*).

These notions on the causation of sciatica, however, were based only on inference or circumstantial evidence. Thus, because arthritic changes could be demonstrated radiologically in patients with sciatic pain, the cause was deemed to be compression of the L5 spinal nerve by lumbosacral "arthritis."[57,58] Later, this notion was superceded by the revelation that herniated intervertebral discs could compress lumbosacral nerve roots.[59] The compressive causes of sciatica, however, were introduced without it being demonstrated that root compression could, in fact, cause pain.

Early investigators were probably drawn to their conclusions by the observations that most of their patients had weakness or numbness in association with their sciatic pain. Because weakness and numbness are features of nerve compression, it was understandably attractive to ascribe the pain to the same cause and mechanism. Moreover, these conclusions were made and the nerve root compression theory established before the earliest experiments on somatic-referred pain.[20,21]

It is surprising that nerve-root compression was sustained as the mechanism for referred pain, because it is known that compression of nerves elsewhere in the body does not cause pain.[60] Indeed, this paradox led to criticisms of the nerve-root compression theory.[61] However, subsequent clinical and laboratory experiments have helped resolve this paradox, albeit at the expense of raising new questions.

MacNab[62] reported that experimental compression of normal nerve roots, using catheters inserted into intervertebral foramina, evoked paresthesia and numbness, but did not cause pain. On the other hand, Smyth and Wright[46] demonstrated that pulling on nerve roots previously affected by disc herniation did evoke sciatic pain. Thus clinically damaged, but not normal, nerve roots are capable of generating pain.

These clinical observations have been corroborated by animal experiments, which showed that activity in nociceptive afferent fibers could be elicited by mechanical stimulation of previously damaged nerve roots, but not by stimulation of normal roots.[63] The questions raised by these experiments are (1) how do normal and damaged roots differ and (2) how soon after a compressive lesion is a normal root sufficiently damaged to become painful? These questions remain unanswered.

Another observation from these same animal experiments[63] is that nociceptive activity could be elicited by stimulation of dorsal root ganglia irrespective of whether they were normal or damaged. Thus dorsal root ganglia are apparently more susceptible to mechanical stimulation than axons, and this difference may explain why root compression is capable of producing pain when compression of nerve trunks is not. Compression of the cell bodies in the dorsal root ganglia seems to be the key difference.

Other issues aside, there is no doubt that under the appropriate circumstances, compression of nerve roots can cause pain, but an unfortunate legacy of the concept of sciatica is the tendency in some circles to interpret all forms of pain in the lower limb as due to nerve-root compression. This is not justified.

The experiments of Smyth and Wright[46] showed that traction on nerve roots produced only a particular form of pain. It was lancinating or shooting in quality, and was felt along a relatively narrow band "no more than one-and-a-half inches wide."[46] This neuralgic type of pain is the only type that has been shown to be produced by root compression. Therefore, only this form of pain can legitimately be called sciatica and ascribed to root compression. In contrast, somatic-referred pain is static, aching in quality, hard to localize, and should be recognized as a different entity.

There are two further irregularities concerning the concepts of sciatica and nerve-root compression. First, there is no known mechanism whereby a compressive lesion can selectively affect only nociceptive axons (i.e., without also affecting large-diameter afferent fibers that convey touch and other sensations). Therefore, there is no mechanism whereby root compression can cause pain without causing other neurologic abnormalities as well. Thus, for root compression to be deemed the cause, radicular pain must be accompanied by other features of nerve compression: numbness, weakness, or paresthesia. In the absence of such accompanying features, it is very difficult to maintain that root compression is the cause of any pain. Pain in the lower limb in the absence of objective neurologic signs is most likely to be somatic-referred pain.

The second irregularity relates to back pain. All the experimental studies on radicular pain emphasize that root compression causes pain in the lower limb. Thus, although radicular pain may feel as if it starts in the back and radiates into the lower limb, there is no evidence that root compression can or should cause isolated low back pain. It is implausible that a compressive lesion could stimulate only those afferents in a root that come from the lumbar spine but spare those from the lower limb. Isolated low back pain suggests a somatic lesion, which should be sought, and the pain should not be dismissed as due to nerve-root compression when no evidence of compression can be found. One reservation, however, must be raised: apparently local back pain may in fact be referred pain from pelvic or abdominal visceral or vascular disease. For this reason, abdominal and pelvic examinations are essential parts of the assessment of any patient presenting with low back pain.

## Combined States

Whereas it is evident that back pain and referred pain may be caused by a variety of disorders and mechanisms, it is critical to realize that a patient's complaints may not be due to a single disorder or a single mechanism. Several disorders may coexist and different mechanisms may be coactive. The simplest examples are the coexistence of zygapophyseal disorders and disc disorders at the same or different segmental levels, with each disorder contributing separately to the patient's overall complaint.

A more complex example relates to nerve-root compression syndromes. The cardinal features of nerve-root compression are the objective neurologic signs of weakness or numbness. In the presence of such signs accompanied by the lancinating pain that is characteristic of radicular pain, the syndrome may legitimately be ascribed to nerve-root compression. However, nerve-root compression may only be part of a patient's complaint. Local somatic and somatic-referred pain may occur in addition to the symptoms of nerve-root compression. In such cases, the most likely source or sources of the somatic pain are the structures immediately adjacent to the compressed root.

The closest relation of a nerve root is its dural sleeve, and it is obvious that any lesion that might compress a root must first affect its dural sleeve. Given that the dura is pain-sensitive,[46,47] it becomes a potent possible source of low back pain and even referred pain,[46] which can occur alone or be superimposed on any radicular pain. However, the mechanism involved is distinctly different from that of any radicular pain, because dural pain is caused by the stimulation of nerve endings in the dural sleeve, not by nerve compression.

Since the dura is mechanosensitive,[46] traction of the dura over a space-occupying lesion, like a herniated disc, could be the possible cause of dural pain. The dura is also chemosensitive,[47] and therefore an additional or alternative process could be chemical irritation of the dura. With regard to the latter, it has been demonstrated that disc material contains potent inflammatory chemicals,[64-66] and when disc material ruptures into the epidural space it seems to elicit an autoimmune inflammatory reaction that can affect not only the roots but the dura as well.[67-70]

The other two possible sources of pain concurrent with root compression are the adjacent disc and zygapophyseal joint. Regardless of any herniation that compresses a root, a disc itself may be an intrinsic source of pain, the pain being mechanical in origin caused by strain of the annulus fibrosus of the diseased disc. In such cases, treating the nerve-root compression may relieve the objective neurologic signs and any radicular pain, but the discogenic pain may continue unless it is treated as well.

A zygapophyseal joint may compress or traumatize the underlying roots by developing osteophytes,[71] but a degenerative zygapophyseal joint may also be independently painful, causing both local and somatic-referred pain. Thus, while resecting the osteophytes may decompress the roots, it may not relieve the intrinsic low back pain and referred pain stemming from the diseased joint. This concept has particular ramifications in the interpretation of spinal stenosis where not all the symptoms are necessarily due to the overt nerve-root compression.

## PATTERNS

It might be expected that different causes of lumbar pain should be distinguishable from one another on the basis of differences in the distribution and behavior of symptoms. Frustratingly, however, this is not so. Because different structures in the lumbar spine share a similar segmental nerve supply, and because different disorders share similar mechanisms, no single disorder has a characteristic distribution of local or referred pain.

Even the classic syndrome of herniated nucleus pulposus is fraught with diagnostic pitfalls. The sensitivity of straight leg raising as a test for this condition has been measured to be between 72 and 97 percent,[72] meaning that between 3 and 28 percent of cases remain undetected. Other, classical features such as weakness of extensor hallucis, weakness of ankle dorsiflexion, and absent ankle reflex have sensitivities for less than this.[72] The specificity of straight leg raise, however, is only 11 to 45 percent,[72] meaning that too often conditions other than herniated nucleus pulposus are the cause of the abnormality.

With respect to zygapophyseal joint disorders, experimental studies have shown that local and referred pain patterns from joints at different levels vary considerably in different individuals and that even in a given individual they overlap greatly.[24,25] Furthermore, the incidence of other clinical features in zygapophyseal syndromes, including various aggravating factors, is insufficiently different from their incidence in other syndromes. Fairbank et al[29] performed diagnostic joint blocks on patients presenting with back pain and referred pain, and analyzed the differences between those who responded and those who did not. Although certain features did occur more commonly in responders, they also occurred so frequently in nonresponders that no clinical feature could be identified that could be held to be indicative or pathognomonic of zygapophyseal joint pain.

Other forms of pain, such as disc pain and muscular-pain syndromes, have not been studied in this same rigorous way. Consequently, there is no scientific evidence that permits any claim that certain pain patterns are characteristic of these syndromes. Only the diagnosis of lumbar-disc herniation has withstood scrutiny, while the diagnosis of zygapophyseal syndromes on the basis of conventional clinical signs has been shown to be impossible. Therefore, the diagnosis of lumbar-pain syndromes, other than those caused by disc herniation, relies on investigations outside the realm of symptomatic and conventional physical examination.

In this regard, plain radiography has little value as a diagnostic tool in low back pain,[44] while electromyography, myelography, and computed tomography are of relevance only in nerve-root compression syndromes. For conditions in which pain alone is the complaint, and there are no objective neurologic signs indicative of nerve-root compression, other investigations are required.

The mainstay for the diagnosis of lumbar pain in the absence of neurologic signs are diagnostic blocks and provocation radiology. These techniques are based on the principles that if a structure is the cause of pain, then stressing that structure should reproduce the pain and anesthetizing the structure should relieve it. Thus zygapophyseal joints suspected of being the source of pain can be infiltrated with local anesthetic,[33] and relief of pain implicates the injected joint as the source. Similarly, intervertebral discs can be injected with saline or contrast medium to reproduce pain or with local anesthetic to relieve pain.[44] Radicular pain and dural pain can be diagnosed by infiltrating the root thought to be responsible with local anesthetic.[73–75] In all of these procedures, failure to provoke or relieve the pain excludes the investigated structure as the source of pain, whereupon other structures or other segmental levels in the lumbar spine may be investigated until the responsible site is identified. Although subject to certain technical limitations,[44] these techniques are the only available means of objectively confirming particular causes of pain suspected on the basis of clinical examination.

In conflict with this conclusion are the claims of manipulative therapists who maintain that they are able to diagnose the source of pain in the vertebral column by manual examination. Elaborate methods of assessment for this purpose have been described in manipulative therapy texts.[76–78] However, no research has been undertaken to validate the purported accuracy of these methods. Thus, although perhaps attractive in principle, manual examination as a diagnostic effort is still open to skepticism from those unconvinced of a manipulative therapist's ability to detect changes in discrete components of the spine, and that these changes are at all diagnostic of any cause of pain.

## REFERENCES

1. Yoshizawa H, O'Brien JP, Smith WT, Trumper M: The neuropathology of intervertebral discs removed for low-back pain. J Pathol 132:95, 1980
2. Bogduk N, Tynan W, Wilson AS: The nerve supply to the human lumbar intervertebral discs. J Anat 132:39, 1981
3. Bogduk N, Wilson AS, Tynan W: The human lumbar dorsal rami. J Anat 134:383, 1982
4. Groen G, Baljet B, Drukker J: The nerves and nerve plexuses of the human vertebral column. Am J Anat 188:282, 1990
5. Bogduk N: The innervation of the intervertebral discs. p. 135. In Ghosh P (ed): The Biology of the Intervertebral Disc. CRC Press, Boca Raton, FL, 1988
6. Bogduk N: The innervation of the discs. In Boyling JD, Palastanga N (eds): Grieve's Modern Manual Therapy of the Vertebral Column, 2nd Ed. Churchill Livingstone, Edingurgh (in press)
7. Johnston HM: The cutaneous branches of the posterior primary divisions of the spinal nerves and their distribution in the skin. J Anat 43:80, 1908
8. Bogduk N: The innervation of the lumbar spine. Spine 8:285, 1983
9. Paris SV: Anatomy was related to function and pain. Orthop Clin North Am 14: 475, 1982
10. Pedersen HE, Blunck CFJ, Gardner E: The anatomy of lumbosacral posterior rami and meningeal branches of spinal nerves (sinu-vertebral nerves). J Bone Joint Surg 38A:377, 1956
11. Lazorthes G, Gaubert J: L'innervation des articulations interapophysaires vertebrales. CR Assoc Anat 43e Reunion:488, 1956
12. Lazorthes G, Juskiewenski S: Etude comparative des branches posterieures des nerfs dorsaux et lombaires et de leurs rapports avec les articulations interapophysaires vertebrales. Bull Assoc Anat 49e Reunion:1025, 1964
13. Edgar MA, Nundy S: Innervation of the spinal dura mater. J Neurol Neurosurg Psychiatry 29:530, 1966
14. Lazorthes G, Pouhles J, Espagne J: Etude sur les nerfs sinu-vertebraux lombaires. Le nerf de Roofe existe-t-il? CR Assoc Anat 34e Reunion:317, 1947
15. Groen G, Baljet B, Drukker J: The innervation of the spinal dura mater: anatomy and clinical implications. Acta Neurochir 92:39, 1988
16. Jung A, Brunschwig A: Recherches histologiques des articulations des corps vertebraux. Presse Med 40:316, 1932
17. Hirsch C, Ingelmark B, Miller M: The anatomical basis for low back pain. Acta Orthop Scand 33:1, 1963
18. Jackson HC, Winkelmann RK, Bickel WH: Nerve endings in the human lumbar spinal column and related structures. J Bone Joint Surg 48A:1272, 1966
19. Malinsky J: The ontogenetic development of nerve terminations in the intervertebral discs of man. Acta Anat 38:96, 1959
20. Kellgren JH: Observations on referred pain arising from muscle. Clin Sci 3:175, 1938

21. Kellgren JH: On the distribution of pain arising from deep somatic structures with charts of segmental pain areas. Clin Sci 4:35, 1939
22. Steindler A, Luck JV: Differential diagnosis of pain low in the back: allocation of the source of pain by procain hydrochloride method. JAMA 110:106, 1938
23. Ghormley RK: Low back pain with special reference to the articular facets with presentation of an operative procedure. JAMA 10:1773, 1933
24. Mooney V, Robertson J: The facet syndrome. Clin Orthop 115:149, 1976
25. McCall IW, Park WM, O'Brien JP: Induced pain referral from posterior lumbar elements in normal subjects. Spine 4:441, 1979
26. Mehta M, Sluijter ME: The treatment of chronic back pain. Anaesthesia 34:768, 1979
27. Carrera GF: Lumbar facet joint injection in low back pain and sciatica. Radiology 137:665, 1980
28. Dory MA: Arthrography of the lumbar facet joints. Radiology 140:23, 1981
29. Fairbank JCT, Park WM, McCall IW, O'Brien JP: Apophyseal injection of local anaesthetic as a diagnostic aid in primary low-back pain syndromes. Spine 6:598, 1981
30. Destouet JM, Gilula LA, Murphy WA, Monsees B: Lumbar facet joint injection: indication, technique, clinical correlation, and preliminary results. Radiology 145:321, 1982
31. Rashbaum RF: Radiofrequency facet denervation. Orthop Clin North Am 14:569, 1983
32. Lippit AB: The facet joint and its role in spine pain. Spine 9:746, 1984
33. Carrera GF, Williams AL: Current concepts in evaluation of the lumbar facet joints. CRC Crit Rev Diagn Imaging 21:85, 1984
34. Pawl RP: Results in the treatment of low back syndrome from sensory neurolysis of the lumbar facets (facet rhizotomy) by thermal coagulation. Proc Inst Med Chicago 30:150, 1974
35. Lora J, Long DM: So-called facet denervation in the management of intractable back pain. Spine 1:121, 1976
36. Ogsbury JS, Simons H, Lehman RAW: Facet "denervation" in the treatment of low back syndrome. Pain 3:257, 1977
37. Sluijter ME, Mehta M: Treatment of chronic back and neck pain by percutaneous thermal lesions. p. 141. In Lipton S, Miles J (eds): Persistent Pain: Modern Methods of Treatment. Vol. 3. Academic Press, London, 1981
38. Wiberg G: Back pain in relation to the nerve supply of the intervertebral disc. Acta Orthop Scand 19:211, 1947
39. Falconer MA, McGeorge M, Begg AC: Observations on the cause and mechanism of symptom production in sciatica and low back pain. J Neurol Neurosurg Psychiatry 11:13, 1948
40. Lindblom K: Technique and results in myelography and disc puncture. Acta Radiol 34:321, 1950
41. Collis JS, Gardner WJ: Lumbar discography—an analysis of 1,000 cases. J Neurosurg 19:452, 1962
42. Wiley JJ, MacNab I, Wortzman G: Lumbar discography and its clinical applications. Can J Surg 11:280, 1968
43. Simmons EH, Segil CM: An evaluation of discography in the localization of symptomatic levels in discogenic disease of the spione. Clin Orthop 108:57, 1975
44. Park WM: The place of radiology in the investigation of low back pain. Clin Rheum Dis 6:93, 1980

45. White AH: Injection techniques for the diagnosis and treatment of low back pain. Orthop Clin North Am 14:553, 1983
46. Smyth MJ, Wright V: Sciatica and the intervertebral disc: an experimental study. J Bone Joint Surg 40A:1401, 1958
47. El Mahdi MA, Latif FYA, Janko M: The spinal nerve root innervation and a new concept of the clinicopathological interrelations in back pain and sciatica. Neurochirurgia 24:137, 1981
48. Cuatico W, Parker JC, Pappert E, Pilsl S: An anatomical and clinical investigation of spinal meningeal nerves. Acta Neurochir 90:139, 1988
49. Cuatico W, Parker JC: Further observations on spinal meningeal nerves and their role in pain production. Acta Neurochir 101:126, 1989
50. Boas RA: Post-surgical low back pain. p. 188. In Peck C, Wallace M (eds): Problems in Pain. Pergamon, Sydney, 1980
51. Bogduk N: The lumbar disc and low back pain. In Loeser J (ed): Neurosurg Clin North Am 2:791, 1991
52. Bogduk N, Twomey LT: Nerves of the lumbar spine. p. 107. Clinical Anatomy of the Lumbar Spine. 2nd Ed. Churchill Livingstone, Melbourne, 1991
53. Bogduk N: Lumbar dorsal ramus syndrome. Med J Aust 2:537, 1980
54. Bogduk N: Lumbar dorsal ramus syndromes. In Boyling JD, Palastanga N (eds): Grieve's Modern Manual Therapy of the Vertebral Column, 2nd Ed. Churchill Livingstone, Edinburgh (in press)
55. Feinstein B, Langton JNK, Jameson RM, Schiller F: Experiments on pain referred from deep structures. J Bone Joint Surg 36A:981, 1954
56. Hockaday JM, Whitty CWM: Patterns of referred pain in the normal subject. Brain 90:481, 1967
57. Danforth MS, Wilson PD: The anatomy of the lumbosacral region in relation to sciatic pain. J Bone Joint Surgery 7:109, 1925
58. Williams PC: Reduced lumbosacral joint space: its relation to sciatic irritation. JAMA 99:1677, 1962
59. Mixter WJ, Barr JS: Rupture of the intervertebral disc with involvement of the spinal canal. N Engl J Med 211:210, 1934
60. Fisher CM: Pain states: a neurological commentary. Clin Neurosurg 31:32, 1984
61. Kelly M: Is pain due to pressure on nerves? Neurology 6:32, 1956
62. MacNab I: The mechanism of spondylogenic pain. p. 89. In Hirsch C, Zotterman Y (eds): Cervical Pain. Pergamon, Oxford, 1972
63. Howe JF, Loeser JD, Calvin WH: Mechano-sensitivity of dorsal root ganglia and chronically injured axons: a physiological basis for the radicular pain of nerve root compression. Pain 3:25, 1977
64. Marshall LL, Trethewie ER, Curtain CC: Chemical radiculitis: a clinical, physiological and immunological study. Clin Orthop 129:61, 1977
65. Saal JS, Franson RC, Dobrow R et al: High levels of inflammatory phospholipase A2 activity in lumbar disc herniation. Spine 15:674, 1990
66. Franson RC, Saal JS, Saal JF: Human disc phospholipase A2 is inflammatory. Spine 17:S129, 1992
67. Gertzbein SD, Tile M, Gross A, Falk R: Autoimmunity and degenerative disease of the lumbar spine. Orthop Clin North Am 6:67, 1975
68. Gertzbein SD: Degenerative disk disease of the lumbar spine. Clin Orthop 129:68, 1977
69. Gertzbein SD, Tai JH, Devlin SR: The stimulation of lymphocytes by nucleus pulposus in patients with degenerative disc disease of the lumbar spine. Clin Orthop 123:149, 1977

70. Murphy RW: Nerve roots and spinal nerves in degenerative disk disease. Clin Orthop 129:46, 1977
71. Epstein JA, Epstein BS, Lavine LS et al: Lumbar nerve root compression at the intervertebral foramina caused by arthritis of the posterior facets. J Neurosurg 39: 362, 1973
72. Andersson GBJ: Sensitivity, specificity and predictive value. p. 277. In Frymoyer JW (ed): The Adult Spine, Principles and Practice. Vol. 1. Raven Press, New York, 1991
73. Stanley D, McLaren MI, Euinton HA, Getty CJM: A prospective study of nerve root infiltration in the diagnosis of sciatica. A comparison with radiculography, computed tomography and operative findings. Spine 15:540, 1990
74. Tajima T, Furukawa K, Kuramochi E: Selective lumbosacral radiculography and block. Spine 5:68, 1980
75. Dooley JF, McBroom RJ, Taguchi T, McNab I: Nerve root infiltration in the diagnosis of radicular pain. Spine 13:79, 1988
76. Maitland GD: Vertebral Manipulation. 4th Ed. Butterworths, London, 1977
77. Grieve GP: Common Vertebral Joint Problems. Churchill Livingstone, Edinburgh, 1982
78. Bourdillon JF: Spinal Manipulation. 3rd Ed. Heinemann, London, 1982

# 4 | Anatomy and Function of the Lumbar Back Muscles and Their Fascia[*]

*Nikolai Bogduk*

The lumbar spine is surrounded by muscles that, for descriptive purposes and on functional grounds, can be divided into three groups. These are (1) psoas major and psoas minor, which cover the anterolateral aspects of the lumbar spine; (2) lateral intertransverse muscles and quadratus lumborum, which connect and cover the front of the transverse processes; and (3) the lumbar back muscles, which lie behind and cover the posterior elements of the lumbar spine.

## PSOAS MAJOR AND MINOR

The psoas major is a long muscle that arises from the anterolateral aspect of the lumbar spine and descends over the brim of the pelvis to insert into the lesser trochanter of the femur. It is essentially a muscle of the thigh whose principal action is flexion of the hip. Some interpretations had maintained that

---

[*] This chapter is from Bogduk N, Twomey LT: The lumbar muscles and their fascia. pp. 83–105. In: Clinical Anatomy of the Lumbar Spine. 2nd Ed. Churchill Livingstone, Melbourne, 1991, with permission.

because it arises from the lumbar spine, the psoas major might have an action on the lumbar spine, either to flex the lumbar spine when the thigh is fixed, as in the exercise of "sit-ups," or at least to "stabilize" the lumbar spine.[1-3] However, these views are not consonant with either its anatomy or its biomechanics.

The psoas major has diverse, but systematic, attachments to the lumbar spine (Fig. 4-1). At each segmental level, it is attached to the medial half or so of the anterior surface of the transverse process, to the intervertebral disc, and to the margins of the vertebral bodies adjacent to the disc.[4] The muscle fibers from the L5–S1 intervertebral disc, the L5 vertebral body, and the L5 transverse process form the deepest and lowest bundle of fibers within the muscle. These fibers are systematically overlapped by fibers from the disc, vertebral margins, and transverse process at L4, and in turn these fibers are overlapped by those from L3, and so on. As a result, the muscle can be seen in cross section to be concentrically layered, with fibers from higher levels forming the outer surface of the muscle and those from lower levels being buried sequentially, deeper within its substance.[4]

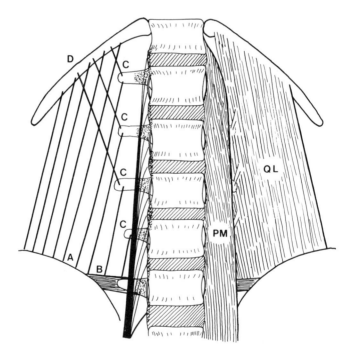

**Fig. 4-1.**   Psoas major *(PM)* and quadratus lumborum *(QL)*. At each segmental level psoas major attaches to the transverse process, the intervertebral disc, and adjacent vertebral margins, and to the tendinous arch covering the vertebral body. The attachments of quadratus lumborum are to the iliac crest *(A)*, the ilio-lumbar ligament *(B)*, the transverse processes *(C)*, and the 12th rib *(D)*. (From Bogduk and Twomey,[92] with permission.)

All the muscular fibers converge to a common tendon that crosses the iliopubic eminence, but within the muscle all muscular fibers are the same length.[4] As a result the fibers from L1 become tendinous before those from L2, and so on. This arrangement constitutes morphologic evidence that the psoas major cannot act on the lumbar spine. It indicates that all fibers are designed to contract in unison to the same extent. This is appropriate for a muscle acting to flex the thigh but inappropriate to move the lumbar spine. During flexion of the lumbar spine (whether in the sagittal or coronal plane), each lumbar vertebra undergoes a different linear excursion than the others; the upper ones move much further than the lower ones. If the psoas was responsible for such movements, the length of its fibers should be proportional to the excursion undergone by their vertebra of origin, which is not the case. However, more compelling evidence arises from the biomechanics of the psoas major.

Plotting the lines of action of each fascicle of psoas reveals that they have a varied and variable relationship to the axes of sagittal rotation of the lumbar vertebrae; some fascicles pass behind the upper axes but cross the middle axes and lie in front of the lower axes; others cross some axes but lie in front of the others.[4] The net effect is that the psoas major tends to extend the upper lumbar spine but flex the lower lumbar spine. However, its capacity to do so is limited by the proximity of the lines of action of its fascicles to the axes of rotation. The fascicles pass so close to the axes that the moments that they exert are next to trivial. Even when the moments of all fascicles are summed, the total is small. In essence, the psoas major, acting at maximum force-capacity, can generate a flexion moment that is barely enough to raise one-quarter of an average body weight, in the exercise of "sit-ups."[4]

The emphasis placed on psoas major as a muscle of the lumbar spine is not justified. Morphologically and mechanically it is simply a flexor of the thigh that has assumed an adventitious origin on the lumbar spine.

The psoas minor is an inconstant small muscle belly that arises from the T12–L1 intervertebral disc and forms a very long narrow tendon that inserts into the region of the iliopubic eminence. Its biomechanical significance is unknown.

## LATERAL INTERTRANSVERSE MUSCLES

The lateral intertransverse muscles consist of two parts: the ventral lateral intertransverse and the dorsal lateral intertransverse. The ventral intertransverse muscles connect the margins of consecutive transverse processes, while the dorsal intertransverse muscles each connect an accessory process to the transverse process below (Fig. 4-2). Both the ventral and dorsal intertransverse muscles are innervated by the ventral rami of the lumbar spinal nerves,[5] and consequently cannot be classified among the back muscles, which are all innervated by the dorsal rami. On the basis of their attachments and their nerve supply, the ventral and dorsal intertransverse muscles are considered to be

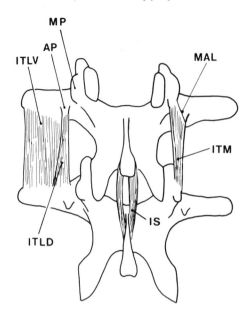

**Fig. 4-2.** The short, intersegmental muscles. *ITLV*, ventral intertransverse laterals; *ITLD*, dorsal intertransverse laterals; *ITM*, medial intertransverse muscles; *IS*, interspinals; *AP*, accessory process; *MP*, mamillary process; *MAL*, mamillo-accessory ligament. (From Bogduk and Twomey,[92] with permission.)

homologous to the intercostal and levator costae muscles of the thoracic region.[5]

The function of the lateral intertransverse muscles has never been determined experimentally. One might presume that on the basis of their attachments they act synergistically with the quadratus lumborum in lateral flexion of the lumbar spine. However, their small size lends doubt to this notion. Instead, it may be that they play a proprioceptive role like the other intersegmental muscles of the lumbar spine (see below).

## QUADRATUS LUMBORUM

The quadratus lumborum is a wide, more or less rectangular muscle that covers the lateral two-thirds or so of the anterior surfaces of the L1 to L4 transverse processes and extends laterally a few centimeters beyond the tips of the transverse processes. In detail, the muscle is a complex aggregation of various oblique and longitudinally running fibers that connect the lumbar transverse processes, the ilium, and the 12th rib[6] (see Fig. 4-1).

Caudally, the muscle arises from the L5 transverse process, the trough formed by the superior and anterior iliolumbar ligaments, and from the iliac crest lateral to the point of attachment of the iliolumbar ligament. From this series of attachments the most lateral fibers pass directly toward the lower, anterior surface of the 12th rib. More medial fibers pass obliquely upward and medially to the anterior surfaces of each of the lumbar transverse processes above L5. These oblique fibers intermingle with other oblique fibers that run upward and laterally from each of the lumbar transverse processes to the 12th rib.

The majority of the fibers of the quadratus lumborum are connected to the 12th rib and one of the functions of this muscle is said to be to fix the 12th rib during respiration.[7] The remaining fibers of quadratus lumborum connect the ilium to the upper four lumbar transverse processes, and these are the only fibers of quadratus lumborum that are suitably disposed to execute lateral flexion of the lumbar spine.

## THE LUMBAR BACK MUSCLES

The lumbar back muscles are those muscles that lie behind the plane of the lumbar transverse processes and that exert an action on the lumbar spine. They include muscles that attach to the lumbar vertebrae and thereby act directly on the lumbar spine, and certain other muscles that although not attaching to the lumbar vertebrae, nevertheless exert an action on the lumbar spine.

For descriptive purposes and on morphologic grounds, the lumbar back muscles can be divided into three groups:

1. The short intersegmental muscles—the interspinals and the medial intertransverse muscles.
2. The polysegmental muscles that attach to the lumbar vertebrae—the multifidus and the lumbar components of longissimus and iliocostalis.
3. The long polysegmental muscles, represented by the thoracic components of longissimus and iliocostalis lumborum, which, in general, do not attach to the lumbar vertebrae but cross the lumbar region from thoracic levels to find attachments on the ilium and sacrum.

The descriptions of the back muscles offered in this chapter, notably those of the multifidus and erector spinae, differ substantially from those given in standard textbooks. Traditionally, these muscles have been regarded as stemming from a common origin on the sacrum and ilium and passing upward to assume diverse attachments to the lumbar and thoracic vertebrae and ribs. However, in the face of several studies of these muscles,[8-12] it is considered more appropriate to view these muscles in the reverse direction: from above downward. Not only is this more consistent with the pattern of their nerve supply,[12,13] but it clarifies the identity of certain muscles and the identity of the erector spinae aponeurosis, and reveals the segmental biomechanical disposition of the muscles.

### Interspinals

The lumbar interspinals are short paired muscles that lie on either side of the interspinous ligament and connect the spinous processes of adjacent lumbar vertebrae (see Fig. 4-2). There are four pairs in the lumbar region. Although disposed to act synergistically with the multifidus to produce posterior sagittal rotation of the vertebra above, the interspinals are quite small and would not contribute appreciably to the force required to move a vertebra. This paradox is similar to that which applies for the medial intertransverse muscles and is discussed further in that context.

## Medial Intertransverse Muscles

The medial intertransverse muscles can be considered to be true back muscles, because, unlike the lateral intertransverse muscles, they are innervated by the lumbar dorsal rami.[5,13] The medial intertransverse muscles arise from an accessory process, the adjoining mamillary process and the mamillo-accessory ligament that connects these two processes.[14] They insert into the superior aspect of the mamillary process of the vertebra below (see Fig. 4-2).

The medial intertransverse muscles lie lateral to the axis of lateral flexion and behind the axis of sagittal rotation. However, they lie very close to these axes and are very small muscles. Therefore, it is questionable whether they could contribute any appreciable force in either lateral flexion or posterior sagittal rotation. It might be argued that perhaps larger muscles might provide the bulk of the power to move the vertebrae, and the intertransverse muscles could act to "fine tune" the movement. However, this suggestion is highly speculative, if not fanciful, and does not take into account their small size and considerable mechanical disadvantage.

A tantalizing alternative suggestion is that the intertransverse muscles act as large, proprioceptive transducers; their value lies not in the force they can exert, but in the muscle spindles they contain. Placed close to the lumbar vertebral column, the intertransverse muscles could monitor the movements of the column and provide feedback that influences the action of the surrounding muscles. Such a role has been suggested for the cervical intertransverse muscles, which have been found to contain a high density of muscle spindles.[15–17] Indeed, all unisegmental muscles of the vertebral column have between two and six times the density of muscles spindles found in the longer, polysegmental muscles, and there is growing speculation that this underscores the proprioceptive function of all short, small muscles of the body.[18–20]

## Multifidus

Multifidus is the largest and most medial of the lumbar back muscles. It consists of a repeating series of fascicles that stem from the laminae and spinous processes of the lumbar vertebrae and exhibit a constant pattern of attachments caudally.[12]

The shortest fascicles of the multifidus are the "laminar fibers," which arise from the caudal end of the dorsal surface of each vertebral lamina and

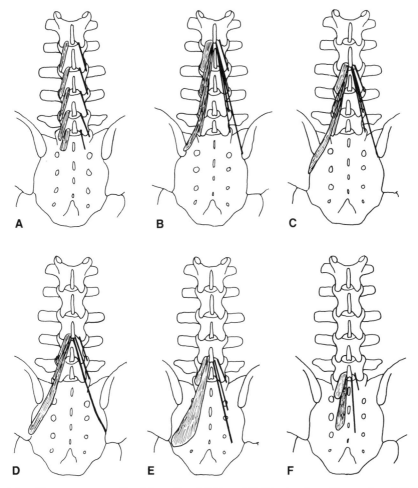

**Fig. 4-3.** The component fascicles of multifidus. (**A**) The laminar fibers of multifidus. (**B–F**) The fascicles from the L1 to L5 spinous processes, respectively. (From Bogduk and Twomey,[92] with permission.)

insert into the mamillary process of the vertebra two levels caudad (Fig. 4-3A). The L5 laminar fibers have no mamillary process into which they can insert, and insert instead into an area on the sacrum just above the first dorsal sacral foramen. Because of their attachments, the laminar fibers may be considered homologous to the thoracic rotatores.

The bulk of the lumbar multifidus consists of much larger fascicles that radiate from the lumbar spinous processes. These fascicles are arranged in five overlapping groups such that each lumbar vertebra gives rise to one of these groups. At each segmental level, a fascicle arises from the base and caudolateral edge of the spinous process, and several fascicles arise, by way of a common tendon, from the caudal tip of the spinous process. This tendon is referred to hereafter as the "common tendon." Although confluent with one another at their origin, the fascicles in each group diverge caudally to assume separate attachments to mamillary processes, the iliac crest, and the sacrum.

The fascicle from the base of the L1 spinous process inserts into the L4 mamillary process, whereas those from the common tendon insert into the mamillary processes of L5, S1, and the posterior superior iliac spine (Fig. 4–3B).

The fascicle from the base of the spinous process of L2 inserts into the mamillary process of L5, whereas those from the common tendon insert into the S1 mamillary process, the posterior superior iliac spine, and an area on the iliac crest just caudoventral to the posterior superior iliac spine (Fig. 4-3C).

The fascicle from the base of the L3 spinous process inserts into the mamillary process of the sacrum, whereas those fascicles from the common tendon insert into a narrow area extending caudally from the caudal extent of the posterior superior iliac spine to the lateral edge of the third sacral segment (Fig. 4-3D). The L4 fascicles insert onto the sacrum in an area medial to the L3 area of insertion, but lateral to the dorsal sacral foramina (Fig. 4-3E), whereas those from the L5 vertebra insert onto an area medial to the dorsal sacral foramina (Fig. 4-3F).

It is noteworthy that while many of the fascicles of multifidus attach to mamillary processes, some of the deeper fibers of these fascicles attach to the capsules of the zygapophyseal joints next to the mamillary processes.[21] This attachment allows the multifidus to protect the joint capsule from being caught inside the joint during the movements executed by the multifidus.

The key feature of the morphology of the lumbar multifidus is that its fascicles are arranged segmentally. Each lumbar vertebrae is endowed with a group of fascicles that radiate from its spinous process, anchoring it below to mamillary processes, the iliac crest, and the sacrum. This disposition suggests that the fibers of multifidus are arranged in such a way that their principal action is focused on individual lumbar spinous processes.[12] They are designed to act in concert on a single spinous process. This contention is supported by the pattern of innervation of the muscle. All the fascicles arising from the spinous processes of a given vertebra are innervated by the medial branch of the dorsal ramus that issues from below that vertebra.[12,13] Thus the muscles that directly act on a particular vertebral segment are innervated by the nerve of that segment.

In a posterior view, the fascicles of multifidus are seen to have an oblique, caudolateral orientation. Their line of action, therefore, can be resolved into two vectors: a large vertical vector, and a considerably smaller horizontal vector[9] (Fig. 4-4A).

The small horizontal vector suggests that the multifidus could pull the spinous processes sideways, and therefore produce horizontal rotation. However, horizontal rotation of lumbar vertebrae is impeded by the impaction of the contralateral zygapophyseal joints. Horizontal rotation occurs after impaction of the joints only if an appropriate shear force is applied to the intervertebral discs, but the horizontal vector of multifidus is so small that it is unlikely that

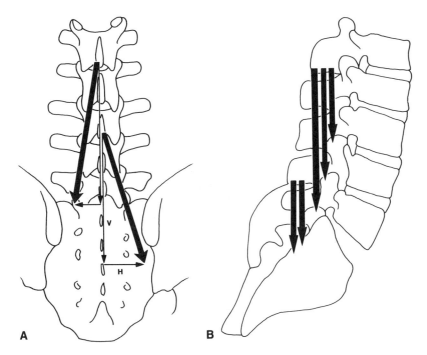

**Fig. 4-4.** The force vectors of multifidus. (**A**) In an anteroposterior view, the oblique line of action of the multifidus at each level *(bold arrows)* can be resolved into a major vertical vector *(V)* and a smaller horizontal vector *(H)*. (**B**) In a lateral view, the vertical vectors of the multifidus are seen to be aligned at right angles to the spinous processes. (From Bogduk and Twomey,[92] with permission.)

multifidus would be capable of exerting such a shear force on the disc by acting on the spinous process. Indeed, electromyographic studies reveal that multifidus is inconsistently active in derotation and that, paradoxically, it is active in both ipsilateral and contralateral rotation.[22] Rotation, therefore, cannot be inferred to be a primary action of multifidus. In this context, multifidus has been said to act only as a stabilizer in rotation,[21,22] but the aberrant movements that it is supposed to stabilize have not been defined (although see below).

The principal action of multifidus is expressed by its vertical vector, and further insight is gained when this vector is viewed in a lateral projection (Fig. 4-4B). Each fascicle of multifidus, at every level, acts virtually at right angles to its spinous process of origin.[9] Thus, using the spinous process as a lever, every fascicle is ideally disposed to produce posterior sagittal rotation of its vertebra. The right-angle orientation, however, precludes any action as a posterior horizontal translator. Therefore, the multifidus can only exert the "rocking" component of extension of the lumbar spine or control this component during flexion.

Having established that multifidus is primarily a posterior sagittal rotator of the lumbar spine, it is possible to resolve the paradox about its activity during horizontal rotation of the trunk.[9] In the first instance, it should be realized that rotation of the lumbar spine is an indirect action. Active rotation of the lumbar spine occurs only if the thorax is first rotated, and is therefore secondary to thoracic rotation. Secondly, it must be realized that a muscle with two vectors of action cannot use these vectors independently. If the muscle contracts, then both vectors are exerted. Thus, multifidus cannot exert axial rotation without simultaneously exerting a much larger posterior sagittal rotation.

The principal muscles that produce rotation of the thorax are the oblique abdominal muscles. The horizontal component of their orientation is able to turn the thoracic cage in the horizontal plane and thereby impart axial rotation to the lumbar spine. However, the oblique abdominal muscles also have a vertical component to their orientation. Therefore, if they contract to produce rotation they will also simultaneously cause flexion of the trunk, and therefore, of the lumbar spine. To counteract this flexion, and maintain pure axial rotation, extensors of the lumbar spine must be recruited, and this is how multifidus becomes involved in rotation.

The role of multifidus in rotation is not to produce rotation, but to oppose the flexion effect of the abdominal muscles as they produce rotation. The aberrant motion stabilized by multifidus during rotation is, therefore, the unwanted flexion unavoidably produced by the abdominal muscles.[9]

Apart from its action on individual lumbar vertebrae, the multifidus, because of its polysegmental nature, can also exert indirect effects on any interposed vertebrae. Since the line of action of any long fascicle of multifidus lies behind the lordotic curve of the lumbar spine, such fascicles can act like bowstrings on those segments of the curve that intervene between the attachments of the fascicle. The bowstring effect would tend to accentuate the lumbar lordosis, resulting in compression of intervertebral discs posteriorly and strain of the discs and longitudinal ligament anteriorly. Thus a secondary effect of the action of multifidus is to increase the lumbar lordosis and the compressive and tensile loads on any vertebrae and intervertebral discs interposed between its attachments.

## Lumbar Erector Spinae

The lumbar erector spinae lies lateral to the multifidus and forms the prominent dorsolateral contour of the back muscles in the lumbar region. It consists of two muscles: the longissimus thoracis and the iliocostalis lumborum. Furthermore, each of these muscles has two components: a lumbar part, consisting of fascicles arising from lumbar vertebrae, and a thoracic part, consisting of fascicles arising from thoracic vertebrae or ribs.[8,10,11] These four parts may be referred to, respectively, as longissimus thoracis pars lumborum, iliocostalis lumborum pars lumborum, longissimus thoracis pars lumborum, and longissimus thoracis pars thoracis.[10]

In the lumbar region, the longissimus and iliocostalis are separated from each other by the lumbar intermuscular aponeurosis, an anteroposterior contin-

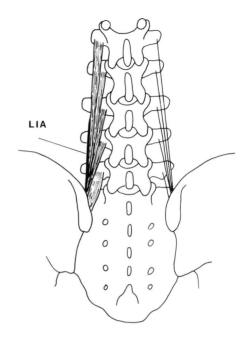

**Fig. 4-5.** The lumbar fibers of longissimus (longissimus thoracis pars lumborum). On the left, the five fascicles of the intact muscle are drawn. The formation of the lumbar intermuscular aponeurosis *(LIA)* by the lumbar fascicles of longissimus is depicted. On the right, the lines indicate the attachments and span of the fascicles. (From Bogduk and Twomey,[92] with permission.)

uation of the erector spinae aponeurosis.[8,10] It appears as a flat sheet of collagen fibers that extend rostrally from the medial aspect of the posterior superior iliac spine for 6 to 8 cm. It is formed mainly by the caudal tendons of the rostral four fascicles of the lumbar component of longissimus (Fig. 4-5).

## Longissimus Thoracis Pars Lumborum

The longissimus thoracis pars lumborum is composed of five fascicles, each arising from the accessory process and the adjacent medial end of the dorsal surface of the transverse process of a lumbar vertebra (see Fig. 4-5).

The fascicle from the L5 vertebra is the deepest and shortest. Its fibers insert directly into the medial aspect of the posterior superior iliac spine. The fascicle from L4 also lies deeply, but lateral to that from L5. Succeeding fascicles lie progressively more dorsally so that the L3 fascicle covers those from L4 and L5, but is itself covered by the L2 fascicle, whereas the L1 fascicle lies most superficially.

The L1 to L4 fascicles all form tendons at their caudal ends, which converge to form the lumbar intermuscular aponeurosis, which eventually attaches to a narrow area on the ilium immediately lateral to the insertion of the L5 fascicle. The lumbar intermuscular aponeurosis thus represents a common tendon of insertion, or the aponeurosis, of the bulk of the lumbar fibers of longissimus.

Each fascicle of the lumbar longissimus has both a dorsoventral and a rostrocaudal orientation.[10] Therefore, the action of each fascicle can be resolved into a vertical vector and a horizontal vector, the relative sizes of which differ from L1 to L5 (Fig. 4-6A). Consequently, the relative actions of longissimus differ at each segmental level. Furthermore, the action of longissimus, as a whole, will differ according to whether the muscle contracts unilaterally or bilaterally.

The large vertical vector of each fascicle lies lateral to the axis of lateral flexion and behind the axis of sagittal rotation of each vertebra. Thus contracting unilaterally the longissimus can laterally flex the vertebral column, but acting bilaterally the various fascicles can act, like multifidus, to produce posterior sagittal rotation of their vertebra of origin. However, their attachments to the accessory and transverse processes lie close to the axes of sagittal rotation, and therefore their capacity to produce posterior sagittal rotation is less efficient than that of multifidus, which acts through the long levers of the spinous processes.[10]

The horizontal vectors of the longissimus are directed backward. Therefore, when contracting bilaterally the longissimus is capable of drawing the

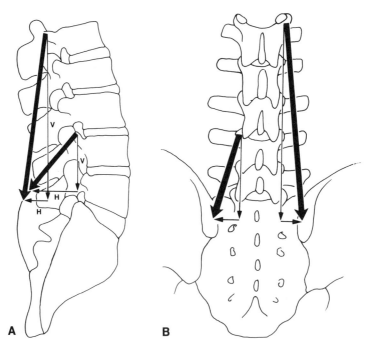

**Fig. 4-6.** The force vectors of the longissimus thoracis pars lumborum. (**A**) In a lateral view, the oblique line of action of each fascicle of longissimus can be resolved into a vertical (*V*) and a horizontal (*H*) vector. The horizontal vectors of lumbar fascicles are larger. (**B**) In an anteroposterior view, the line of action of the fascicles can be resolved into a major vertical vector and a much smaller horizontal vector. (From Bogduk and Twomey,[92] with permission.)

lumbar vertebrae backward. This action of posterior translation can restore the anterior translation of the lumbar vertebrae that occurs during flexion of the lumbar column. The capacity for posterior translation is greatest at lower lumbar levels where the fascicles of longissimus assume a greater dorsoventral orientation (Fig. 4-6B).

Reviewing the horizontal and vertical actions of longissimus together, it can be seen that longissimus expresses a continuum of combined actions along the length of the lumbar vertebral column. From below upward, its capacity as a posterior sagittal rotator increases, while reciprocally, from above downward, the fascicles are better designed to resist or restore anterior translation. It is emphasized that the longissimus cannot exert its horizontal and vertical vectors independently. Thus whatever horizontal translation it exerts must occur simultaneously with posterior sagittal rotation. The resolution into vectors simply reveals the relative amounts of simultaneous translation and sagittal rotation exerted at different segmental levels.

It might be deduced that because of the horizontal vector of longissimus, this muscle, acting unilaterally, could draw the accessory and transverse processes backward and therefore produce axial rotation. However, in this regard, the fascicles of longissimus are oriented almost directly toward the axis of axial rotation and so are at a marked mechanical disadvantage to produce axial rotation.

## Iliocostalis Lumborum Pars Lumborum

The lumbar component of iliocostalis lumborum consists of four overlying fascicles arising from the L1 to L4 vertebrae.[10] Rostrally, each fascicle attaches to the tip of the transverse process and to an area extending 2 to 3 cm laterally onto the middle layer of the thoracolumbar fascia (Fig. 4-7).

The fascicle from L4 is the deepest, and caudally it is attached directly to the iliac crest just lateral to the posterior superior iliac spine. This fascicle is covered by the fascicle from L3 that has a similar but more dorsolaterally located attachment on the iliac crest. In sequence, L2 covers L3 and L1 covers L2 with insertions on the iliac crest becoming successively more dorsal and lateral. The most lateral fascicles attach to the iliac crest just medial to the attachment of the "lateral raphe" of the thoracolumbar fascia (see below). The most medial fibers of iliocostalis contribute to the lumbar intermuscular aponeurosis, but only to a minor extent.

Although an L5 fascicle of iliocostalis lumborum is not described in the literature, it is represented in the iliolumbar "ligament." In neonates and children this "ligament" is completely muscular in structure. By the third decade of life the muscle fibers are entirely replaced by collagen, giving rise to the familiar iliolumbar ligament.[23] On the basis of sites of attachment and relative orientation, the posterior band of the iliolumbar ligament would appear to be derived from the L5 fascicle of iliocostalis, whereas the anterior band of the ligament is a derivative of the quadratus lumborum.

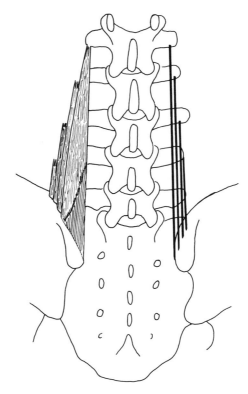

**Fig. 4-7.**   The lumbar fibers of iliocostalis (iliocostalis lumborum pars lumborum). On the left, the four lumbar fascicles of iliocostalis are shown. On the right, their span and attachments are indicated by the lines. (From Bogduk and Twomey,[92] with permission.)

The disposition of the lumbar fascicles of iliocostalis is similar to that of the lumbar longissimus, except that the fascicles are situated more laterally. Like that of the lumbar longissimus, their action can be resolved into horizontal and vertical vectors (Fig. 4-8A).

The vertical vector is still predominant, and therefore the lumbar fascicles of iliocostalis contracting bilaterally can act as posterior sagittal rotators (Fig. 4-8B), but because of the horizontal vector, a posterior translation will be exerted simultaneously, principally at lower lumbar levels where the fascicles of iliocostalis have a greater forward orientation. Contracting unilaterally, the lumbar fascicles of iliocostalis can act as lateral flexors of the lumbar vertebrae, for which action the transverse processes provide very substantial levers.

Contracting unilaterally, the fibers of iliocostalis are better suited to exert axial rotation than the fascicles of lumbar longissimus, because their attachment to the tips of the transverse processes displaces them from the axis of horizontal rotation and provides them with substantial levers for this action. Because of this leverage, the lower fascicles of iliocostalis are the only intrinsic muscles of the lumbar spine reasonably disposed to produce horizontal rotation. Their

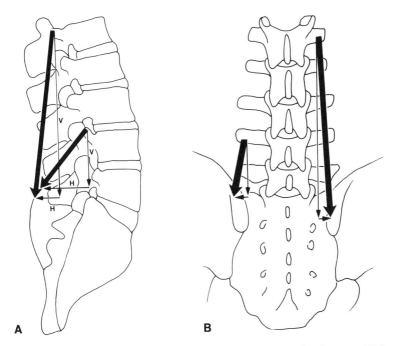

**Fig. 4-8.** The force vectors of the iliocostalis lumborum pars lumborum. **(A)** In a lateral view, the line of action of the fascicles can be resolved into vertical *(V)* and horizontal *(H)* vectors. The horizontal vectors are larger at lower lumbar levels. **(B)** In an anteroposterior view, the line of action is resolved into a vertical vector and a very small horizontal vector. (From Bogduk and Twomey,[92] with permission.)

effectiveness as rotators, however, is dwarfed by the oblique abdominal muscles that act on the ribs and produce lumbar rotation indirectly by rotating the thoracic cage. However, because iliocostalis cannot exert axial rotation without simultaneously exerting posterior sagittal rotation, the muscle is well suited to cooperate with multifidus to oppose the flexion effect of the abdominal muscles when they act to rotate the trunk.

## Longissimus Thoracis Pars Thoracis

The thoracic fibers of longissimus thoracis typically consist of 11 or 12 pairs of small fascicles arising from the ribs and transverse processes of T1 or T2 down to T12 (Fig. 4-9). At each level, two tendons can usually be recognized: a medial one from the tip of the transverse process, and a lateral one from the rib, although in the upper 3 or 4 levels, the latter may merge medially with the fascicle from the transverse process. Each rostral tendon extends 3 to 4 cm before forming a small muscle belly measuring 7 to 8 cm in length. The muscle bellies from the higher levels overlap those from lower levels. Each muscle

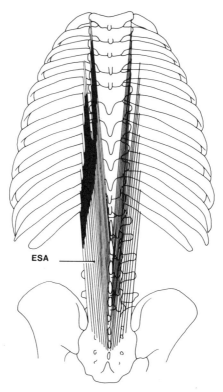

**Fig. 4-9.**   The thoracic fibers of longissimus (longissimus thoracis pars thoracis). The intact fascicles are shown on the left. The darkened areas represent the short muscle bellies of each fascicle. Note the short rostral tendons of each fascicle, and the long caudal tendons, which collectively constitute most of the erector spinae aponeurosis *(ESA)*. The span of the individual fascicles is indicated on the right. (From Bogduk and Twomey,[92] with permission.)

belly eventually forms a caudal tendon that extends into the lumbar region. The tendons run in parallel, with those from higher levels being most medial. The fascicles from the T2 level attach to the L3 spinous process, whereas the fascicles from the remaining levels insert into spinous processes at progressively lower levels. For example, those from T5 attach to L5 and those from T7 attach to S2 or S3. Those from T8 to T12 diverge from the midline to find attachment to the sacrum along a line extending from the S3 spinous process to the caudal extent of the posterior superior iliac spine.[10] The lateral edge of the caudal tendon of T12 lies alongside the dorsal edge of the lumbar intermuscular aponeurosis formed by the caudal tendon of the L1 longissimus bundle.

The side-to-side aggregation of the caudal tendons of longissimus thoracis pars thoracis forms much of what is termed the erector spinae aponeurosis, which covers the lumbar fibers of longissimus and iliocostalis, but affords no attachment to them.

The longissimus thoracis pars thoracis is designed to act on thoracic vertebrae and ribs. Nonetheless, when contracting bilaterally it acts indirectly on the lumbar vertebral column, and uses the erector spinae aponeurosis to produce an increase in the lumbar lordosis. However, not all of the fascicles of longissimus thoracis span the entire lumbar vertebral column. Those from the second rib and T2 reach only as far as L3, and only those fascicles arising between the T6 or T7 and the T12 levels actually span the entire lumbar region. Consequently, only a portion of the whole thoracic longissimus acts on all the lumbar vertebrae.

The oblique orientation of the longissimus thoracis pars thoracis also permits it to laterally flex the thoracic vertebral column and thereby indirectly flex the lumbar vertebral column laterally.

## Iliocostalis Lumborum Pars Thoracis

The iliocostalis lumborum pars thoracis consists of fascicles from the lower seven or eight ribs that attach caudally to the ilium and sacrum[10] (Fig. 4-10). These fascicles represent the thoracic component of iliocostalis lumborum, and should not be confused with the iliocostalis thoracis, which is restricted to the thoracic region between the upper six and lower six ribs.

Each fascicle of the iliocostalis lumborum pars thoracis arises from the angle of the rib via a ribbonlike tendon measuring some 9 to 10 cm in length. It then forms a muscle belly of 8 to 10 cm in length. Thereafter, each fascicle continues as a tendon, contributing to the erector spinae aponeurosis, and ultimately attaching to the posterior superior iliac spine. The most medial tendons, from the more rostral fascicles, often attach more medially to the dorsal surface of the sacrum, caudal to the insertion of multifidus.

The thoracic fascicles of iliocostalis lumborum have no attachment to lumbar vertebrae. They attach to the iliac crest and thereby span the lumbar region. Consequently, by acting bilaterally, it is possible for them to exert an indirect "bowstring" effect on the vertebral column, causing an increase in the lordosis of the lumbar spine. Acting unilaterally, the iliocostalis lumborum pars thoracis can use the leverage afforded by the ribs to laterally flex the thoracic cage and thereby laterally flex the lumbar vertebral column indirectly. The distance between the ribs and ilium does not shorten greatly during rotation of the trunk, and therefore the iliocostalis lumborum pars thoracis can have little action as an axial rotator. However, contralateral rotation greatly increases this distance, and the iliocostalis lumborum pars thoracis can serve to derotate the thoracic cage and, therefore, the lumbar spine.

## ERECTOR SPINAE APONEUROSIS

One of the cardinal revelations of recent studies of the lumbar erector spinae[8,10] is that this muscle consists of both lumbar and thoracic fibers. Modern textbook descriptions largely do not recognize the lumbar fibers, especially

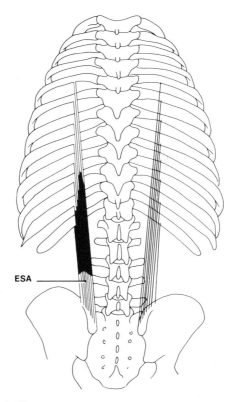

**Fig. 4-10.**   The thoracic fibers of iliocostalis lumborum (iliocostalis lumborum pars thoracis). The intact fascicles are shown on the left, and their span is shown on the right. The caudal tendons of the fascicles collectively form the lateral parts of the erector spinae aponeurosis *(ESA).* (From Bogduk and Twomey,[92] with permission.)

those of iliocostalis[8]; moreover, they do not note that the lumbar fibers (of both longissimus and iliocostalis) have attachments quite separate from those of the thoracic fibers. The lumbar fibers of the longissimus and iliocostalis pass between the lumbar vertebrae and the ilium. Thus, through these muscles, the lumbar vertebrae are anchored directly to the ilium. They do not gain any attachment to the erector spinae aponeurosis, which is the implication of all modern textbook descriptions that deal with the erector spinae.

The erector spinae aponeurosis is described as a broad sheet of tendinous fibers that is attached to the ilium, the sacrum, and the lumbar and sacral spinous processes, and which forms a common origin for the lower part of erector spinae. However, as described above, the erector spinae aponeurosis is formed virtually exclusively by the tendons of the longissimus thoracis pars thoracis and iliocostalis pars thoracis.[8,10] The medial half or so of the aponeurosis is formed by the tendons of longissimus thoracis, and the lateral half is formed by the iliocostalis lumborum (Fig. 4-11). The only additional contribution comes from the most superficial fibers of multifidus from upper lumbar

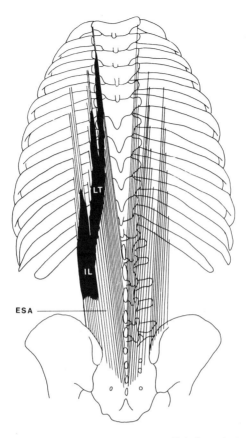

**Fig. 4-11.**   The erector spinae aponeurosis *(ESA)*. This broad sheet is formed by the caudal tendons of the thoracic fibers of longissimus thoracis *(LT)* and iliocostalis lumborum *(IL)*. (From Bogduk and Twomey,[92] with permission.)

levels, which contribute a small number of fibers to the aponeurosis[12] (see Figs. 4-9 and 4-10). Nonetheless, the erector spinae aponeurosis is essentially formed only by the caudal attachments of muscles acting from thoracic levels.

The lumbar fibers of erector spinae do not attach to the erector spinae aponeurosis. Indeed, the aponeurosis is free to move over the surface of the underlying lumbar fibers, and this suggests that the lumbar fibers, which form the bulk of the lumbar back musculature, can act independently from the rest of the erector spinae.

## THORACOLUMBAR FASCIA

The thoracolumbar fascia consists of three layers of fascia that envelop the muscles of the lumbar spine, effectively separating them into three compartments. The anterior layer of thoracolumbar fascia is quite thin, and is derived from the fascia of quadratus lumborum. It covers the anterior surface of quadratus lumborum, and is attached medially to the anterior surfaces of the lumbar transverse processes. In the intertransverse spaces it blends with the intertransverse ligaments, and may be viewed as one of the lateral extensions of the intertransverse ligaments. Lateral to the quadratus lumborum, the anterior layer blends with the other layers of the thoracolumbar fascia.

The middle layer of thoracolumbar fascia lies behind the quadratus lumborum. Medially, it is attached to the tips of the lumbar transverse processes, and is directly continuous with the intertransverse ligaments. Laterally, it gives rise to the aponeurosis of the transversus abdominis. Its actual identity is debatable. It may represent a lateral continuation of the intertransverse ligaments, a medial continuation of the transversus aponeurosis, a thickening of the posterior fascia of the quadratus, or a combination of any or all of these.

The posterior layer of thoracolumbar fascia covers the back muscles. It arises from the lumbar spinous processes in the midline posteriorly, and wraps around the back muscles to blend with the other layers of the thoracolumbar fascia along the lateral border of the iliocostalis lumborum. The union of the fasciae is quite dense at this site, and the middle and posterior layers in particular form a dense raphe that, for purposes of reference, has been called the lateral raphe.[24]

Traditionally, the thoracolumbar fascia has been ascribed no other function than to invest the back muscles and to provide an attachment for the transversus abdominis and the internal oblique muscles.[7] However, in recent years there has been considerable interest in its biomechanical role in the stability of the lumbar spine, particularly in the flexed posture and in lifting. This has resulted in anatomic and biomechanical studies of the anatomy and function of the thoracolumbar fascia, notably its posterior layer.[24–26]

The posterior layer of thoracolumbar fascia covers the back muscles from the lumbosacral region through to the thoracic region as far rostrally as the splenius muscle. In the lumbar region, it is attached to the tips of the spinous processes in the midline. Lateral to the erector spinae, between the 12th rib and the iliac crest, it unites with the middle layer of thoracolumbar fascia in the lateral raphe. At sacral levels, the posterior layer extends from the midline to the posterior superior iliac spine and the posterior segment of the iliac crest.

On close inspection, the posterior layer exhibits a cross-hatched appearance, manifest because it consists of two laminae: a superficial lamina with fibers oriented caudomedially and a deep lamina with fibers oriented caudolaterally.[24]

The superficial lamina is formed by the aponeurosis of latissimus dorsi, but the disposition and attachments of its constituent fibers differ according to the portion of latissimus dorsi from which they are derived (Fig. 4-12). Those fibers derived from the most lateral 2 to 3 cm of the muscle are short and insert directly into the iliac crest without contributing to the thoracolumbar fascia. Fibers from the next most lateral 2 cm of the muscle approach the iliac crest near the lateral margin of the erector spinae, but then deflect medially, bypassing the crest to attach to the L5 and sacral spinous processes. These fibers form the

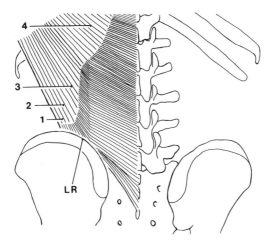

**Fig. 4-12.** The superficial lamina of the posterior layer of thoracolumbar fascia. *1,* Aponeurotic fibers of the most lateral fascicles of latissimus dorsi insert directly into the iliac crest. *2,* Aponeurotic fibers of the next most lateral part of latissimus dorsi glance past the iliac crest and reach the midline at sacral levels. *3,* Aponeurotic fibers from this portion of the muscle attach to the underlying lateral raphe *(LR)*, and then deflect medially to reach the midline at the L3 to L5 levels. *4,* Aponeurotic fibers from the upper portions of latissimus dorsi pass directly to the midline at thoracolumbar levels. (From Bogduk and Twomey,[92] with permission.)

sacral portion of the superficial lamina. A third series of fibers become aponeurotic just lateral to the lumbar erector spinae. At the lateral border of the erector spinae they blend with the other layers of thoracolumbar fascia in the lateral raphe, but they they deflect medially, continuing over the back muscles to reach the midline at the levels of the L3, L4, and L5 spinous processes. These fibers form the lumbar portion of the superficial lamina of the posterior layer of thoracolumbar fascia.

The rostral portions of the latissimus dorsi cross the back muscles and do not become aponeurotic until some 5 cm lateral to the midline at the L3 and higher levels. These aponeurotic fibers form the thoracolumbar and thoracic portions of the thoracolumbar fascia.

Beneath the superficial lamina, the deep lamina of the posterior layer consists of bands of collagen fibers emanating from the midline, principally from the lumbar spinous processes (Fig. 4-13). The bands from L4, L5, and S1 spinous processes pass caudolaterally to the posterior superior iliac spine. Those from the L3 spinous process and L3–L4 interspinous ligament wrap around the lateral margin of the erector spinae to fuse with the middle layer of thoracolumbar fascia in the lateral raphe. Above L3 the deep lamina progressively becomes thinner, consisting of sparse bands of collagen that dissipate laterally over the erector spinae. A deep lamina is not formed at thoracic levels.

Collectively, the superficial and deep laminae of the posterior layer of thoracolumbar fascia form a retinaculum over the back muscles. Attached to

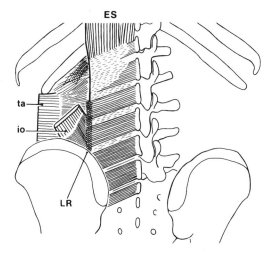

**Fig. 4-13.** The deep lamina of the posterior layer of thoracolumbar fascia. Bands of collagen fibers pass from the midline to the posterior superior iliac spine and to the lateral raphe *(LR)*. Those bands from the L4 and L5 spinous processes form alarlike ligaments that anchor these processes to the ilium. Attaching to the lateral raphe laterally are the aponeurosis of transversus abdominis *(ta)*, and a variable number of the most posterior fibers of internal oblique *(io)*. *ES*, erector spinae. (From Bogduk and Twomey,[92] with permission.)

the midline medially and the posterior superior iliac spine and lateral raphe laterally, the fascia covers or ensheaths the back muscles preventing their displacement dorsally. Additionally, the deep lamina alone forms a series of distinct ligaments. When viewed bilaterally, the bands of fibers from the L4 and L5 spinous processes appear like alar ligaments anchoring these spinous processes to the ilia. The band from the L3 spinous process anchors this process indirectly to the ilium via the lateral raphe. Thirdly, the lateral raphe forms a site where the two laminae of the posterior layer fuse not only with the middle layer of thoracolumbar fascia, but also with the transversus abdominis, whose middle fibers arise from the lateral raphe (see Fig. 4-13). The posterior layer of thoracolumbar fascia thereby provides an indirect attachment for the transversus abdominis to the lumbar spinous processes. The mechanical significance of these three morphologic features is explored below.

## FUNCTIONS OF THE BACK MUSCLES AND THEIR FASCIA

Each of the lumbar back muscles is capable of several possible actions. No action is unique to a muscle and no muscle has a single action. Instead, the back muscles provide a pool of possible actions that may be recruited to suit the needs of the vertebral column. Therefore, the functions of the back muscles need to be considered in terms of the observed movements of the vertebral column. In this regard, three types of movements can be addressed: (1) minor active movements of the vertebral column, (2) postural movements, and (3) major movements in forward bending and lifting. In this context *postural movements* refers to movements, usually subconscious, that occur to adjust and maintain a desired posture when this is disturbed, usually by the influence of gravity.

## Minor Active Movements

In the upright position, the lumbar back muscles play a minor, or no active role in executing movement, because gravity provides the necessary force. During extension, the back muscles contribute to the initial tilt, drawing the line of gravity backward,[27,28] but are unnecessary for further extension. Muscle activity is recruited when the movement is forced or resisted,[29] but is restricted to muscles acting on the thorax. The lumbar multifidus, for example, shows little or no involvement.[30]

The lateral flexors can bend the lumbar spine sideways, but once the center of gravity of the trunk is displaced, lateral flexion can continue under the influence of gravity. However, the ipsilateral lateral flexors are used to direct the movement, and the contralateral muscles are required to balance the action of gravity and control the rate and extent of movement. Consequently, lateral flexion is accompanied by bilateral activity of the lumbar back muscles, but the contralateral muscles are relatively more active, because they must balance the load of the laterally flexing spine.[27,28,31–34] If a weight is held in the hand on the side to which the spine is laterally flexed, a greater load is applied to the spine, and the contralateral back muscles show greater activity to balance this load.[31,33]

## Maintenance of Posture

The upright vertebral column is well stabilized by its joints and ligaments, but it is still liable to displacement by gravity or when subject to asymmetrical weightbearing. The back muscles serve to correct such displacements, and depending on the direction of any displacement, the appropriate back muscles will be recruited.

During standing at ease, the back muscles may show slight continuous activity,[22,27,29,32,34–45] intermittent activity,[27,29,34,45,46] or no activity,[38,41–43,45] and the amount of activity can be influenced by changing the position of the head or allowing the trunk to sway.[27]

The explanation for these differences probably lies in the location of the line of gravity in relation to the lumbar spine in different individuals.[29,38,43,45,47] In about 75 percent of individuals the line of gravity passes in front of the center of the L4 vertebra, and therefore essentially in front of the lumbar spine.[38,43] Consequently, gravity will exert a constant tendency to pull the thorax and lumbar spine into flexion. To preserve an upright posture, a constant level of activity in the posterior sagittal rotators of the lumbar spine will be needed to oppose the tendency to flexion. Conversely, when the line of gravity passes behind the lumbar spine, gravity tends to extend it, and back muscle activity is not required. Instead, abdominal muscle activity is recruited to prevent the spine from extending under gravity.[38,43]

Activities that displace the center of gravity of the trunk sideways will tend to cause lateral flexion. To prevent undesired lateral flexion, the contralateral lateral flexors will contract. This occurs when weights are carried in one hand.[27,41] Carrying equal weights in both hands does not displace the line of gravity, and back muscle activity is not increased substantially on either side of the body.[27,41]

During sitting, the activity of the back muscles is similar to that during standing,[36,37,48,49] but in supported sitting, as with the elbows resting on the knees, there is no activity in the lumbar back muscles,[27,34] and with arms resting on a desk, back muscle activity is substantially decreased.[36,37,48] In reclined sitting, the back rest supports the weight of the thorax, lessening the need for muscular support. Consequently, increasing the recline of the back rest of a seat decreases lumbar back muscle activity.[36,37,48,50]

## Major Active Movements

Forward flexion and extension of the spine from the flexed position are movements during which the back muscles have their most important function. As the spine bends forward, there is an increase in the activity of the back muscles,[22,27,29–32,34,35,44,46,51–54] and this increase is proportional to the angle of flexion and the size of any load carried.[31,33,55,56] The movement of forward flexion is produced by gravity, but the extent and the rate at which it proceeds is controlled by the eccentric contraction of the back muscles. Movement of the thorax on the lumbar spine is controlled by the long thoracic fibers of longissimus and iliocostalis. The long tendons of insertion allow these muscles to act around the convexity of the increasing thoracic kyphosis and anchor the thorax to the ilium and sacrum. In the lumbar region, the multifidus and the lumbar fascicles of longissimus and iliocostalis act to control the anterior sagittal rotation of the lumbar vertebrae. At the same time the lumbar fascicles of longissimus and iliocostalis also act to control the associated anterior translation of the lumbar vertebrae.

At a certain point during forward flexion, the activity in the back muscles ceases, and the vertebral column is braced by the locking of the zygapophyseal joints and tension in its posterior ligaments (Ch. 7). This phenomenon is known as "critical point".[44,45,47,57] However, critical point does not occur in all individuals, or in all muscles.[22,27,34,45,51] When it does occur, it does so when the spine has reached about 90 percent maximum flexion, even though at this stage, the hip flexion that occurs in forward bending is still only 60 percent complete.[47,57]

Carrying weights during flexion causes the critical point to occur later in the range of vertebral flexion.[47,57]

The physiologic basis for critical point is still obscure. It may be due to reflex inhibition initiated by proprioceptors in the lumbar joints and ligaments, or in muscle stretch and length receptors.[57] Whatever the mechanism, the significance of critical point is that it marks the transition of spinal loadbearing from muscles to the ligamentous system.

Extension of the trunk from the flexed position is characterized by high levels of back muscle activity.[22,27,44,46,54] In the thoracic region, the iliocostalis and longissimus, acting around the thoracic kyphosis, lift the thorax by rotating it backward. The lumbar vertebrae are rotated backward, principally by the lumbar multifidus, causing their superior surfaces to be progressively tilted upward to support the rising thorax.

## Compressive Loads of the Back Muscles

Because of the downward direction of their action, as the back muscles contract they exert a longitudinal compression of the lumbar vertebral column, and this compression raises the pressure in the lumbar intervertebral discs. Any activity that involves the back muscles, therefore, is associated with a rise in nuclear pressure. As measured in the L3–L4 intervertebral disc, the nuclear pressure correlates with the degree of myoelectric activity in the back muscles.[31,33,57,58] As muscle activity increases, disc pressure rises.

Disc pressures and myoelectric activity of the back muscles have been used extensively to quantify the stresses applied to the lumbar spine in various postures and by various activities.[36,49,50,59–64] From the standing position, forward bending causes the greatest increase in disc pressure. Lifting a weight in this position raises disc pressure even further, and the pressure is greatly increased if a load is lifted with the lumbar spine both flexed and rotated. Throughout these various maneuvers, back muscle activity increases in proportion to the disc pressure.

One of the prime revelations of combined discometric and electromyographic studies of the lumbar spine during lifting relates to the comparative stresses applied to the lumbar spine by different lifting tactics. In essence, it has been shown that, on the basis of changes in disc pressure and back muscle activity, there are no differences between using a "stoop" lift or a "leg" lift (i.e., lifting a weight with a bent back versus lifting with a straight back).[31,50,65] The critical factor is the distance of the load from the body. The further the load is from the chest the greater the stresses on the lumbar spine, and the greater the disc pressure and back muscle activity.[65]

### Strength of the Back Muscles

The strength of the back muscles has been determined in experiments on normal volunteers.[28] Two measures of strength are available: the absolute maximum force of contraction in the upright posture and the moment generated on the lumbar spine. The absolute maximum strength of the back muscles as a whole is about 4000 N. Acting on the short moment arms provided by the spinous processes and pedicles of the lumbar vertebrae, this force converts to an extensor moment of 200 Nm. These figures apply to average males under the age of 30 years; young females exhibit about 60 percent of this strength, whereas individuals over the age of 30 years are about 10 to 30 percent weaker, respectively.[28]

By comparing these values with the detailed morphology of the back muscles, modeling studies have revealed the extent to which individual muscles contribute to the overall strength of the back muscles.[24,66] It emerges that with respect to extension moments, about half the total, maximum moment exerted on the L5–S1 joint is generated by the thoracic fibers of longissimus thoracis and iliocostalis lumborum. The remainder is generated by those fibers of multifidus, longissimus, and iliocostalis that arise from the lumbar vertebrae, with multifidus contributing about half of this remainder.[66]

## Lifting

In biomechanical terms, the act of lifting constitutes a problem in balancing moments. When an individual bends forward to execute a lift, flexion occurs at the hip joint and in the lumbar spine. Indeed most of the forward movement seen during trunk flexion occurs at the hip joint.[57] The flexion forces are generated by gravity acting on the mass of the object to be lifted and on the mass of the trunk above the level of the hip joint and lumbar spine (Fig. 4-14). These forces exert flexion moments on both the hip joint and the lumbar spine. In each case the moment will be the product of the force and its perpendicular distance from the joint in question. The total flexion moment acting on each joint will be the sum of the moments exerted by the mass to be lifted and the mass of the trunk. For a lift to be executed these flexion moments have to be overcome by a moment acting in the opposite direction. This could be exerted by longitudinal forces acting downward behind the hip joint and vertebral column or by forces acting upward in front of the joints pushing the trunk upward.

There are no doubts as to the capacity of the hip extensors to generate large moments and overcome the flexion moments exerted on the hip joint even by the heaviest of loads that might be lifted.[67,68] However, the hip extensors are only able to rotate the pelvis backward on the femurs; they do not act on the lumbar spine. Thus, regardless of what happens at the hip joint, the lumbar spine still remains subject to a flexion moment that must be overcome in some other way. Without an appropriate mechanism the lumbar spine would stay flexed as the hips extended; indeed, as the pelvis rotated backward, flexion of the lumbar spine would be accentuated as its bottom end was pulled backward with the pelvis while its top end remained stationary under the load of the flexion moment. A mechanism is required to allow the lumbar spine to resist this deformation or to cause it to extend in unison with the hip joint.

Despite much investigation and debate, the exact nature of this mechanism

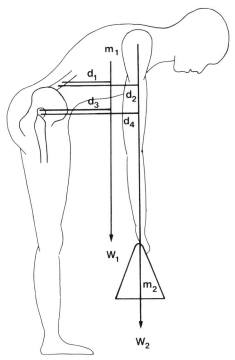

**Fig. 4-14.** The flexion moments exerted on a flexed trunk. Forces generated by the weight of the trunk and the load to be lifted act vertically in front of the lumbar spine and hip joint. The moments they exert on each joint are proportional to the distance between the line of action of each force and the joint in question. The mass of the trunk $(m_1)$ exerts a force $(W_1)$ that acts a measurable distance in front of the lumbar spine $(d_1)$ and the hip joint $(d_3)$. The mass to be lifted $(m_2)$ exerts a force $(W_2)$ that acts a measurable distance from the lumbar spine $(d_2)$ and hip joint $(d_4)$. The respective moments acting on the lumbar spine will be $W_1d_1$ and $W_1d_3$; those on the hip joint will be $W_2d_2$ and $W_2d_4$. (From Bogduk and Twomey,[92] with permission.)

remains unresolved. In various ways the back muscles, intraabdominal pressure, the thoracolumbar fascia, and the posterior ligamentous system have been believed to participate.

For light lifts the flexion moments generated are relatively small. In the case of a 70-kg man lifting a 10-kg mass in a fully stooped position, the upper trunk weighs about 40 kg and acts about 30 cm in front of the lumbar spine while the arms holding the mass to be lifted lie about 45 cm in front of the lumbar spine. The respective flexion moments are therefore $40 \times 9.8 \times 0.30 = 117.6$ Nm and $10 \times 9.8 \times 0.45 = 44.1$ Nm, for a total of 161.7 Nm. This load is well within the capacity of the back muscles (200 Nm, see Strength of the Back Muscles). Thus, as the hips extend, the lumbar back muscles are capable of resisting further flexion of the lumbar spine, and indeed, could even actively extend it, and the weight would be lifted.

Increasing the load to be lifted to over 30 kg increases the flexion moment to 132.2 Nm, which when added to the flexion moment of the upper trunk exceeds the capacity of the back muscles. To remain within the capacity of the back muscles such loads must be carried closer to the lumbar spine (i.e., they must be borne with a much shorter moment arm). Even so, decreasing the moment arm to about 15 cm limits the load to be carried to about 90 kg. The back muscles are simply not strong enough to raise greater loads. Such realizations have generated concepts of several additional mechanisms that serve to aid the back muscles in overcoming large flexion moments.

In 1957 Bartelink[69] raised the proposition that intraabdominal pressure could aid the lumbar spine in resisting flexion by acting upward on the diaphragm—the so-called intraabdominal balloon mechanism. Bartelink himself was circumspect and reserved in raising this conjecture, but the concept was rapidly popularized, particularly among physiotherapists. Even though it was never validated, the concept seemed to be treated as proven fact. It received early endorsement in orthopedic circles,[30] and intraabdominal pressure was adopted by ergonomists and others as a measure of spinal stress and safe lifting standards.[70–76] In more contemporary studies, intraabdominal pressure has been monitored during various spinal movements and lifting tasks.[31,65]

Reservations about the validity of the abdominal balloon mechanism have arisen from several quarters. Studies of lifting tasks reveal that unlike myoelectric activity, intraabdominal pressure does not correlate well with the size of the load being lifted or the applied stress on the vertebral column as measured by intradiscal pressure.[57,58,77,78] Indeed, deliberately increasing intraabdominal pressure by a Valsalva maneuver does not relieve the load on the lumbar spine but actually increases it.[79] Clinical studies have shown that although abdominal muscles are weaker than normal in patients with back pain, intraabdominal pressure is not different.[80] Furthermore, strengthening the abdominal muscles both in normal individuals[81] and in patients with back pain[82] does not influence intraabdominal pressure during lifting.

The most strident criticism of the intraabdominal balloon theory comes from bioengineers and others who maintain that (1) to generate any significant antiflexion moment the pressure required would exceed the maximum hoop tension of the abdominal muscles[83–85]; (2) such a pressure would be so high as to obstruct the abdominal aorta[83] (a reservation raised by Bartelink himself)[69]; and (3) because the abdominal muscles lie in front of the lumbar spine and connect the thorax to the pelvis, whenever they contract to generate pressure they must also exert a flexion moment on the trunk, which would negate any antiflexion value of the intraabdominal pressure.[67,85–87]

These reservations inspired an alternative explanation of the role of the abdominal muscles during lifting. Farfan, Gracovetsky, and colleagues[26,67,85–88] noted the crisscross arrangement of the fibers in the posterior layer of thoracolumbar fascia and surmised that if lateral tension was applied to this fascia it would result in an extension moment being exerted on the lumbar spinous processes. Such tension could be exerted by the abdominal muscles that arise from the thoracolumbar fascia, and the trigonometry of the fibers in the thoracolumbar fascia was such that they could convert lateral tension into an appreciable extension moment—the so-called gain of the thoracolumbar fascia.[85] The role of the abdominal muscles during lifting was thus to brace, if not actually extend, the lumbar spine by pulling on the thoracolumbar fascia. Any rises in intraabdominal pressure were thereby only coincidental, occurring because of the contraction of the abdominal muscles acting on the thoracolumbar fascia.

Subsequent anatomic studies revealed several liabilities of this mode.[89] First, the posterior layer of thoracolumbar fascia is well developed only in the lower lumbar region, but nevertheless its fibers are appropriately oriented to enable lateral tension exerted on the fascia to produce extension moments at least on the L2 to L5 spinous processes (Fig. 4-15). However, dissection reveals that of the abdominal muscles internal oblique offers only a few fibers that irregularly attach to the thoracolumbar fascia; transversus abdominis is the only muscle that consistently attaches to the thoracolumbar fascia, but only its very middle fibers do so. The size of these fibers is such that even on maximum contraction the force they exert is very small. Calculations revealed that the extensor moment they could exert on the lumbar spine amounted to less than 6 Nm.[89] Thus the contribution that abdominal muscles might make to antiflexion moments is trivial, a conclusion also borne out by subsequent, independent modeling studies.[90]

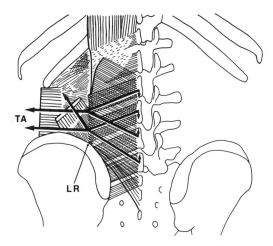

**Fig. 4-15.** The mechanics of the thoracolumbar fascia. From any point in the lateral raphe *(LR)*, lateral tension in the posterior layer of thoracolumbar fascia is transmitted upward through the deep lamina of the posterior layer, and downward through the superficial layer. Because of the obliquity of these lines of tension, a small downward vector is generated at the midline attachment of the deep lamina, and a small upward vector is generated at the midline attachment of the superficial lamina. These mutually opposite vectors tend to approximate or oppose the separation of L2 and L4 and of L3 and L5 spinous processes. Lateral tension on the fascia can be exerted by the transversus abdominis *(TA),* and to a lesser extent by the few fibers of internal oblique when they attach to the lateral raphe. (From Bogduk and Twomey,[92] with permission.)

A totally different model of lifting was elaborated by Farfan and Gracovetsky.[26,67,85] Noting the weakness of the back muscles, these authors proposed that extension of the lumbar spine was not required to lift heavy loads or loads with long moment arms. They proposed that the lumbar spine should remain fully flexed in order to engage (i.e., maximally stretch), what they referred to as the "posterior ligamentous system," namely the capsules of the zygapophyseal joints, the interspinous and supraspinous ligaments, and the posterior layer of thoracolumbar fascia, the latter acting passively to transmit tension between the lumbar spinous processes and ilium.

Under such conditions the active energy for a lift was provided by the powerful hip extensor muscles. These rotated the pelvis backward. Meanwhile, the external load acting on the upper trunk kept the lumbar spine flexed. Tension would develop in the posterior ligamentous system, which bridged the thorax and pelvis. With the posterior ligamentous system so engaged, as the pelvis rotated backward the lumbar spine would be passively raised while remaining in a fully flexed position. In essence, the posterior sagittal rotation of the pelvis would be transmitted through the posterior ligaments first to the L5 vertebra, then to L4, and so on, up through the lumbar spine into the thorax. All that was required was that the posterior ligamentous system be sufficiently strong to withstand the passive tension generated in it by the movement of the pelvis at one end and the weight of the trunk and external load at the other. The lumbar spine would thereby be raised like a long, rigid arm rotating on the pelvis and raising the external load with it.

Contraction of the back muscles was not required if the ligaments could take the load. Indeed, muscle contraction was distinctly undesirable, because any active extension of the lumbar spine would disengage the posterior ligaments and preclude them from transmitting tension. The back muscles could be recruited only once the trunk had been raised sufficiently to shorten the moment arm of the external load, reducing its flexion moment to within the capacity of the back muscles.

The attraction of this model was that it overcame the problem of the relative weakness of the back muscles by dispensing with their need to act, which in turn was consistent with the myoelectric silence of the back muscles at full flexion of the trunk and the recruitment of muscle activity only once the trunk had been elevated and the flexion moment arm had been reduced. Support for the model also came from surgical studies that reported that if the midline ligaments and thoracolumbar fascia were conscientiously reconstructed after multilevel laminectomies, the postoperative recovery and rehabilitation of patients were enhanced.[91]

However, although attractive in a qualitative sense, the mechanism of the posterior ligamentous system was not validated quantitatively. The model requires that the ligaments be strong enough to sustain the loads applied. In this regard, data on the strength of the posterior ligaments are scant and irregular, but sufficient data are available to permit an initial appraisal of the feasibility of the posterior ligament model.

The strength of spinal ligaments varies considerably, but average values

**Table 4-1.** Strength of the Posterior Ligamentous System

| Ligament | Reference | Average Force at Failure[a] (N) | Moment Arm[b] (m) | Maximum Moment (Nm) |
|---|---|---|---|---|
| PLL | 94 | 90 | 0.02 | 1.8 |
| LF | 94 | 244 | 0.03 | 7.3 |
| ZJC | 94 | 680 | 0.04 | 27.2 |
|  | 95 | 672 |  |  |
| ISL | 94 | 107 | 0.05 | 5.4 |
| TLF | 94 | 500 | 0.06 | 30.0 |
| Total |  |  |  | 51.7 |

*Abbreviations:* ISL, interspinous ligament; LF, ligmentum flavum; PLL, posterior longitudinal ligament; TLF, the posterior layer of thoracolumbar fascia and the erector spinae aponeurosis that forms the so-called supraspinous ligament; ZJC, zygapophyseal joint capsules (bilaterally).

[a] Average force at failure has been calculated using raw data provided in the references cited.

[b] Moment arms are estimates based on inspection of a representative vertebra measuring the perpendicular distance between the location of the instantaneous axis of rotation and the sites of attachment of the various ligaments.

(From Bogduk and Twomey,[92] with permission.)

can be calculated. Table 4-1 summarizes some of the available data. The strongest posterior "ligaments" of the lumbar spine are the zygapophyseal joint capsules and the thoracolumbar fascia forming the midline "supraspinous ligament." However, when the relatively short moment arms over which these ligaments act are considered, it transpires that the maximum moment they can sustain is relatively small. Even the sum total of all their moments is considerably less than that required for heavy lifting and is some four times less than the maximum strength of the back muscles. Of course, it is possible that the data quoted may not be representative of the true mean values of the strength of these ligaments, but it does not seem likely that the literature quoted underestimated their strength by a factor of four or more. Under these conditions, it is evident that posterior ligamentous system alone is not strong enough to perform the role required of it in heavy lifting. The posterior ligamentous system is not strong enough to replace the back muscles as a mechanism to prevent flexion of the lumbar spine during lifting. Some other mechanisms must operate.

One such mechanism is that of the hydraulic amplifier effect.[88] Originally set forth by Gracovetsky et al,[88] it proposed that because the thoracolumbar fascia surrounded the back muscles as a retinaculum it could serve to brace these muscles and enhance their power. The engineering basis for this effect is complicated, and the concept remained unexplored until very recently. A mathematical proof has been published that suggests that by investing the back muscles the thoracolumbar fascia enhances the strength of the back muscles by some 30 percent.[95] This is an appreciable increase and an attractive mechanism for enhancing the antiflexion capacity of the back muscles. However, the validity of this proof is still being questioned on the grounds that the principles used, although applicable to the behavior of solids, may not be applicable to muscles; the concept of the hydraulic amplifier mechanism still remains under scrutiny.

Quite a contrasting model has been proposed to explain the mechanics of the lumbar spine in lifting. It is based on arch theory and maintains that the behavior, stability, and strength of the lumbar spine during lifting can be explained by viewing the lumbar spine as an arch braced by intraabdominal pressure.[96,97] This intriguing concept, however, has not met with any degree of acceptance, and indeed, has been challenged from some quarters.[98]

## SUMMARY

Despite much effort over recent years the exact mechanism of heavy lifting still remains unexplained. The back muscles are too weak to extend the lumbar spine against large flexion moments; the intraabdominal balloon has been refuted; the abdominal mechanism and thoracolumbar fascia has been refuted; and the posterior ligamentous system appears too weak to replace the back muscles. Engineering models of the hydraulic amplifier effect and the arch model are still subject to debate.

What remains to be explained is what provides the missing force to sustain heavy loads, and why intraabdominal pressure is so consistently generated during lifts if it is neither to brace the thoracolumbar fascia nor to provide an intraabdominal balloon. At present these questions can only be addressed by conjecture, but certain concepts appear worthy of consideration.

With regard to intraabdominal pressure, one concept that has been overlooked in studies of lifting is the role of the abdominal muscles in controlling axial rotation of the trunk. Investigators have focused their attention on movements in the sagittal plane during lifting and have ignored the fact that when bent forward to address an object to be lifted the trunk is liable to axial rotation. Unless the external load is perfectly balanced and lies exactly in the midline, it will cause the trunk to twist to the left or the right. Thus, to keep the weight in the midline and in the sagittal plane, the lifter must control any twisting effect. The oblique abdominal muscles are the principal rotators of the trunk and would be responsible for this bracing. In contracting to control axial rotation, the abdominal muscles would secondarily raise intraabdominal pressure. This pressure rise is therefore an epiphenomenon and would reflect not the size of any external load but its tendency to twist the flexed trunk.

With regard to loads in the sagittal plane, the passive strength of the back muscles has been neglected in discussions of lifting. From the behavior of isolate muscle fibers it is known that as a muscle elongates its maximum contractile force diminishes, but its passive elastic tension rises; this is to such an extent that in an elongated muscle the total passive and active tension generated is at least equal to the maximum contractile capacity of the muscle at resting length. Thus, although they become electrically silent at full flexion, the back muscles are still capable of providing passive tension equal to their maximum contractile strength. This would allow the silent muscles to supplement the engaged posterior ligamentous system. With the back muscles providing some 200 Nm and the ligaments some 50 Nm or more, the total antiflexion capacity of the lumbar spine rises to about 250 Nm, which would allow some 30 kg to be safely lifted at 90° trunk flexion. Larger loads could be sustained by proportionally shortening the moment arm. Consequently, the mechanism of lifting may well be essentially as proposed by Farfan and Gracovetsky,[26,67,88] except that the passive tension in the back muscles constitutes the major component of the "posterior ligamentous system."

# REFERENCES

1. Basmajian JV: Electromyography of iliopsoas. Anat Rec 132:127, 1958
2. Nachemson A: Electromyographic studies on the vertebral portion of the psoas muscle. Acta Orthop Scand 37:177, 1966
3. Nachemson A: The possible importance of the psoas muscle for stabilization of the lumbar spine. Acta Orthop Scand 39:47, 1968
4. Bogduk N, Pearcy M, Hadfield G: Anatomy and biomechanics of psoas major. Clin Biomech 7:109, 1992
5. Cave AJE: The innervation and morphology of the cervical intertransverse muscles. J Anat 71:497, 1937
6. Poirier P: Myologie. p. 139. In Poirier P, Charpy A (eds): Traite d'Anatomie Humaine. 3rd Ed. Vol. 2, Fasc 1. Masson, Paris, 1912
7. Williams PL, Warwick R: Gray's Anatomy. 37th Ed. Churchill Livingstone, London, 1989
8. Bogduk N: A reappraisal of the anatomy of the human lumbar erector spinae. J Anat 131:525, 1980
9. Macintosh JE, Bogduk N: The biomechanics of the lumbar multifidus. Clin Biomech 1:205, 1986
10. Macintosh JE, Bogduk N: The morphology of the lumbar erector spinae. Spine 12: 658, 1986
11. Macintosh JE, Bogduk N: The attachments of the lumbar erector spinae. Spine 16: 783, 1991
12. Macintosh JE, Valencia F, Bogduk N, Munro RR: The morphology of the lumbar multifidus muscles. Clin Biomech 1:196, 1986
13. Bogduk N, Wilson AS, Tynan W: The human lumbar dorsal rami. J Anat 134:383, 1982
14. Bogduk N: The lumbar mamillo-accessory ligament. Its anatomical and neurosurgical significance. Spine 6:162, 1981
15. Abrahams VC: The physiology of neck muscles; their role in head movement and maintenance of posture. Can J Physiol Pharmacol 55:332, 1977
16. Abrahams VC: Sensory and motor specialization in some muscles of the neck. Trends Neuosci 4:24, 1981
17. Cooper S, Danial PM: Muscles spindles in man, their morphology in the lumbricals and the deep muscles of the neck. Brain 86:563, 1963
18. Bastide G, Zadeh J, Lefebvre D: Are the "little muscles" what we think they are? Surg Radiol Anat 11:255, 1989
19. Nitz AJ, Peck D: Comparison of muscle spindle concentrations in large and small human epaxial muscles acting in parallel combinations. Am Surg 52:273, 1986
20. Peck D, Buxton DF, Nitz A: A comparison of spindle concentrations in large and small muscles acting in parallel combinations. J Morphol 180:243, 1984

21. Lewin T, Moffet B, Viidik A: The morphology of the lumbar synovial intervertebral joints. Acta Morphol Neere-Scand 4:299, 1962
22. Donisch EW, Basmajian JV: Electromyography of deep back muscles in man. Am J Anat 133:25, 1972
23. Luk KDK, Ho HC, Leong JCY: The iliolumbar ligament. A study of its anatomy, development and clinical significance. J Bone Joint Surg 68B:197, 1986
24. Bogduk N, Macintosh J: The applied anatomy of the thoracolumbar fascia. Spine 9:164, 1984
25. Fairbank JCT, O'Brien JP: The abdominal cavity and thoracolumbar fascia as stabilisers of the lumbar spine in patients with low back pain. Engineering Aspects of the Spine 2:83, 1980
26. Gracovetsky S, Farfan HF, Lamy C: The mechanism of the lumbar spine. Spine 6:249, 1981
27. Floyd WF, Silver PHS: The function of the erectores spinae muscles in certain movements and postures in man. J Physiol 129:184, 1955
28. McNeill T, Warwick D, Andersson G, Schultz A: Trunk strengths in attempted flexion, extension and lateral bending in healthy subjects and patients with low back disorders. Spine 5:529, 1980
29. Ortengren R, Andersson GBJ: Electromyographic studies of trunk muscles with special reference to the functional anatomy of the lumbar spine. Spine 2:44, 1977
30. Morris JM, Lucas DB, Bresler B: Role of the trunk in stability of the spine. J Bone Joint Surg 43A:327, 1961
31. Andersson GBJ, Ortengren R, Nachemson A: Intradiscal pressure, intra-abdominal pressure and myoelectric back muscle activity related to posture and loading. Clin Orthop 129:156, 1977
32. Carlsoo S: The static muscle load in different work positions: an electromyographic study. Ergonomics 4:193, 1961
33. Ortengren R, Andersson G, Nachemson A: Lumbar loads in fixed working postures during flexion and rotation. p. 159. In Asmussen E, Jorgensen K (eds): Biomechanics VI-B, International Series on Biomechanics, Vol. 2B. University Park Press, Baltimore, 1978
34. Portnoy H, Morin F: Electromyographic study of the postural muscles in various positions and movements. Am J Physiol 186:122, 1956
35. Allen CEL: Muscle action potentials used in the study of dynamic anatomy. Br J Phys Med 11:66, 1948
36. Andersson BJG, Ortengren R: Myoelectric activity during sitting. Scand J Rehabil Med, suppl. 3:73, 1974
37. Andersson BJG, Jonsson B, Ortengren R: Myoelectric activity in individual lumbar erector spinae muscles in sitting: a study with surface and wire electrodes. Scand J Rehabil Med, suppl. 3:91, 1974
38. Asmussen E, Klausen K: Form and function of the erect human spine. Clin Orthop 25:55, 1962
39. Carlsoo S: Influence of frontal and dorsal loads on muscle activity and on the weight distribution in the feet. Acta Orthop Scand 34:299, 1964
40. De Vries HA: Muscle tonus in postural muscles. Am J Phys Med 44:275, 1965
41. Jonsson B: The functions of the individual muscles in the lumbar part of the spinae muscle. Electromyography 10:5, 1970
42. Joseph J, McColl I: Electromyography of muscles of posture: posterior vertebral muscles in males. J Physiol 157:33, 1961
43. Klausen K: The form and function of the loaded human spine. Acta Physiol Scand 65:176, 1965

44. Morris JM, Benner G, Lucas DB: An electromyographic study of the intrinsic muscles of the back in man. J Anat 96:509, 1962
45. Valencia FP, Munro RR: An electromyographic study of the lumbar multifidus in man. Electromyogr Clin Neurophysiol 25:205, 1985
46. Floyd WF, Silver PHS: Function of erectores spinae in flexion of the trunk. Lancet 1:133, 1951
47. Kippers V, Parker AW: Electromyographic studies of erectores spinae: symmetrical postures and sagittal trunk motion. Aust J Physiother 31:95, 1985
48. Andersson BJG, Ortengren R: Lumbar disc pressure and myoelectric back muscle activity during sitting. II. Studies of an office chair. Scandinav J Rehab Med 6:115, 1974
49. Andersson BJG, Ortengren R, Nachemson AL et al: The sitting posture: an electromyographic and discometric study. Orthop Clin North Am 6:105, 1975
50. Nachemson AL: The lumbar spine. An orthopaedic challenge. Spine 1:59, 1976
51. Okada M: Electromyographic assessment of the muscular load in forward bending postures. J Fac Sci Univ Tokyo 8:311, 1970
52. Golding JSR: Electromyography of the erector spinae in low back pain. Postgrad Med J 28:401, 1952
53. Koreska J, Robertson D, Mills RH: Biomechanics of the lumbar spine and its clinical significance. Orthop Clin North Am 8:121, 1977
54. Pauly JE: An electromyographic analysis of certain movements and exercises. I. Some deep muscles of the back. Anat Rec 155:223, 1966
55. Andersson GBJ, Ortengren R, Herberts P: Quantitative electromyographic studies of back muscle activity related to posture and loading. Orthop Clin North Am 8:85, 1977
56. Schulz A, Andersson GBJ, Ortengren R et al: Analysis and quantitative myoelectric measurements of loads on the lumbar spine when holding weights in standing postrues. Spine 7:390, 1982
57. Kippers V, Parker AW: Posture related to myoelectric silence of erectores spinae during trunk flexion. Spine 7:740, 1984
57. Andersson GBJ: Loads on the lumbar spine: in vivo measurements and biomechanical analyses. p. 32. In Winter DA, Norman RW, Wells RP et al (eds): Biomechanics IX-B, International Series on Biomechanics. Human Kinetics, Champaign, IL, 1983
58. Ortengren R, Andersson GBJ, Nachemson AL: Studies of relationships between lumbar disc pressure, myoelectric back muscle activity, and intra-abdominal (intragastric) pressure. Spine 6:98, 1981
59. Andersson GBJ, Ortengren R, Nachemson A: Quantitative studies of the back in different working postures. Scand J Rehabil Med, suppl. 6:173, 1978
60. Andersson BJG, Ortengren R, Nachemson A, Elfstron G: Lumbar disc pressure and myoelectric activity during sitting. I. Studies on an experimental chair. Scand J Rehabil Med 6:104, 1974
61. Andersson BJG, Ortengren R, Nachemson A, Elfstrom G: Lumbar disc pressure and myoelectric back muscle activity during sitting. IV. Studies on a car driver's seat. Scand J Rehabil Med 6:128, 1974
62. Nachemson A: The load on lumbar disks in different positions of the body. Clin Orthop 45:107, 1966
63. Nachemson AL, Elfstron G: Intravital dynamic pressure measurements in lumbar discs. A study of common movements, maneuvers and exercises. Scand J Rehabil Med suppl. 1:1, 1970
64. Nachemson A, Morris JM: In vivo measurements of intradiscal pressure. J Bone Joint Surg 46:1077, 1964

65. Andersson GBJ, Ortengren R, Nachemson A: Quantitative studies of back loads in lifting. Spine 1:178, 1976
66. Bogduk N, Macintosh JE, Pearcy MJ: A universal model of the lumbar back muscles in the upright posture. Spine 17:897, 1992
67. Farfan HF: Muscular mechanism of the lumbar spine and the position of power and efficiency. Orthop Clin North Am 6:135, 1975
68. Farfan HF: A reorientation in the surgical approach to degenerative lumbar intervertebral joint disease. Orthop Clin North Am 8:9, 1977
69. Bartelink DL: The role of abdominal pressure in relieving the pressure on the lumbar intervertebral discs. J Bone Joint Surg 39B:718, 1957
70. Davis PR: Posture of the trunk during the lifting of weights. Br Med J 1:87, 1959
71. Davis PR: The use of intra-abdominal pressure in evaluating stresses on the lumbar spine. Spine 6:90, 1981
72. Davis PR, Stubbs DA: Safe levels of manual forces for young males. Appl Ergon 8:141, 1977
73. Davis PR, Troup JDG: Pressures in the trunk cavities when pulling, pushing and lifting. Ergonomics 7:465, 1964
74. Troup JDG: Dynamic factors in the analysis of stoop and crouch lifting methods: a methodological approach to the development of safe materials handling standards. Orthop Clin North Am 8:201, 1977
75. Troup JDG: Biomechanics of the vertebral column. Physiotherapy 65:238, 1979
76. Kumar S, Davis PR: Lumbar vertebral innervation and intra-abdominal pressure. J Anat 114:47, 1973
77. Granhed H, Johnson R, Hansson T: The loads on the lumbar spine during extreme weight lifting. Spine 12:146, 1987
78. Leskinen TPJ, Stalhammar HR, Kuorinka IAA, Troup JDG: Hip torque, lumbosacral compression, and intraabdominal pressure in lifting and lowering tasks. p. 55. In Winter DA, Norman RW, Wells RP et al (eds): Biomechanics IXB, International Series on Biomechanics. Human Kinetics, Champaign, IL 1983
79. Nachemson AL, Andersson GBJ, Schultz AB: Valsalva maneuver biomechanics. Effects on trunk load of elevated intraabdominal pressure. Spine 11:476, 1986
80. Hemborg B, Mortiz U: Intra-abdominal pressure and trunk muscle activity during lifting II: chronic low-back patients. Scand J Rehabil Med 17:5, 1985
81. Hemborg B, Moritz U, Hamberg J et al: Intra-abdominal pressure and trunk muscle activity during lifting—effect of abdominal muscle training in healthy subjects. Scand J Rehabil Med 15:183, 1983
82. Hemborg B, Moritz U, Hamberg J et al: Intra-abdominal pressure and trunk muscle activity during lifting III: effects of abdominal muscle training in chronic low-back patients. Scand J Rehabil Med 17:15, 1985
83. Farfan HF, Gracovetsky S: The abdominal mechanism. Paper presented at the International Society for the Study of the Lumbar Spine Meeting, Paris, May 16–20, 1981
84. Farfan HF, Gracovetsky S, Helleur C: The role of mathematical models in the assessment of task in the workplace. p. 38. In Winter DA, Norman RW, Wells RP et al (eds): Biomechanics IXB, International Series on Biomechanics. Human Kinetics, Champaign, IL, 1983
85. Gracovetsky S, Farfan HF, Helleur C: The abdominal mechanism. Spine 10:317, 1985
86. Bearn JG: The significance of the activity of the abdominal muscles in weight lifting. Acta Anat 45:83, 1961

87. Farfan HF: The biomechanical advantage of lordosis and hip extension for upright activity. Man as compared with other anthropoids. Spine 3:336, 1978

88. Gracovetsky S, Farfan HF, Lamy C: A mathematical model of the lumbar spine using an optimal system to control muscles and ligaments. Orthop Clin North Am 8:135, 1977

89. Macintosh JE, Bogduk N, Gracovetsky S: The biomechanics of the thoracolumbar fascia. Clin Biomech 2:78, 1987

90. McGill SM, Norman RW: Potential of lumbodorsal fascia forces to generate back extension moments during squat lifts. J Biomed Eng 10:312, 1988

91. Crock HV, Crock MC: A technique for decompression of the lumbar spinal canal. Neuro-orthopaedics 5:96, 1988

92. Bogduk N, Twomey LT: The lumbar muscles and their fascia. pp. 83–105. In: Clinical Anatomy of the Lumbar Spine. 2nd Ed. Churchill Livingstone, Melbourne, 1991

93. Mykelbust JB, Pintar F, Yoganandan N et al: Tensile strength of spinal ligaments. Spine 13:526, 1988

94. Cyron BM, Hutton WC: The tensile strength of the capsular ligaments of the apophyseal joints. J Anat 132:145, 1981

95. Hukins DWL, Aspden RM, Hickey DS: Thoracolumbar fascia can increase the efficiency of the erector spinae muscles. Clin Biomech 5:30, 1990

96. Aspden RM: Intra-abdominal pressure and its role in spinal mechanics. Clin Biomech 2:168, 1987

97. Aspden RM: The spine as an arch. A new mathematical model. Spine 14:266, 1989

98. Adams M: Letter to the editor. Spine 14:1272, 1989

# 5 | The Maitland Concept: Assessment, Examination, and Treatment by Passive Movement

*Geoffrey D. Maitland*

It would be difficult for me, as one who has been involved in the practice of manipulative physical therapy in Australia for the past four decades, to objectively assess my particular contribution to the discipline. I therefore begin this chapter, by way of explanation and justification, with a relevant and pertinent quotation from Lance Twomey, who asked me to write it.

> In my view, the Maitland approach to treatment differs from others, not in the mechanics of the technique, but rather in its approach to the patient and his particular problem. Your attention to detail in examination, treatment, and response is unique in physical therapy, and I believe is worth spelling out in some detail:
> The development of your concepts of assessment and treatment
> Your insistence on sound foundations of basic biologic knowledge
> The necessity for high levels of skill
> The evolution of the concepts: it did not "come" to you fully developed, but is a living thing, developing and extending
> The necessity for detailed examination and for the examination/treatment/re-examination approach

(This last area is well worth very considerable attention because, to me, it is the essence of "Maitland".)

Although the text of this chapter deals with "passive movement," it must be very clearly understood that I do not believe that passive movement is the only form of treatment that will alleviate neuromusculoskeletal disorders. What the chapter *does* set out to do is to provide a conceptual framework for treatment, which is considered by many to be unique. Thus, for want of a better expression, the particular approach to assessment, examination, and treatment outlined in this paper is described as "the Maitland concept," and referred to hereafter as "the concept."

To portray all aspects of the concept by the written word alone is difficult because so much of it depends on a particular clinical pattern of reasoning. The approach is methodical and involved, and therefore difficult to describe adequately without clinical demonstration. *The Maitland concept requires open-mindedness, mental agility, and mental discipline linked with a logical and methodical process of assessing cause and effect. The central theme demands a positive personal commitment (empathy) to understand what the person (patient) is enduring.* The key issues of the concept that require explanation are personal commitment, mode of thinking, techniques, examination, and assessment.

## PERSONAL COMMITMENT TO THE PATIENT

All clinicians would claim that they have a high level of personal commitment to every patient. True as that may be, many areas of physical therapy require that a deeper commitment to certain therapeutic concepts be developed than is usual. Thus the therapist must have a personal commitment to care, reassure, communicate, listen and believe, and inspire confidence.

All therapists must make a conscious effort (particularly during the first consultation), to gain the patient's confidence, trust, and relaxed comfort in what may be at first an anxious experience. The achievement of this trusting relationship requires many skills, but it is essential if proper *care* is to be provided.

Within the first few minutes, we clinicians must make the patient believe that we want to know what the patient feels; not what the doctor or anyone else feels, but what the patient feels is the main issue. This approach immediately puts patients at ease by showing that we are concerned about their symptoms and the effect they are having.

We must use the patient's terminology in our discussions; we must adapt our language (and jargon) to that of the patient. We must make our *concern* for the patient's symptoms show in a way that matches the patient's feelings about the symptoms. In other words, we should adapt our approach to match the patient's mode of expression, not make or expect the patient to adapt to our personality and our knowledge. The patient also needs to be *reassured* of the belief and understanding of the therapist.

*Communication* is another skill that clinicians must learn to use effectively and appropriately. As far as personal commitment is concerned, this involves understanding the nonverbal as well as the verbal aspects of communication, so that it can be used to further enhance the relationship between patient and clinician. Some people find that this is a very difficult skill to acquire, but however much effort is required to learn it, it must be learned and used.

*Listening* to the patient must be done in an open-minded and nonjudgmental manner. It is most important to accept the story the patient weaves, while at the same time being prepared to question it closely. Accepting and listening are very demanding skills, requiring a high level of objectivity.

It is a very sad thing to hear patients say that their doctor or physical therapist does not listen to them carefully enough or with enough sympathy, sensitivity, or attention to detail. The following quotation from *The Age,*[1] an Australian daily newspaper, sets out the demands of "listening" very clearly:

> Listening is itself, of course, an art: that is where it differs from merely hearing. Hearing is passive; listening is active. Hearing is involuntary; listening demands attention. Hearing is natural; listening is an acquired discipline.

Acceptance of the patient and his or her story is essential if trust between patient and clinician is to be established. We must accept and note the subtleties of the patient's comments about a disorder even if they may sound peculiar. Expressed in another way, the patient and his or her symptoms are "innocent until proven guilty" (i.e., the patient's report is true and reliable until found to be unreliable, biased or false). In this context, the patient needs to be guided to understand that the body can tell things about a disorder and its behavior that we (the clinicians) cannot know unless the patient expresses them. This relationship should inspire confidence and build up trust between both parties.

This central core of the concept of total commitment must begin at the outset of the first consultation and carry through to the end of the total treatment period.

Other important aspects of communication are discussed under Examination and Assessment.

## MODE OF THINKING: THE PRIMACY OF CLINICAL EVIDENCE

As qualified physical therapists, we have absorbed much scientific information and gained a great deal of clinical experience, both of which are essential for providing effective treatment. The "science" of our discipline enables us to make diagnoses and apply the appropriate "art" of our physical skill. However, the accepted theoretical basis of our profession is continually developing and changing. The gospel of yesterday becomes the heresy of tomorrow. It is essential that we remain open to new knowledge and open-minded in areas of uncertainty, so that inflexibility and tunnel vision do not result in a misapplication of our "art." Even with properly attested science applied in its right context, with precise information concerning the patient's history of disorder, symptoms, and signs, a correct diagnosis is often difficult. Matching of the clinical findings to particular theories of anatomic, biomechanical, and pathologic knowledge, so as to attach a particular "label" to the patient's condition, may not always be appropriate. Therapists must remain open-minded so that as treatment progresses, the patient is reassessed in relation to the evolution of the condition and the responses to treatment.

In summary, the scientific basis underlying the current range of diagnoses of disorders of the spine is incompletely understood. It is also changing rapidly with advances in knowledge and will continue to do so. In this context, the therapist may be sure of the clinical evidence from the patient's history and clinical signs, but should beware of the temptation to "fit the diagnosis" to the inflexible and incomplete list of options currently available. The physical therapist must remain open-minded, not only at the initial consultation, but also as noting the changing responses of the patient during assessment and treatment. When the therapist is working in a relatively "uncharted area" like human spinal disorders, one should not be influenced too much by the unreliable mass of inadequately understood biomechanics, symptomatology, and pathology.

This section, in essence, is the most important aspect of the concept that makes it different from that which others teach. It leaves one's mind totally open and not blocked by the theoretical compartment, the medical diagnostic titles, and the rigid philosophies of some manipulators (both medical and lay).

Consequently, I have drawn up a list of practical steps to follow. In the early era of its evolution, the Maitland concept had as its basis the following stages within a treatment:

1. Having assessed the effect of a patient's disorder, perform a single treatment technique
2. Take careful note of what happens during the performance of the technique
3. Having completed the technique, assess the effect of the technique on the patient's symptoms including movements
4. Having completed steps 2 and 3, and taken into account the available theoretical knowledge, plan the next treatment approach and repeat the cycle from step 1 again

**Table 5-1.** One Diagnosis with Many Presentations

| Theory | Clinical |
|---|---|
| Diagnosis: disc herniation | $H_1$ (history); $Sy_1$ (symptoms); $S_1$ (signs)<br>$H_2$; $Sy_2$; $S_3$<br>$H_3$; $Sy_3$; $S_3$<br>Etc. |

**Table 5-2.** Different Diagnoses for One Set of Symptoms and Signs

| Theory | Clinical |
|---|---|
| Diagnosis 1 | |
| Diagnosis 2 | H; Sy; S |
| Diagnosis 3 | |
| Diagnosis 4 | |

*Abbreviations:* H, history; Sy, symptoms; S, signs.

It becomes obvious that this sequence can only be useful and informative if both the clinical history taking and physical examinations have been accurate.

The actual pattern of the concept requires us to keep our thoughts in two separate but interdependent compartments: the *theoretical* framework and the *clinical* assessment. An example may help to clarify these concepts. We know that a lumbar intervertebral disc can herniate and cause pain, which can be referred into the leg. However, there are many presentations that can result from such a herniation (Table 5-1).

The reverse is also true: a patient may have one set of symptoms for which more than one diagnostic title can be applied[2] (Table 5-2).

Because of the circumstances shown in Tables 5-1 and 5-2, it is obvious that it is not always possible to have a precise diagnosis for every patient treated. The more accurate and complete our theoretical framework, the more appropriate will be our treatment. If the theoretical framework is faulty or deficient (as most are admitted to be), a full and accurate understanding of the patient's disorder may be impossible. The therapist's humility and open-mindedness are therefore essential, and inappropriate diagnostic labels must not be attached to a patient prematurely. The theoretical and clinical components must, however, influence one another. With this in mind, I have developed an approach separating theoretical knowledge from clinical information by what I have called the *symbolic, permeable brick wall* (Table 5-3). This serves to separate theory and practice, and to allow each to occupy (although not exclusively) its own compartment. That is, information from one side is able to filter through to the other side. In this way, theoretical concepts influence

**Table 5-3.** Symbolic, Permeable Brick Wall

| Theory | | | Clinical |
|---|---|---|---|
| Diagnosis | B | W | H; Sy; S |
| | R | A | |
| | I | L | |
| | C | L | |
| | K | | |

*Abbreviations:* H, history; Sy, symptoms; S, signs.

examination and treatment, while examination and treatment lead one back to a reconsideration of theoretical premises.

Using this mode of thinking, the brick-wall concept frees the clinician's mind from prejudice, allowing the therapist to ponder the possible reasons for a patient's disorder; to speculate, consider a hypothesis, and discuss with others the possibilities regarding other diagnoses without anyone really knowing all the answers, yet all having clear understanding of the patient's symptoms and related signs (Fig. 5-1).

This mode of thinking requires the use of accurate language, whereas inaccurate use of words betrays faulty logic. The way in which an individual makes a statement provides the listener with an idea both of the way that person is thinking and of the frame of reference for the statement.

A simple example may help to make this point clear. Imagine a clinician presenting a patient at a clinical seminar, and on request the patient demonstrates his area of pain. During the ensuing discussion, the clinician may refer to the patient's pain as "sacroiliac pain." This is a wrong choice of words. To be true to concept we have outlined, of keeping clinical information and theoretical interpretations separate, one should describe the pain simply as a "pain in the sacroiliac area." It would be an unjustified assumption to suggest that pathology in the sacroiliac joint was the source of pain, but the former description above could be interpreted in this way. On the other hand, describing the pain as "in the sacroiliac area" indicates that we are considering other possible sites of origin for the pain besides the sacroiliac joints, thereby keeping our diagnostic options open until we have more evidence. This is an essential element to the concept. Some readers may believe that attention to this kind of detail is unnecessary and pedantic. Quite the opposite is true. The correct and careful choice of words indicates a discipline of mind and an absence of prejudice, which influences all our diagnostic procedures including the whole process of examination, treatment, and interpretation of the patient's response.

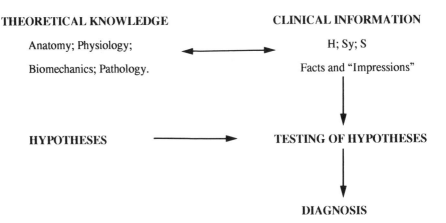

**Fig. 5-1.**    Flow chart demonstrating relationships and contexts for theoretical and clinical knowledge with related hypotheses. H, history; Sy, symptoms; S, signs.

A clinician's written record of a patient's examination and treatment findings also shows clearly whether the therapist's thinking processes are right or wrong. A genuine scientific approach involves logical thinking, vertical and lateral thinking, and inductive and deductive reasoning. It requires a mind that is uncluttered by confused and unproven theory, which is at the same time able to use proven facts, and has the critical ability to distinguish between well-attested facts and unsubstantiated opinions. It requires a mind that is honest, methodical, and self-critical. It also requires a mind that has the widest possible scope in the areas of improvisation and innovation.

## TECHNIQUES

### Therapy

Many physical therapy clinicians are continually seeking new techniques of joint mobilization. When they hear a new name or when a new author has written a book on manipulation, they attempt to acquire the "new" technical skills, and immediately apply them. In reality, the techniques are of secondary importance. Of course, if they are poorly performed or misapplied, treatment may fail and the therapist may lose confidence in the techniques. However, there are many acceptable techniques each of which can be modified to suit a patient's disorder and the clinician's style and physique. Accordingly, there is no absolute set of techniques that can belong or be attributed to any one person. There should be no limit to the selection of technique: the biomechanically based techniques of Kaltenborn; the "shift" techniques of McKenzie; the combined-movements technique of Edwards; the neural techniques of Elvey and Butler; the osteopathic and chiropractic technique; the Cyriax techniques; the Stoddard technique; the bonesetters' techniques; the Maigne techniques; and the Mennell techniques. All of these techniques are of the present era. Every experienced practitioner must feel totally free to make use of any of them. The most important consideration is that the technique chosen be appropriate to the particular patient or situation, and that its effect should be carefully and continually assessed.

### Management

Within the broad concept of this chapter, there are certain techniques of management that are continually used, but are not described by other authors. These techniques are as follows.

When treating patients having very painful disorders, passive-treatment movements can be used in an oscillatory fashion ("surface stirring" as described by Maitland[3]), but with two important provisos: (1) the oscillatory movement is performed without the patient experiencing any pain whatsoever, or even any discomfort; and (2) the movement is performed only in that part of the range of movement where there is no resistance (i.e., where there is no stiffness or muscle spasm restricting the oscillations).

One may question how a pain free oscillatory movement, which avoids every attempt to stretch structures, can produce any improvement in a patient's symptoms. A scientific answer to this question has been suggested[3] but there is a far more important clinical conclusion. It has been repeatedly shown clinically that such a technique does consistently produce a measurable improvement in range of movement with reduction in pain and disability and no demonstrable harmful effects. This demonstrates that the treatment is clinically, and therefore "scientifically," correct even though an adequate theoretical explanation for its effectiveness may not yet be available. Reliable and repeated demonstration of effectiveness must validate a treatment method. To know how the method achieves the result is a theoretical problem for science to solve. The "scientific" examination must match the primary clinical observation, the latter being the aspect of which we can be sure.

This example demonstrates once more how this mode of thinking, so essential to the concept, is so necessary for the further development of treatment methods. Without this mode of thinking we would never have found that passive-movement treatment procedures can successfully promote union in non-uniting fractures.[4,5]

Oscillatory movements as an important component of passive movement are referred to above in relation to the treatment of pain. There is another treatment procedure that requires oscillatory movement to be effective. This is related to the intermittent stretching of ligamentous and capsular structures. There are clearly defined areas of application for this treatment, which are described elsewhere.[3]

There are occasions when a passive treatment movement needs to be performed with the opposing joint surfaces compressed together.[6] Without the compression component, the technique would fail to produce any improvement in the patient's symptoms.

Using the movements and positions by which a patient is able to reproduce his symptoms as an initial mandatory test is essential to the concept. This tactic, like the formalized examination of combined movements (the original contribution in cooperation with Edwards[7]) is very special to the concept.

Although it is frequently recognized that straight-leg raising can be used as a treatment technique for low lumbar disorders, it is not widely appreciated that the technique can be made more effective by using straight-leg raising in the "slump test" position.[8] In the same slumped position, the neck flexion component of the position can be effectively used when such movement reproduces a patient's low back pain.

Sometimes a patient is able to guide the therapist as to what to do because his body tells him what it wants (and what it does not want). Figure 5-2 is a perfect example of such circumstances. The disorder had been very difficult to treat because progress gained at a treatment would not be retained well enough. The disorder was at the level of T6–T7 and had been responding to extremely gentle traction. Then one day the patient came in saying that he needed the traction but he also needed to have the vertebra pushed backward

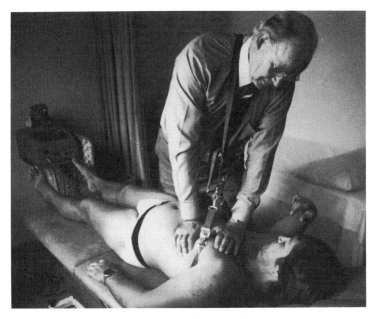

**Fig. 5-2.** Thoracic mobilization via the sternum.

and toward the left while having the levels above being twisted to the right. Figure 5-2 shows how the position was obtained while the mobilizing was produced through his sternum. He claimed he was 60 percent better after the first such treatment, and 80 percent better after the second. At his suggestion treatment was discontinued and on review 12 months later he showed no signs of slipping back.

"Accessory" movements produced by applying alternating pressure on palpable parts of the vertebrae are also very important in terms of techniques and the Maitland concept. Any treatment concept that does not include such techniques is missing a critical link essential to a full understanding of the effects of manipulation on patients with low lumbar disorders.

It is important to remember that there is no dogma or clear set of rules that can be applied to the selection and use of passive-movement techniques; the choice is open-ended. A technique is the brainchild of ingenuity. "The achievements are limited to the extent of one's lateral and logical thinking" (K. Hunkin, unpublished data, 1985).

## EXAMINATION

### History Taking

The care, precision, and scope of examination required by those using this concept are greater and more demanding than other clinical methods I have observed. The concept's demands differ from those of other methods in many respects.

The history taking and examination demand a total commitment to understanding what the patient is suffering and the effects of the pain and disability on the patient. Naturally, one is also continually attempting to understand the cause of the disorder (the theoretical compartment of the concept).

Examination must include a sensitive elucidation of the person's symptoms in relation to (1) precise area(s) indicated on the surface of the body; (2) the depth at which symptoms are experienced; (3) whether there is more than one site of pain, or whether multiple sites overlap or are separate; and (4) changes in the symptoms in response to movements or differences in joint positions in different regions of the body.

The next important and unique part of the examination is for the patient to re-enact the movement that best reveals the disorder or, if applicable, to re-enact the movement that produced the injury. The function or movement is then analyzed by breaking it into components in order to make clinical sense of particular joint-movement pain responses, which are applicable to the complaint.

The routine examination of physiologic movements is performed with a degree of precision rarely used by other practitioners. If the person's disorder is an "end-of-range" type of problem, the details of the movement examination required are as follows:

1. At which point in the range are the symptoms first experienced; how do they vary with continuation of the movement; and in what manner do the symptoms behave during the symptomatic range?

2. In the same way and with the same degree of precision, how does muscle spasm or resistance vary during the symptomatic range?

3. Finally, what is the relationship of the symptom to the resistance or spasm and during that same movement? There may be no relationship whatsoever, in which case the stiffness is relatively unimportant. However, if the behavior of the symptoms matches the behavior of the stiffness, both should improve in parallel during treatment.

An effective method of recording the findings of all components of a movement disorder is to depict them in a "movement diagram." These also are an innovative part of the concept. The use of movement diagrams facilitates demonstration of changes in the patient's condition in a more precise and objective manner. They are discussed at length in the fifth edition of *Vertebral Manipulation*.[9]

If the patient's disorder is a "pain through range" type of problem, the details of the movement examination required are as follows:

1. At what point in the range does discomfort or pain first increase?

2. How do the symptoms behave if movement is taken a short distance beyond the onset of discomfort? Does intensity markedly increase or is the area of referred pain extended?

3. Is the movement a normal physiologic movement in the available range

or is it protected by muscle spasm or stiffness? Opposing the abnormal movement and noting any change in the symptomatic response compared with entry
2 is performed to assess its relevance to the course of treatment.

## Palpatory Techniques

The accessory movements are tested by palpation techniques and seek the
same amount and type of information as described above. They are tested in
a variety of different joint positions. The three main positions are: (1) the neutral
mid-range position for each available movement (i.e., midway between flexion/
extension, rotation left and right, lateral flexion left and right, and distraction/
compression; (2) the joint in a "loose-packed position,"[10] at the particular position where the person's symptoms begin, or begin to increase; and (3) position
at the limits of the available range.

These palpatory techniques of examination and treatment have been peculiar to this concept from its beginnings. As well as seeking symptomatic responses to the movement as described above, the palpation is also used to
assess positional anomalies and soft-tissue abnormalities, which are at least as
critical to the concept as the movement tests.

The testing of physiologic and accessory movement can be combined in a
variety of ways in an endeavor to find the comparable movement sign most
closely related to the person's disorder. Edwards[11,12] originally described a
formal method of investigating symptomatic responses and treating appropriate
patients using "combined movement" techniques. In addition, joint surfaces
may be compressed, both as a prolonged, sustained firm pressure, and as an
adjunct to physiologic and accessory movement. These are two further examples of examination developed as part of the Maitland concept.

Differentiation tests are perfect examples of physical examination procedures that demonstrate the mode of thinking so basic to the Maitland concept.
When any group of movements reproduces symptoms, the concept requires a
logical and thoughtful analysis to establish which movement of which joint is
affected. The simplest example of this is passive supination of the hand and
forearm, which when held in a stretched position, reproduces the patient's
symptoms. The stages of this test are as follows:

1. Hold the fully supinated hand/forearm in the position that is known to
reproduce the pain.

2. Hold the hand stationary and pronate the distal radioulnar joint 2°
or 3°.

3. If the pain arises from the wrist, the pain will increase because in pronat-
ing the distal radioulnar joint, added supination stress is applied at the radiocar-
pal and midcarpal joints.

4. While in the position listed in stage 1, again hold the hand stationary,
but this time increase supination of the distal radioulnar joint. This decreases
the supination stretch at the wrist joints and will reduce any pain arising from

the wrist. However, if the distal radioulnar joint is the source of pain, the increased supination stretch will cause the pain to increase.

All types of differentiation tests require the same logically ordered procedure. These objective tests follow the same logic as the subjective modes of assessment described at the beginning of this chapter, and provide additional evidence leading to accurate diagnosis.

## ASSESSMENT

In the last few years it would appear that physical therapists have discovered a new "skill," with the lofty title of "problem solving." This is, and always should be, the key part of all physical therapy treatment. Being able to solve the diagnostic and therapeutic problems and thus relieve the patient of the complaint is just what physical therapists are trained to do. For many years, manipulative physical therapy has been rightly classified as empirical treatment. However, since manipulative physical therapists began to be more strongly involved in problem-solving skills, treatment has become less empirical and more logical. On the basis that the pathology remains unknown in the majority of cases and the effects of the treatment on the tissues (as opposed to symptoms) are unknown, the treatment remains empirical in form. This is true with almost all of the medical science. Nevertheless, the approach to the patient and to physical treatment has become more logical and scientific within the Maitland concept.

Minds existed before computers were developed, and manipulative therapists are trained to sort out and access "input" so that appropriate and logical "output" can be produced. Appropriate problem-solving logic will relate clinical findings to pathology and mechanical disorders. We have called this process of "sorting out" *assessment*. Assessment is the key to successful, appropriate, manipulative treatment, which, because of the reliability of its careful and logical approach, should lead to better treatment for our patients.

Assessment is used in six different situations: (1) analytical assessment at a first consultation; (2) pretreatment assessment; (3) reassessment during every treatment session proving the efficacy of a technique at a particular stage of treatment; (4) progressive assessment; (5) retrospective assessment; (6) final analytical assessment.

## Analytical Assessment

A first consultation requires skills in many areas, but the goals require decisions and judgments from the following five areas: (1) the diagnosis; (2) the phase of the disorder; (3) the degree of stability and irritability of the disorder at the time of treatment; (4) the presenting symptoms and signs; (5) the characteristics of the person.

The answers to the different assessment procedures (1 to 5) cannot be reliably determined without communication and an atmosphere of trust. By using one's own frame of reference, and endeavoring to understand the patient's frame of reference, the characteristics of the patient can be judged. By making use of nonverbal skills, picking out key words or phrases, knowing what type of information to listen for, and recognizing and using "immediate-automatic response" questions (all described later), accurate information can be gained at this first consultation. The physical examination is discussed in the Examination section.

## Pretreatment Assessment

At the beginning of each treatment session a specific kind of assessment is made of the effect of the previous session on the patient's disorder, its symptoms, and changes in movement. Since the first consultation includes both examination of movements and treatment of movements, the assessment at the second treatment session will not be as useful for therapy as it will be at the following treatment sessions.

When the patient attends subsequent treatment sessions, it is necessary to make both subjective and physical assessments (i.e., subjective in terms of how they feel; physical in terms of what changes can be found in quality and range of movement, and in related pain response). When dealing with the subjective side of assessment, it is important to seek spontaneous comment. It is wrong to ask, "How did it feel this morning when you got out of bed, compared with how it used to feel?" The start should be "How have you been?" or some such general question, allowing the patient to provide some information that seems most important to him. This information may be more valuable because of its spontaneous nature.

Another important aspect of the subjective assessment is that statements of fact made by a patient must always be converted to comparisons to previous statements. Having made the subjective assessment, the comparative statement should be the first item recorded on the patient's case notes. And it must be recorded as a *comparison-quotation* of his opinion of the effect of treatment. (The second record in the case notes is the comparative changes determined by the physical movement tests). To attain this subjective assessment, communication skills are of paramount importance. There are many components that make up the skill, but two are of particular importance:

1. *Key words or key phrases:* Having been asked the question, "How has it been?" a patient may respond in a very general and uninformative way. However, during his statements he may include, for example, the word *Monday*. Latch on to Monday, because Monday meant something to him. Find out what it was and use it. "What is it that happened on Monday? Why did you say Monday?"

2. *The immediate-automatic response:* A patient frequently says things

that demand an immediate-automatic response question. As a response to the opening question given above, the patient may respond by saying, "I am feeling better." The immediate-automatic response to that statement, even before he has had a chance to take a breath and say anything else, is "Better than what?" or "Better than when?" It may be that after treatment he was worse and that he is better than he was then, but that he is not better than he was before the treatment.

One aspect of the previous treatment is that it (often intentionally) provokes a degree of discomfort. This will produce soreness, but if the patient says he has more pain, the clinician needs to determine if it is treatment soreness or disorder soreness. For example, a patient may have pain radiating across his lower back and treatment involves pushing on his lumbar spine. He is asked to stand up and is asked, "How do you feel now compared with before I was pushing on your back?" He may say, "it feels pretty sore." He is then asked, "Where does it feel sore?" If he answers, "It's sore in the center," the clinician may consider that it is likely to be treatment soreness. But if he answers, "It's sore across my back," then the clinician may conclude that it is disorder soreness. If it were treatment soreness it would only be felt where the pressure had been applied. If the soreness spreads across his back, the treatment technique must have disturbed the disorder.

In making subjective assessments, a process is included of educating the patient in how to reflect. If a patient is a very good witness, the answers to questions are very clear, but if the patient is not a good witness, then subjective assessment becomes difficult. Patients should learn to understand what the clinician needs to know. At the end of the first consultation, patients need to be instructed in how important it is for them to take notice of any changes in their symptoms. They should report all changes, even ones they believe are trivial. The clinician should explain, "Nothing is too trivial. You can't tell me too much; if you leave out observations that you believe to be unimportant, this may cause me to make wrong treatment judgments." People need to be reassured that they are not complaining, they are informing. Under circumstances when a patient will not be seen for some days or if full and apparently trivial detail is needed, they should be asked to write down the details. The criticism that is made of asking patients to write things down is that they become hypochondriacs. This is a wrong assessment in my experience, because the exercise provides information that might otherwise never be obtained.

There are four specific times when changes in the patient's symptoms can indicate the effect of treatment. They are as follows:

1. *Immediately after treatment:* The question can be asked, "How did you feel when you walked out of here last time compared with when you walked in?" A patient can feel much improved immediately after treatment yet experience exacerbation of symptoms 1 or 2 hours later. Any improvement that does not last longer than 1 hour indicates that the effect of the treatment was only pallia-

tive. Improvement that lasts more than 4 hours indicates a change related to treatment.

2. *Four hours after treatment:* The time interval of 4 hours is an arbitrary time and could be any time from 3 to 6 hours. It is a "threshold" time interval beyond which any improvement or examination can be taken to indicate the success or failure of the treatment. Similarly, if a patient's syndrome is exacerbated by treatment, the patient will be aware of it at about this time.

3. *The evening of the treatment:* The evening of the day of treatment provides information in regard to how well any improvement from treatment has been sustained. Similarly, an exacerbation immediately following treatment may have further increased by evening. This is unfavorable. Conversely, if the exacerbation has decreased, it is then necessary to know whether it decreased to its pretreatment level or decreased to a level that was better than before that day's treatment. This would be a very favorable response, clearly showing that the treatment had alleviated the original disorder.

4. *On rising the next morning:* This is probably the most informative time of all for signaling a general improvement. A patient may have no noticeable change in his symptoms on the day or night of the treatment session, but may notice that on getting out of bed the next morning that the usual lower back stiffness and pain are less, or that they may pass more quickly than usual. Even at this time span, any changes can be attributed to treatment. However, changes that are noticed *during* the day after treatment, or on getting out of bed the second morning after treatment, are far less likely to be a result of treatment. Nevertheless, the patient should be questioned in depth to ascertain what reasons exist, other than treatment, to which the changes might be attributed.

Because accurate assessment is so vitally and closely related to treatment response, each treatment session must be organized in such a way that the assessments are not confused by changes in treatment. For example, if a patient has a disorder that is proving very difficult to treat, and at the eighth treatment session he reports that he feels there may have been some slight favorable change from the last treatment, the clinician has no alternative in planning the eighth treatment session. In the eighth treatment, that which was done at the seventh must be repeated in exactly the same manner in every respect. To do otherwise could render the assessment at the ninth treatment confusing. If the seventh treatment is repeated at the eighth session, there is nothing that the patient can say or demonstrate that can confuse the effect attributable to that treatment. If there was an improvement between the seventh and eighth treatment (and the eighth treatment was an identical repetition of the seventh treatment), yet no improvement between the eighth and the ninth treatment, the improvement between treatments seven and eight could not have been due to treatment.

There is another instance when the clinician must recognize that there can be no choice as to what the eighth treatment must be. If there had been no improvement with the first six treatments, and at the seventh treatment session a totally new technique was used, the patient may report at the eighth session that there had been a surprisingly marked improvement in symptoms. It may be that this unexpected improvement was due to treatment or it may have been due to some other unknown reason. There is only one way that the answer can be found—the treatment session should consist of no treatment techniques at all. Physical assessment may be made but no treatment techniques should be performed. At the ninth session, if the patient's symptoms have worsened considerably, the treatment cannot be implicated in the cause because none had been administered. The clinician can then repeat the seventh treatment and see if the dramatic improvement is achieved again. If it is, then the improvement is highly likely to have been due to that treatment.

Whatever is done at one treatment session is done in such a way that when the patient comes back the next time, the assessment cannot be confusing.

Another example of a different kind is that a patient may say at each treatment session that he is "the same," yet assessment of his movement signs indicates that they are improving in a satisfactory manner, and therefore that one would expect an improvement in his symptoms. To clarify this discrepancy, specific questions must be asked. It may be that he considers he is "the same" because his back is still just as stiff and painful on first getting out of bed in the morning as it was at the outset of treatment. The specific questioning may divulge that he now has no problems with sitting, and that he can now walk up and down the stairs at work without pain. Although his sitting, climbing, and descending stairs have improved, his symptoms on getting out of bed are the same, and this explains his statement of being "the same." The physical movement tests will have improved in parallel with his sitting and stair-climbing improvements.

## Assessment During Every Treatment Session

Proving the value or failure of a technique applied through a treatment session is imperative. Assessment (problem solving) should be part of all aspects of physical therapy. In this chapter it is related to passive movement. There are four kinds of assessment, and probably the one that most people think of first is the one in which the clinician is trying to prove the value of a technique that is being performed on a patient.

### Proving the Value of a Technique

Before even choosing the technique to be used it is necessary to know what symptoms the patient has and how his movements are affected in terms of both range and the pain response during the movement. Selection of a treatment technique depends partly on knowing what that technique should achieve while it is being performed. In other words, is it the aim to provoke discomfort and, if so, how much "hurt" is permissible? It is also necessary to have an expectation of what the technique should achieve after it has been performed.

With these considerations in mind, it is necessary to keep modifying the treatment technique until it achieves the expected goal during its performance. Assuming that this is achieved and that the technique has been performed for the necessary length of time, the patient is then asked to stand, during which time he is watched to see if there are any nuances that may provide a clue as to how his back is feeling. The first thing to ask him is, "How do you feel now compared with when you were standing there before the technique?" It is then necessary to clarify any doubts concerning the interpretation of what he says he is feeling. It is important to understand what the patient means to say if the subjective effect of the technique is to be determined usefully.

Having subjectively assessed the effect of the technique, it is then necessary to re-examine the major movements that were faulty, to compare them with their state before the technique. An important aspect of checking and rechecking the movements is that there may be more than one component to the patient's problems. For example, a patient may have back pain, hip pain, and vertebral-canal pain. Each of these may contribute to the symptoms in his lower leg. On reassessing him after a technique, it is necessary to assess at least one separate movement for *each* of the components, so it can be determined what the technique has achieved for each component. It is still necessary to check all of the components even if it is expected that a change will only be effected in one of the components. Having completed all of these comparison assessments, the effect of that technique at that particular stage of the disorder is now recorded in detail.

## Progressive Assessment

At each treatment session the symptoms and signs are assessed for changes for their relation to the previous treatment session and to "extracurricular" activities. At about each fourth treatment session a subjective assessment is made, comparing how the patient feels today with how he felt four treatments previously. The purpose of this progressive assessment is to clarify and confirm the treatment by assessment of the treatment response. One is often surprised by the patient's reply to a question, "How do you feel now compared with 10 days (i.e., four treatments) ago?" The goal is to keep the treatment-by-treatments assessment in the right perspective in relation to the patient's original disorder.

## Retrospective Assessment

The first kind of retrospective assessment is that made routinely at each group of three or four treatment sessions when the patient's symptoms and signs are compared with before treatment began, as described above.

A second kind of retrospective assessment is made toward the end of treatment when the considerations relate to a final assessment. This means that the clinician is determining (1) whether treatment should be continued; (2) whether spontaneous recovery is occurring; (3) whether other medical treatments or investigations are required; (4) whether medical components of the disorder are preventing full recovery; (5) what the patient's future in terms of prognosis is likely to be.

A third kind of retrospective assessment is made when the patient's disorder has not continued to improve over the last few treatment sessions. Under these circumstances, it is the subjective assessment that requires the greatest skill, and its findings are far more important than the assessment of the physical-movement tests. The clinician needs to know what specific information to look for. This is not a facetious remark, since it is the most common area where mistakes are made, thereby ruining any value in the assessment. The kinds of question the clinician should ask are as follows:

"During the whole time of treatment, is there anything I have done that has made you worse?"

"Of the things I have done to you, is there any one particular thing (or more) that you feel has helped you?"

"Does your body tell you anything about what it would like to have done to it to make it start improving?"

"My record of your treatment indicates that after the lumbar-traction treatment last Friday, you had a bad day Saturday, but that by Monday the pain had subsided and you thought you might have been better than you were before the traction. Looking back to that weekend now, do you feel that the traction did help you? Do you feel that if the traction had been gentler and of shorter duration that you might not have had the recurrence of symptoms, and that you might then have been more sure of the treatment's effect?"

"Do your symptoms tell you that it might be a good plan to stop treatment for say, 2 weeks, after which a further assessment and decision could be made?"

And so the probing interrogation continues until two or three positive answers emerge, which will guide the further measures that should be taken. The questions are the kind that involve the patient in making decisions, and that guide the clinician in making a final decision regarding treatment.

There is a fourth kind of retrospective assessment. If treatment is still producing improvement but its rate is less than anticipated, a good plan is to stop treatment for 2 weeks and to then reassess the situation. If the patient has improved over the 2-week period, it is necessary to know whether the improvement has been a day-to-day affair, thus indicating a degree of spontaneous improvement. If the improvement only occurred for the first 2 days after the last treatment, then it would seem that the last treatment session was of value and that three or four additional treatments should be given followed by another 2-week break and reassessment.

### Final Analytical Assessment

When treatment has achieved all it can, the clinician needs to make an assessment in relation to the possibility of recurrence, the effectiveness of any prophylactic measures, the suggestion of any medical measures that can be carried out, and finally an assessment of the percentage of remaining disability. The answers to these matters are to be found analyzing all the information derived from (1) the initial examination; (2) the behavior of the disorder throughout treatment; (3) the details derived from retrospective assessments; and (4) the state of affairs at the end of treatment, taking into account the subjective and physical changes.

This final analytical assessment is made easier as a clinician gains experience. It is necessary for this experience to be based on a self-critical approach and on analysis of the results, with the reasons for these results.

## CONCLUSIONS

The question has often been asked, "How did this method of treatment evolve?" The attributes necessary to succeed in this treatment method are an analytical, self-critical mind and a talent for improvisation.

With this as a basis, the next step is to learn to understand how a patient's disorder affects him. Coupled with this is the need to have sound reasons for trying a particular technique and then the patience to assess its effect. In the Maitland concept, this has developed over the years into a complex interrelated series of assessments:

Q: Why are painless techniques used to relieve pain?

A: Experience with patients who have had manipulative treatment elsewhere allows us to inquire as to which kind of technique was used and to observe its effect. When patients emphasize the extreme gentleness of some successful clinicians, one is forced to the conclusion that there must be ways of moving a joint extremely gently and thus improving patients' symptoms. Having accepted this fact (and that is not always easy), the obvious next step is to reproduce these techniques. For example, a technique one patient may describe can then be used on other patients who fit into the same kind of category. The clinician can learn what its possibilities are via the assessment process.

Q: Why, conversely, are some of the techniques quite vigorous and painful?

A: When treatment reaches a stage when nothing seems to help, a useful axiom is "Find the thing that hurts them, and hurt them." This should not be interpreted as being cruel to a patient, or that one is "out to hurt them," come what may. The hurting is a controlled progressive process with a strong emphasis on assessment. From using this kind of treatment on appropriate patients, it has become obvious that some disorders need to be pushed to the point of eliciting pain in order to aid recovery. This approach may be seriously questioned by some practitioners, but it can be a most useful technique in appropriate circumstances.

Q:   How did treating joints using strong compression of the joint surfaces come about?

A:   If, for example, a patient has shoulder symptoms, felt only when lying on it, and if normal examination methods reveal very little, then the thought processes go something like this:

"I believe him when he says he has a shoulder problem."

"There is nothing to indicate any serious or sinister disorder."

"He has not responded to other treatments."

"So it *must* be possible to find something on examination that relates to his problem."

"How can I find that something? What lead is there?"

"He says, 'I cannot lie on it.'"

"So I will ask him to lie on it and then move it around and see what happens."

By experiment with techniques (improvisation) until the patient's pain can be reproduced, and having found the thing that hurts him, treatment should then aim to hurt him in this *controlled* manner:

"As the patient doesn't move his shoulder around when he's asleep and lying on it, why is my examination using compression only, without movement, *not* painful?"

One would expect it to be painful!

"However, he has to lie on it for half an hour before pain forces him to change his position, so try compression again but make it stronger and sustain it longer." After half a minute or so of sustained maximum compression without movement his pain will certainly appear.

Q:   How did the slump test and treatment evolve?

A:   Some patients who have low back pain complain about difficulty getting into a car. By re-enacting the action and analyzing it, it is found that it was not the flexing of the lumbar spine that made getting into the car difficult; it was the head/neck flexion that provoked the low back symptoms. Examination using standard movement tests for structures between the head and the sacrum do not reveal anything; therefore, re-enact the particular movements and remember that the only structure connecting both areas must be in the vertebral column, most likely within the vertebral canal. To put these structures on stretch was the only method that *reproduced* the complaint. The maximum stretch position is the position now referred to as the slump position.

Q:   We now read of using mobilizing techniques to make a nonuniting fracture unite. How did this come about?

A:   In the past, traditional methods used to stimulate union have been (1) remove all support for the fracture site and allow the patient to take weight through the fracture, and (2) surgically explore the area and make both ends of the fracture site bleed, and then splint them in apposition again. If such things can promote union, then why not try passively moving the fracture site? Based on this reasoning and linking it with our axiom "find the thing that hurts and hurt them," it was found that it was possible to cause "fracture-site pain." This characteristic pain was found to have two other characteristics: (1) the pain stopped immediately when the treating movement was stopped, and (2) no side effects were provoked. This then meant that the treatment could be repeated, and in fact pain became harder to provoke (union took place).

## REFERENCES

1. *The Age.* p. 5. 21 August 1982
2. McNab I: Negative disc exploration: an analysis of the causes of nerve root involvement in 68 patients. J Bone Joint Surg 53A:891, 1971
3. Maitland GD: Passive movement techniques for intra-articular and periarticular disorders. Aust J Physiother 31:3, 1985
4. McNair JFS: Non-uniting fractures management by manual passive mobilization. Proceedings Manipulative Therapists' Association of Australia, p. 88, Brisbane, 1985
5. McNair JFS, Maitland GD: The role of passive mobilization in the treatment of a nonuniting fracture site—a case study. International Conference on Manipulative Therapy, Perth, 1983
6. Maitland GD: The hypothesis of adding compression when examining and treating synovial joints. Orthop Sports Phys Ther 2:7, 1980
7. Edwards BC: Combined movements of the lumbar spine: examination and clinical significance. Aust J Physiother 25:147, 1979
8. Maitland GD: Negative disc exploration: positive canal signs. Aust J Physiother 25: 6, 1979
9. Maitland GD: Vertebral manipulation. 5th Ed. Butterworths, London, 1986
10. MacConaill MA, Basmajian SV: Muscles and Movements. Waverly Press, Baltimore, 1969
11. Edwards BC: Movement patterns. International Conference on Manipulative Therapy, Manipulative Therapists' Association of Australia, Perth, 1983
12. Edwards BC: Manual of Combined Movements. Churchill Livingstone, London, 1992

# 6 | Mechanical Diagnosis and Therapy for Disorders of the Low Back

*Robin A. McKenzie*

In the first edition of this book,[1] I wrote, "Over the next few years, physical therapy will have the opportunity to become the key profession within medicine responsible for the delivery of conservative care for mechanical disorders of the spine. If appropriate steps are not taken now we may never again have another such opportunity."

Since 1987 the practice of physical therapy has changed little. Assessment methods and therapies are lamentably outdated. Time is running out. Chiropractors in the United States already see more patients with mechanical back pain than the combined total of patients seen by all other health providers. Scientific support for chiropractic is accumulating at a very creditable rate. Conversely, the scientific literature contains little to support the controlled use by physical therapists of such modalities as heat, cold,[2] laser therapy,[3] transcutaneous electrical stimulation,[4] infrared, short-wave diathermy, interferential therapy, or magnetic therapy.[5] Although Nwuga[6] found a benefit from the use of ultrasound in treating herniated discs, the experiment has not been successfully repeated by others.

On the other hand, Gnatz[7] documented case studies of two patients with disc herniation where paraspinal ultrasound following hot pack application caused severe increase in low back and radicular pain during application.

In the United States, legislative and scientific advances by chiropractors

171

suggest that physical therapists are falling further behind in the race for the patient's spine. Medical tolerance of chiropractors, if not actual support, is growing worldwide.[8] Since the study by Meade et al,[9] chiropractic is taking on a new and confident profile. Education of chiropractors is moving toward the traditional medical training model, and more medical professionals are involved in their education.

Physical therapists in general are not specially trained, nor are they skilled in the delivery of treatment for spinal disorders. Only those physical therapists with special training in mechanical procedures and manual techniques can expect to attain the skills necessary to compete successfully with chiropractors. Some institutions now provide postgraduate training in manual and manipulative techniques for physical therapists. Even so, doubts sometimes remain as to the level of expertise dispensed.

Although a myriad of techniques may be taught for each and every skeletal articulation, the indications for the use of such techniques are frequently based on findings derived from palpation of intersegmental motion or from radiologic screening. Neither palpation nor radiographs[5] are helpful in determining diagnosis in nonspecific mechanical low back pain. Failure to obtain consistent results with manual or manipulative procedures frequently drives manual therapists and chiropractors down the long road in the never ending search for the ultimate technique that surely must somewhere exist, and that must surely succeed when all else has failed.

A major obstacle to the attainment of excellence in the delivery of spinal therapy is the requirement that physical therapists become expert in the treatment of all musculoskeletal disorders. Such expertise is difficult if not impossible to acquire when spread so widely. Chiropractors, on the other hand, devote the greater part of their training solely to the study of knowledge related to spinal disorders and their treatment.

Perhaps the time has come for the political forces within the profession of physical therapy to make a stand and insist that only those with specialist skills and qualifications should be permitted to treat activity-related spinal disorders. It is now common for orthopedic surgeons to specialize in specific surgical techniques for specific anatomic regions. Thus there are surgeons specializing in hip replacements or knee replacements, as well as those devoting their entire skills to spinal surgery. If physical therapists are to compete in the current environments they must likewise establish soundly based specialties. Such specialists must have the ability to critically analyze the scientific literature. The evidence is there for all to see. Adopt scientifically valid methods of assessment and treatment or perish. Society will no longer permit the dispensation of useless treatment. Our treatment methods must be directed at improving the pathologic condition rather than modulating pain.

Increasingly, for the treatment of mechanical back disorders, the scientific literature is recommending that active care replace passive; that modalities are out; that exercise, activity, and movement are the means by which we are most likely to improve the health of injured spinal structures.

## PATHOLOGY

Modern medicine has advanced with such rapidity that it can be fairly stated that in the past 20 years we have learned more of the precise nature of the causes of spinal pain than in all of previous recorded history, and the search has narrowed to two structures likely to be involved in the production of most mechanical back pain.[5]

The intervertebral disc, with its strong annulus fibrosus retaining the gel-like nucleus, probably attracts the most attention.[10-17] Indeed, Mooney[18] has recently stated that, "In summary, what is the answer to the question of where is the pain coming from in the chronic low back pain patient? I believe its source ultimately, is in the disc."

The journal *Spine* has published the results of many studies aimed at the examination of intervertebral disc structure, function, pathology, and treatment. The other mobile structures to capture the attention of those investigating back pain are the zygapophyseal joints. These are also probable sources of pain, but the precise pathology causing the pain is unknown. The frequency of "facet" joint pain, however, has been challenged in two recent studies.[19,20]

Disorders of the sacroiliac joint occur without doubt, but most are inflammatory in origin. That true mechanical lesions occur is also recognized. They are, however, uncommon and usually only occur following pregnancy.[21] Physical therapists, especially in the United States,[22] or wherever therapists are receiving instruction from osteopaths, are "discovering" sacroiliac pathology in many of their patients. It is likely that either the proponents are wrong or the literature is in error.

The historical obsession of physical therapists with the musculature as the main source of backache has already been exposed.[23-25] Although orthopedic opinion does not support the proposal,[26] muscle imbalance as well as muscle strain are still considered by some physical therapists to be common causes of persistent back pain.

It appears now to be generally accepted within medicine that many low-back problems are mechanical in origin, probably arising in the intervertebral disc early in life and in the apophyseal joints much later in life.[27-30] Therefore, the treatment for these particular problems should mainly be mechanical. This fact has been recognized through 2500 years of recorded history,[31] and most treatments today given for the alleviation of back pain contain mechanical components.

Physical therapists have widely adopted (as occurred with the chiropractors and osteopaths) a system of "pathology" quite separate and contrary to that which exists within medicine as a whole, and orthopedics in particular. Medicine has always been able to exert control over and put pressure on its wayward practitioners in order to protect the public from outrageous claims and methods of treatment.

Is it not time to adopt those controls within physical therapy, especially when we see such fringe concepts as craniosacral technique and myofascial release techniques being taught without the slightest scientific evidence to support their consideration as tools for the treatment of spinal disorders? If we fail to curb the development of unscientific cultism, we deserve to lose what should be our rightful place within the medical team.

## MECHANICAL TREATMENT

By adopting active mechanical procedures for treating mechanical low back pain, physical therapists have much to gain. In the 1950s physiotherapists, especially in British Commonwealth countries, began incorporating manipulative procedures in their treatments. Prior to this, mechanical therapy within physiotherapy consisted of techniques of massage and exercise in which the proponents were particularly adept. Then along came spinal manipulative therapy (SMT), but there was no amalgamation between the exercise of physiotherapy and the manipulation of the osteopath and chiropractor. The conceptual model for the dispensing of exercise was completely different from the conceptual model for the use of manipulative therapy. There was no marriage between patient-generated and therapist-generated force. The two partners were incompatible.

Presently all over the world enthusiastic physiotherapists, frustrated and stifled by years of control by medicine or disillusioned by the use of ineffectual methods of physiotherapy, are "discovering" mobilization and manipulation and are delivering SMT as the treatment of choice for most patients with spinal pain. This initial enthusiasm, although understandable, must be tempered and brought into perspective. Those of us well experienced in the use of manipulative therapy still derive that unique satisfaction whenever a spectacular improvement is obtained. There is no doubt that many patients benefit from SMT. Several studies demonstrate that there is a short-term benefit obtained from SMT.[32–37]

A recent study[9] has found that a long-term benefit may be obtained from SMT administered by a chiropractor. The study has attracted much attention by chiropractors who obviously find much that is pleasing in the conclusions drawn. The study has many flaws however, which are elegantly described by Assendelft et al.[38] SMT nevertheless has a particular and important part to play in the treatment of spinal pain. Those in the profession who, due to long experience with SMT, are fully aware of the limitations as well as the benefits of this form of treatment, must utilize this experience to moderate the excesses that emerge from the overuse of manipulative techniques.

Until we have learned to distinguish between improvement that occurs directly as a result of treatment, and improvement that results from spontaneous healing or the natural history, our credibility is at risk. When our patients improve over a period of 3 to 4 months, can we seriously attribute their recovery to our manipulative or mechanical prowess applied over this period? Failure to recognize and understand the natural history and the self-limiting characteristics of the nonspecific spinal disorder will perpetuate the inability of so many to critically review their treatment methods and results.

Finally, we must be increasingly concerned that all currently prescribed mechanical treatments for mechanical spinal disorders create dependence on such therapies. Whenever we do something *to* or *for* the patient, the patient, and very often the therapist, attributes any improvement to the treatment dispensed. Ignorance or disregard of the natural history of mechanical back disorders allows all health providers to claim a success rate of over 90 percent!

In the future, because of the ever-rising cost of health care, society will demand that treatments for musculoskeletal disorders contain "self-treatment concepts" that will allow the patient future independence from therapy and therapists. If there is the slightest chance that patients can be educated in a method of treatment that enables them to reduce their own pain and disability using their own understanding and resources, they should receive that education. Every patient is entitled to this information, and every therapist should be obliged to provide it. It is appropriate at this point to quote directly from Nachemson[39]:

> In the therapeutic field today, it is virtually impossible to introduce a new drug without clinical and laboratory tests to prove its effectiveness and we are increasingly alert to and critical of different types of pharmacological side effects. The same approach should be used for the different forms of treatment of low back pain and we should critically re-assess our present methods.

## THE QUEBEC TASK FORCE REPORT

The findings and recommendations of the Quebec Task Force[5] (QTF) are important to all health providers involved with the diagnosis and treatment of mechanical spinal disorders.

Published in *Spine*, the Report of the Quebec Task Force on Activity Related Spinal Disorders was commissioned and funded by the Institute for Workers Health and Safety of Quebec, which was concerned about the increasing cost of treating spinal disorders, especially the cost of physical therapy. The problems of diagnosis are highlighted in some of the following excerpts.

> Pain is the primordial, and often the only, symptom of the vast majority of spinal disorders.
>
> Of the numerous pathologic conditions of the spine, nonspecific ailments of back pain in the lumbar, dorsal, and cervical regions, with or without radiation of pain, comprise the vast majority of problems found among workers (and the incidence in general populations can only be greater).

It is estimated that 85 percent of back pain episodes are nonspecific.[5] Thus only 15 percent of patients can be specifically diagnosed with our present technology and understanding.

Although there are considerably more clinical studies on patients suffering from problems of the lumbar area than there are on patients with problems in the cervical region, pain develops because of the irritation of structures sensitive to pain, and these are the same for all segments of the spine. These structures are bones, discs, joints, nerves, muscles and soft tissues.

It is difficult to identify precisely the origin of the pain, because even if its characteristics may sometimes point to a given structure, the pain often remains unspecific. In addition, it is generally impossible to corroborate clinical observations through histologic studies, because on one hand the usual benignity of spinal disorders does not justify that tissue be removed and on the other, there is often no modification of tissue identifiable through current methods.

Nachemson[39] confirms our dilemma: "With one exception, we are not yet in a position to positively identify precisely the structures involved in the production of common low back problems. The great majority of these problems are mechanical in origin but defy identification as to the structure involved or the nature of the fault."

In spite of the technological advances that have provided computed tomography (CT) scanning and magnetic resonance imaging (MRI), positive findings from these imaging techniques are found in large numbers of normal asymptomatic subjects.

In order to promote a better system of identification of spinal disorders, the QTF made several recommendations. It was felt that it would be helpful if all professions involved in the care of spinal disorders were able to better communicate with one another. The following recommendations were made with regard to the development of the ideal system of classification:

*Reliability:* A given case of a vertebral disorder shall be classified in the same manner by two or several practitioners.

*Clinical usefulness:* It will facilitate the making of clinical decisions as well as the evaluation of care.

*Simplicity:* Its use will be simple and will neither call for complete paraclinical examinations nor encourage superfluous investigations.

Using these criteria as a guide, the QTF has recommended the following categories be adopted by all health-related professions involved in the treatment of back pain:

1. Pain in the lumbar, dorsal, or cervical areas, without radiation below the gluteal fold or beyond the shoulder, respectively, and in the absence of neurologic signs

2. Pain in the lumbar dorsal, or cervical areas, with radiation proximally (i.e., to an upper or lower limb but not beyond the elbow or the knee, respectively) and not accompanied by neurologic signs

3. Pain in the lumbar, dorsal, or cervical areas, with radiation distally (i.e., beyond the knee or the elbow, respectively) but without neurologic signs

4. Pain in the lumbar, dorsal, or cervical areas, with radiation to a limb and with the presence of neurologic signs (e.g., focal muscular weakness, asymmetry of reflexes, sensory loss in a dermatome, or specific loss of intestinal, bladder, or sexual function)

"This category includes the radicular syndromes, which are well described in classic textbooks. These radicular syndromes may be due to various affections, the most frequent one being the discal hernia. However, other mechanical distortions of the spine may trigger an irritation or a radicular deficit."

The conditions described in the first four categories of the QTF represent 90 percent of activity-related low-back disorders. They also represent progressively complex pathologies. As the symptoms radiate further from the midline, a pathology evolves that is more likely to be resistant to simple treatment methods. Thus, category 1 is the least complex disorder and category 4, representing compression or interference of the conductivity of spinal nerves, is the most complex and potentially disabling entity.

In recommending the use of pain patterns to classify nonspecific mechanical disorders, the QTF attempts to avoid the perpetuation of meaningless diagnoses that are more likely to be wrong than right.

We may not know the precise nature of the injury or the exact location of the structure affected, but in simple terms, mechanical pain arises only from trauma (which will be of limited duration), internal derangement of the intervertebral disc (which may often appear as a recurring and episodic injury), or contracture or adaptive shortening, causing persistent pain long after repair is complete. A further cause of mechanical pain, and probably the most frequently encountered, is that arising from prolonged static loading in the absence of injury.

If we confine ourselves to the mechanical disorders of the back, there are relatively few atypical pathologies occurring in our daily patient caseload. Most problems can be related to either internal or external disruption and/or displacement of the interverbetral disc, or to damage and consequent repair of ligamentous or capsular periarticular soft tissues. Each disorder causes pain to behave in a typically characteristic fashion. Pain location and intensity can change, and the manner in which this occurs allows us to separate problems caused by internal disc displacement from problems arising from contractures and fibrosis. This is necessary because the former require different treatment than the latter.

## THE USE OF PAIN PATTERNS IN DIAGNOSIS AND THERAPY

The use of pain patterns to identify varying categories in the nonspecific spectrum of mechanical back pain, as contained in the QTF report, is also a key feature of the McKenzie classification of mechanical spinal disorders developed in the early 1960s.[40,41] Indeed, the McKenzie system of treatment originally evolved from an ability to systematically alter pain location by applying repeated movements, which caused pain to move from a distal to a central location. "Centralization of pain" is indicative of good outcome and is a prognostic sign in all patients with radiating or referred symptoms.[42]

By repeating movements that cause pain to move from a distal to a more proximal location, a QTF classification can be changed from a more to a less complex pathology. Expressed in another way, rapid nonsurgical treatment of referred and radiating symptoms is frequently possible using specifically customized end-range repeated movements that centralize pain. The McKenzie system provides a logical and compatible treatment protocol that fits well with the QTF recommendations. The McKenzie protocols are described elsewhere.[1,40–52]

## Mechanical Diagnosis

After 40 years of experience in treating mechanical disorders of the spine, I still consider it preferable that the patient's general practitioner or a specialist establish a differential diagnosis. Thus serious pathologies should be excluded from the patient population. Radiologic information eliminates most serious disorders and exposes architectural faults unsuitable for the mechanical approach.

There are many differing views regarding the best method of establishing a mechanical diagnosis. It is agreed almost universally that it is necessary to obtain detailed information from the patient by way of history, but there is often disagreement about the importance and relevance of much of this information. Some therapists attach much importance to one particular response, whereas others will consider the same response to be irrelevant.

Clinicians have a simple choice. If a large range of detailed information is to be gathered, much of it will be irrelevant or unreliable.[53] If clinicians are prepared to limit the information, then they will increase its reliability and relevance.

There are those, mainly osteopathically oriented, who decide the nature of the mechanical problem principally by palpatory means; some even claim to be able to determine by palpation alone the levels of existing pathology. However, intertherapist reliability using palpation alone has yet to be demonstrated.[54,55]

Chiropractors rely on a combination of diagnostic criteria, but mainly on information obtained from radiologic and palpatory findings. These have always been their main tools of diagnosis and remain so today. Their treatments, however, have expanded significantly as they have embraced more of orthodox medicine in recent years.

In the long run, the most appropriate mechanical procedure for any given condition will be identified from the patient's description of pain responses to the applied mechanical forces. If the implications of these responses are considered within the conceptual models described here, successful application of the McKenzie methods of treatment should follow.

My conclusions on completion of the evaluation process are based on the effects on pain resulting from the application of static and dynamic loading forces. Alteration in pain intensity and location following static loading in flexed or extended postures are correlated with pain responses obtained from repetitive end-range sagittal and frontal plane movements performed in loaded and unloaded positions.

Following the performance of these movements, a subdivision of patients within the nonspecific spectrum of back pain is possible.

## Subgroups in Nonspecific Low Back Pain

Three categories can be identified: postural, dysfunction, and derangement syndrome. Patients in the derangement group are by far the most frequently encountered. The precise means of identification and the concepts and methods of treatment of these syndromes are described in detail elsewhere.[40]

### Postural Syndrome

Patients with the postural syndrome are usually under 30 years of age, have sedentary occupations, and frequently are underexercised. As a result of prolonged end-range static loading, such as occurs in sitting and bending, they develop pain locally, adjacent to the midline of the spinal column. Such patients frequently complain of pain felt separately or simultaneously in the cervical, thoracic, and lumbar areas.

Pain from the postural syndrome is never induced by movement, rarely referred, and never constant. There is no pathology, no loss of movement, and symptoms are entirely subjective.[40]

### Dysfunction Syndrome

Pain in the dysfunction syndrome usually develops insidiously, appearing locally, adjacent to the midline of the spinal column, and is provoked on attempting full movement that deforms adaptively shortened or contracted soft tissues. Pain is always felt at end range and does not occur during the movement. With the exception of a patient with nerve-root adherence, pain from dysfunction is never referred.

Loss of movement in the dysfunction syndrome has two common causes. The most common cause of reduced spinal mobility is poor postural habits and lack of exercise. Poor postural habits allow adaptive shortening of certain structures. The result is a gradual reduction of mobility with aging. The movements reduced are usually those extension movements essential for the maintenance of the very erect posture.

The second cause of reduced spinal mobility is contracture of fibrous repair following trauma. Thus an inextensible scar forms within or adjacent to otherwise healthy structures, and will cause reduced mobility. The pain resulting from stretching of this inextensible scar appears only on attempting full end-range movements. The pain does not occur during the movement or before the scar is stretched. Surrounding healthy structures capable of further extensibility are restricted by the scar tissue itself. Thus the persisting pain results from the repair process itself.

It is not possible to identify the structure causing the pain of dysfunction, but any of the soft tissues adjacent to the vertebral column may adaptively shorten or may be damaged. Thus the pain may result from injury to any of the ligamentous structures in the segment from the intervertebral disc, the zyga-pophyseal joints, or the superficial or deep muscles or their attachments. The pain may also result from adherence of the spinal nerve root or dura following intervertebral disc prolapse or herniation. Described simply, the pain of dysfunction is produced immediately when stretching of shortened tissue occurs. Conversely, the pain ceases immediately when stretching ceases.[40]

### Derangement Syndrome

By far the most common cause of back pain, the derangement syndrome affects those between 20 and 55 years of age. Those affected develop pain, usually of sudden onset; that is, in a matter of a few hours or over a day or two they change from completely normal to significantly disabled beings. Very often this syndrome appears for no apparent reason. The symptoms may be felt locally, in the midline or adjacent to the spinal column, and may radiate or be referred distally in the form of pain, parasthesia, or numbness. The symptoms are produced or abolished, increased or reduced, may centralize or periph-eralize, or remain better or worse following the repetition of certain movements or the maintenance of certain positions.

Pain from the derangement syndrome may alter and change both in regard to the location of the pain, or the extent of the area affected, which may increase or decrease. Pain from the derangement syndrome may cross the midline, for example, and move from the right of the low back to the left.

Discogenic pathology should always be suspected when the patient describes that symptoms change location with repeated movements or prolonged positioning.

Change in the distribution or location of fluid nucleus or sequestrum within the intact annulus may in turn alter the location of pain according to the site of deformation.[56] Posterocentral bulging will cause central or bilateral pain, whereas posterolateral bulging will cause unilateral pain.[57,58]

Pain from the derangement syndrome will be constant as long as tissue within the intact annulus remains displaced. There may be no position in which the patient can find relief. The pain may be present whether movement is performed or not and this pain is usually described as an ache. That ache is then made worse by movement in certain directions and reduced by movement in other directions.

In the derangement syndrome, especially in severe cases, gross loss of movement may occur. Displaced tissue obstructs movement in the direction of the displacement. In severe cases the degree of displacement is such that postural deformities, such as kyphosis and scoliosis, are forced. Sudden loss of spinal mobility and the sudden appearance of postural deformity in acute low back and neck pain may be likened to the sudden locking that may occur in the knee joint where internal derangement of the meniscus is common.

The mechanism of internal derangement of the intervertebral disc is not fully understood. That the nucleus pulposus can be displaced toward and escape through a damaged annular wall is inarguable.[59,60] It is highly likely that this will follow as a consequence of sudden or violent movement, or with sustained postures in younger patients. Older patients have a stiffer, less fluid nucleus,[61] which is less likely to be displaced from within its annular envelope.[59,60,62] It is also hypothesized that prior to a frank annular lesion with nuclear herniation, there exists incomplete tears into which nuclear material may be displaced. This alters the joint biomechanics and may be responsible for the postural deformities (e.g., localized scoliosis) observed.

Creep of the fluid nucleus/annulus complex will disturb the normal alignment of adjacent vertebrae[63] and change the resting shape of the disc.[62] This change of shape will also affect the ability of the joint surface to move in its normal pathway[63] and movement deviation to the right or left of the sagittal plane will result on attempting flexion or extension.

Described simply, the pain of derangement occurs as a consequence of a change in disc shape with related misalignment of the mobile segment and its associated abnormal stresses.[40]

Identification of the different syndromes is based on the effects that repeated movements have on the initiation of the pain: the point in the movement pathway where pain is first perceived; the site of the pain and subsequent change of location of the pain; the increasing or decreasing intensity of the pain; and finally abolition of the pain. Mechanical pain can arise from a limited number of events or combination of events causing force to be applied to innervated soft tissues. Those soft tissues may be in a normal state, a contracted state, or in an anatomically altered state with a change in the shape of the disc. Any of these events can be identified by the response of the patient's pain to the deliberate application of certain mechanical stresses.

Patients with inflammatory disorders, with spondylolisthesis or other undetected minor fracture, and with pathologies unsuited to mechanical therapies will behave atypically and be quickly exposed and recognized when tested in the manner I have described.

## MECHANICAL THERAPY

### Postural Syndrome

Normal tissues can become painful in everyday life by the application of prolonged stresses commonly appearing during static postural loading conditions, such as prolonged sitting, standing, or bending.

Correction of faulty postural habits removes inappropriate causative stresses. No other treatment is required. In order to remove the cause of pain, the therapist must educate the patient.

## Dysfunction Syndrome

Shortened structures cause limited movement and simultaneously cause pain when the shortened structure is stretched.

Treatment would include remodeling short structures by the regular application of stretching exercises. Dysfunction is not rapidly reversible; weeks are required to remodel and lengthen. Structures that have adaptively shortened over weeks and months cannot suddenly lengthen by the application of high velocity thrusts without incurring damage. Regular end-range exercise must be considered as the most likely therapy to influence shortened structures. It remains to be seen whether exercise (REPEX, repeated end-range passive exercise) therapy or manual mobilization is superior in regards to the recovery of function by remodeling.

## Derangement Syndrome

An example of derangement syndrome is frank tears of the annulus fibrosus with nuclear displacement or annular bulging. The patient experiences aching without movement, increased pain with movement in certain directions as displacement increases, and reduced pain in other directions as displacement decreases.

This syndrome is subject to mostly rapid reversal. The use of patient self-treatment methods using repeated end-range movement has been successful in the reduction of derangement within the lower lumbar segments. The rate of reduction of derangement can be accelerated significantly in a large number of cases with the use of REPEX associated with appropriate self-treatment protocols; maintaining reduction by correcting posture and avoiding wrong positions; restoring function before adaptive changes are established; and teaching prevention of recurrence and self-treatment. Mobilization and SMT now become important and may be required if self-treatment provides insufficient reductive pressures.

Mechanical forces used to treat mechanical disorders of the low back should be applied in a graduated form, first using patient self-treatment repeated movements, progressing through mobilization, and finally the application of manipulative procedures.

The time to apply our special techniques of mobilization and manipulation arrives when the patient, having exhausted all possibilities of self-treatment, requires an increase in the degree of pressure in the appropriate direction; that direction, having already been determined during exercise, allows mobilizing procedures to commence. Failing improvement with the use of mobilization, then and only then is manipulation indicated. Thus the gradual development of increasing force to bring about change is a logical and safe method of applying mechanical therapies, assuming that vertebral and vascular pathology are excluded. The ultimate weapon we have is the manipulative thrust technique. Why use that weapon on day 1 when it may well be that the patient without being approached by the therapist is capable of causing the change himself (and learning an important self-management lesson)?

I have, therefore, proposed since that time that we should postpone or avoid mobilization and manipulation until we have determined that resolution of the problem is impossible using the patient's own positions and movements. This concept offers up to 70 percent of people referred to physical therapists with mechanical low back pain the opportunity to treat and manage their own problem and thus become independent of therapists.[46,64]

The remaining 30 percent, including patients categorized by myself as having derangement 4 or 6 and therefore unable to apply self-treatment procedures with lasting benefit, will always require the special skills of the manipulative therapist for correction of any lumbar or sciatic list.[40–65] Others will require techniques in the form of mobilization and some of those will additionally require manipulative thrust procedures.

This is not to suggest that mobilization and manipulation are no longer required in our armamentarium. Spinal manipulative therapy has a particular and important part to play in the treatment of mechanical spinal pain but its dispensation is greatly misused. I am proposing that the time has come when we must rationalize the use of such methods. We are now able to determine within at least 48 hours from commencement of assessment whether manipulative therapy will be necessary at all. It should no longer be ethical to apply the technique in order to find out retrospectively if the procedure was indicated. Spinal mobilization and manipulation should not be dispensed to the entire population with back pain in order to ensure that the very few who really need it actually receive it.

When all mechanical therapies fail to improve the patient's condition, and modulation of pain is considered necessary, physical therapists must ask whether modulating pain with physical therapy "gadgetry" is better for the patient and society as a whole than dispensation of rather inexpensive medication.

## LITERATURE REVIEW

As reported by the Quebec Task Force, the literature is sadly lacking in well-controlled, randomized studies evaluating the various treatments for low back and neck pain. Studies of the McKenzie approach were absent at the time of that report but are now beginning to appear. The McKenzie system is in use worldwide and is the subject of increasing scrutiny.[42–45,50–52,66–82]

Many clinical studies have been completed, and many more are required. The system lends itself to research because the conceptual models of pathology established to identify subgroups in the nonspecific spectrum of back pain relate to the common pathologic processes well described in the literature and encountered daily in orthopedic clinics.

It has now been demonstrated that several different patient populations can be taught to manage their own back problems using self-applied movement as described here and elsewhere. Studies by McKenzie,[64] Ponte et al,[68] Nwuga and Nwuga,[69] Kopp et al,[70] DiMaggio and Mooney,[43] Williams et al,[71] Donelson et al,[42] Alexander et al,[72] Stankovic,[73] Spratt et al,[74] Roberts,[75] and McKinney,[76] have all demonstrated the benefits of this approach to the assessment and treatment of mechanical spinal disorders.

Three studies (Ponte et al,[68] Nwuga and Nwuga,[69] and Elnaggar et al[77]) have compared the use of Williams' flexion exercises with McKenzie treatment in small patient populations. All patients were acute, but patients in one study (Nwuga and Nwuga[69]) all had confirmed disc lesions by myelogram and with reflex changes. Both studies demonstrated a significant difference in favor of the McKenzie approach in terms of the rate of decreasing the pain, restoration of full range of motion, increasing straight-leg-raising comfort, and increasing sitting comfort. The average number of treatment sessions was also significantly lower with the McKenzie approach than with the approach of Williams. Of course, Williams' approach typically has little or no assessment portion but treats all patients essentially the same. The McKenzie system, however, defines the treatment on the basis of the patient's individualized mechanical needs identified by monitoring pain behavior during the assessment.

One of these studies (Nwuga and Nwuga[69]) followed patients for 2 months and noted a clear reduction in the number of recurrences after the McKenzie method. This would seem to reflect the ability of these patients to prevent further problems, thus defeating the high incidence of recurrences.

Elnaggar[77] compared flexion with extension exercises and not surprisingly found no difference in the outcomes between the two groups. By inference, the authors attempted to relate their results to a lack of effectiveness of the McKenzie protocols. The authors were generally unaware of the requirements of the McKenzie treatment methods and incorrectly related the extension exercises used in their study to those described in the McKenzie protocol.

In a randomized, blind study comparing the use of McKenzie with two other treatments (back school and 90/90 traction), 97 percent of the patients treated with McKenzie had improved after 1 week, whereas less than 50 percent improved with either of the other two treatments.[78] The results of both of the latter treatments were similar to, or lower than, what might be expected with no treatment at all. The study attrition rate after the first week of treatment invalidated further conclusions, but the first week's results were felt to be valid.

In a Swedish study[73] the McKenzie system was compared to a mini-back school program in treating acute low back pain in a working population. The McKenzie-treated workers had a median sick leave of 10 days versus 17.5 days in the comparison group and a mean sick-listing for recurrences the first year of 27 days versus 40 days with mini-back school. Only 45 percent of the McKenzie-treated workers had first year relapses versus 80 percent of the comparison group. The average number of McKenzie treatments during the acute episode was only 5.5. It would appear that the McKenzie patients resolved their acute episode and disability faster, were better able to prevent recurrences, and were able to minimize disability when symptoms did recur.

Donelson et al[42] have found that centralization of pain is a reliable predictor of outcome in treating low back and referred pain. In applying repeated sagittal movement testing according to the McKenzie protocols, they found that patients consistently demonstrated a directional preference, the majority centralizing or reducing pain with extension movements. Conversely flexion was found to increase pain.[42]

In a further study on centralization of pain, Donelson et al[79] found that a similar directional preference was shown in a majority of patients tested in the frontal plane, most experiencing centralization or reduction of symptoms when laterally flexing toward the painful side.

Williams[71] found that the adoption of extended lumbar sitting postures reduced or centralized pain in patients with nonspecific low back and referred pain. The effects were most marked in those with leg symptoms. Flexed postures, on the other hand, showed no similar reduction in pain intensity or location change.

Roberts[75] compared McKenzie treatment with nonsteroidal antiinflammatory drug therapy. His patients were recruited prospectively and were treated within 3 weeks of onset of an attack of low back pain. Both groups of patients were encouraged to mobilize actively. Rest, after the first 2 days, was discouraged.

The major measure of outcome was a widely used disability questionnaire. At 7 weeks after onset of the attack, the McKenzie-treated patients were less disabled compared with the drug treatment patients. This difference became significant when those McKenzie patients who could not be diagnosed according to McKenzie's classification at *the time of first assessment* by the physiotherapist were excluded. This suggests that if a definite diagnosis cannot be made on initial assessment the result will be less certain, and that more experienced practitioners will have greater success when treating groups of patients, because correct assessment seems to be a key part of treatment.[75]

The patients in the McKenzie group who had not recovered after six treatments were found to represent a very difficult group to treat—at least by the physiotherapists involved in the study.[75] This limit of six treatments matches the experience of Rath et al[80] in America and Stankovic and Johnell[73] in Scandinavia.

Patients who received McKenzie therapy were, however, away from work for longer than the drug patients and it is suggested that a directive to return to work from the physiotherapist is an important element to the regimen.[75]

Careful psychological assessment was performed on all patients in connection with their personal responsibility for pain control. Patients undergoing McKenzie therapy were significantly more responsible for personal pain control than the drug treatment patients 7 weeks after the onset of the low back pain.

This responsibility alteration was still significantly different when measured 6 months later. McKenzie therapy alters the way patients think about pain.[75]

The mechanism of centralization was examined in detail, and again those patients who could be diagnosed on their first attendance with the physiotherapist showed better responses than the patients whose syndrome was unclear. Scores of pain intensity matched a score for peripheralization with a very significant degree of correlation.[75]

In 1986 Kopp et al[70] reported that of 67 patients with herniated nucleus pulposus (HNP) treated with the McKenzie extension protocol, 35 patients were able to achieve normal lumbar extension within 3 days of admission to the hospital. The remaining 32 patients all required surgery and of these only two were able to achieve extension before surgery. All 67 had failed 6 weeks of conservative treatment prior to being treated by the McKenzie protocol. Kopp and co-workers concluded that the ability of patients with HNP and radiculopathy to achieve full passive lumbar extension is a useful predictor to select patients who can be expected to respond favorably to conservative management. They further reported that the inability to achieve extension (positive extension sign) is an early predictor of the need for surgical intervention, and recommended extension exercises as a therapeutic modality.

In 1990 Alexander et al[72] reported on a followup of the patients in the Kopp study. It was found that after an average of almost 6 years from onset, 33 of the 35 patients who did not require surgery were satisfied with the result and 82 percent had been able to resume their old jobs. At long-term followup, Alexander and co-workers found that a negative extension sign was confirmed as a predictor of a favorable response to nonoperative treatment of HNP in 91 percent of the nonsurgical group in Kopp's study.

Only one study has assessed the long-term value of this treatment approach for mechanical problems in the cervical spine.[76] In a single-blind randomized prospective study, McKinney[76] found that advice to exercise and correct posture in the early phase after injury was superior to outpatient physiotherapy consisting of hot and cold applications, pulsed short-wave diathermy, hydrotherapy, traction, and active and passive repetitive movements. At 2-year followup fewer patients in the exercise group had persisting symptoms. McKinney suggests that the reason for the superior results in the exercise group is that patients given responsibility for their own treatment may become self-sufficient at managing episodes of a minor nature, and there may be psychological advantages in making patients responsible for their own treatment rather than victims of their own symptoms.

Riddle[81] studied a much abbreviated version of the McKenzie system of assessment for low back pain and found the system to have low intertherapist reliability. The therapists used in the Riddle study, unfortunately, did not receive training in the McKenzie protocol, even to a minimum level of competency.

The procedures described in the McKenzie protocol are relatively uncomplicated and safe when applied by persons with the appropriate training. Recently, however, cauda equina lesions have been reported following inappropriate application of the McKenzie protocols by untrained persons.[83] This reinforces the need for adequate training and qualifications for those therapists wishing to claim competence in the use of the McKenzie system.

## REPEATED END-RANGE PASSIVE EXERCISE

Specific customized exercises for individual patient needs can be identified and successfully delivered for self-treatment of low back pain. There are, however, limitations to the system in some cases, usually involving patient fatigue and lack of compliance.

Ideally, to obtain the best results, patient self-treatment exercises should be applied 10 to 15 repetitions every 2 hours. A total number of 80 to 100 end-range movements per day can be achieved with this formula. Most patients with acute and subacute low back pain experience reduction or centralization of pain following the practice of customized self-treatment exercises. They remain better and rapidly and progressively improve with practice. Even so, there remain some whose pain reduces or centralizes for a short period only, and who do not progressively improve daily.

Several possibilities account for lack of response to repeated movements. It can be that the patients condition is irreversible using mechanical therapy. This is not always clear at the first evaluation. It could be the wrong mechanical diagnosis. For instance, the patient may have dysfunction but has been classi-fied as having derangement syndrome. This can be confirmed by reassessing and applying alternative testing procedures.

Lack of response to self-treatment exercises could also indicate that al-though the chosen direction of movement is correct, the frequency, force, or degree of motion applied is inadequate. Would the application of large numbers of cycles to end range accelerate the recovery in such resistant cases?

To enable this question to be answered, a continuous passive motion device has been developed that enables unlimited cycles of progressive end-range exer-cise to be applied to the lumbar spine. REPEX (Howard Wright Ltd, New Plymouth, New Zealand) has now been well trialed clinically at four McKenzie Institute Clinics in New Zealand. With the advent of REPEX, a new concept and dimension in the treatment of spinal therapy has emerged. Findings thus far indicate that REPEX is as effective as the McKenzie exercise protocols in resolving certain mechanical disorders of the lower back, and is superior to exercise in certain other categories (Fig. 6-1).

REPEX enables fine incremental progressions to be made in the applied range of flexion or extension. The equipment delivers 10 cycles/min of end-range motion, which in the case of patients with the derangement syndrome is progressively increased as reduction of the derangement is achieved. Differen-tiation between dysfunction and derangement is imperative and such differentia-tion must be made *prior* to the application of REPEX. The patient should be assessed and the nature of the derangement determined using the McKenzie assessment protocol.

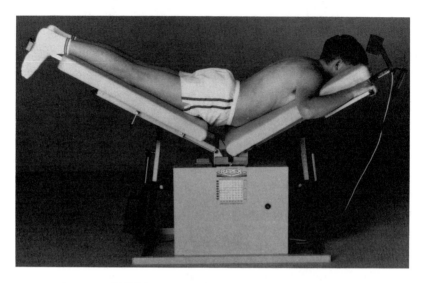

**Fig. 6-1.** REPEX: repeated end-range passive movements.

## REPEX in Acute and Subacute Low Back Pain

Clinical experience indicates that in patients with acute and subacute low back pain, use of REPEX accelerates the rate of recovery significantly. Centralization, reduction, or abolition of symptoms is achieved in one treatment session more frequently and at a faster rate when using REPEX than is possible using patient self-treatment methods alone.

With the use of REPEX it is possible to achieve centralization, reduction, or abolition of pain in cases where patient-generated exercises carried out over several days have failed to produce change. We believe it is also significant that the frequency of application of spinal manipulative thrust techniques by staff at the McKenzie Institute clinics has further reduced since the advent of REPEX.

REPEX has the ability to rapidly reduce derangement even when movement is significantly obstructed, such as occurs in patients fixed in flexion with acute lumbago. Prior to the advent of REPEX, curve reversal from kyphosis to lordosis in this acute disorder was achieved slowly over a period of time using careful positioning and mild-range movement as behavior of pain allowed. With the correct use of REPEX, it is now possible in most cases to restore full movement within 20 to 30 minutes.

A most significant finding from the use of REPEX is the total absence of beneficial effect on pain or range of motion when patient motion is limited to repetition in midrange. Only when applied progressively to end range does pain reduce and motion improve.

## REPEX and Remodeling

The aim of treatment for patients with the dysfunction syndrome is to remodel contracted or adherent tissue to a functional length, thus restoring mobility to the greatest extent possible considering the nature of the injury.[21,27,84] Clinical experience to date suggests that the remodeling process may be significantly accelerated with REPEX.

The fine control of REPEX and the unlimited number of delivery cycles provide a remodeling process previously unobtainable by patient self-generated exercises.

It is important that spinal segments restricted by contracture or fibrosis are not overstretched. REPEX has the capacity to overstretch, and treatment of dysfunction should be progressed slowly in comparison to the rapid progressions applied to patients with the derangement syndrome.

Never before has a therapy been available that applies unlimited cycles of end-range movement to the lumbar spine. *REPEX is a potent tool for the alleviation of pain and the recovery of function in mechanical spinal disorders. As such it also has the potential to cause harm if used improperly.*

## REHABILITATION FOR CHRONIC LOW BACK PAIN

The McKenzie Institute International established a residential spinal therapy and rehabilitation center in 1990 for the treatment of chronic and recurrent mechanical spinal disorders. In light of our experience to date, we believe that the definition of chronic low back pain should be amended to specifically exclude those patients who experience recurrent episodic low back pain. Large numbers of patients in this category are inappropriately classified as having chronic low back pain.

Low back pain chronicity implies that those affected suffer more or less continuous pain, and have few if any, pain-free periods. The view is also widely held that these patients must learn to live with their problem and the chances for recovery are remote. The diagnosis of chronicity implies a hopelessness that creates and perpetuates both physical and mental distress.

We have found that a majority of patients referred to the rehabilitation center, perhaps as many as 60 percent, do not have *continuous* low back pain as such. Instead, they suffer recurring episodes so frequently that the impression is given that pain is continuous. In reality there may be some days or even weeks when no pain is experienced. Because their symptoms are so frequent, patients state that their symptoms are "always present." Thus, instead of receiving appropriate treatment for recurring internal derangement (which requires education in self-reduction procedures), the patient is referred to a chronic pain center.

Management strategies for patients with recurrent episodic low back pain must take into account the rapid reversibility of derangement pathologies, and must include education in procedures of self-reduction and self-treatment. Once identified and treated appropriately, many of these patients are able to resume normal activities and manage their own problem. Only those patients with truly long-standing and unremitting symptoms should be placed in the chronic category.

It does not seem appropriate to insist that patients with recurrent derangement should be forced to undergo work-hardening programs and "work through the pain." No health provider would force such activity on a patient with an internally deranged cartilage within the knee!

Some centers treating chronic pain patients advise reduction of activity levels by either cutting out activity entirely, or restricting motion by attempting to stabilize segments of the spine during activity. The consequences of such advice create in the patient's mind the idea that activities and movement are harmful. Unfortunately, this advice is all too frequently adhered to; chronic back pain patients afraid of moving lose mobility, and soft tissues contract, joints stiffen, and the muscles weaken. Thus, with progressive deterioration of the spinal musculoskeletal system, segments above the affected area become stiff and painful with neck and thoracic symptoms developing long after the onset of low back pain.

For patients with chronic low back symptoms who experience truly constant pain and who have contractures or fibrosis causing loss of function and movement, we have developed a treatment and rehabilitation program in which REPEX is a prime factor in the remodeling process, the recovery of mobility, and reduction of internal derangement. Rehabilitation following REPEX consists of self-treatment procedures to maintain mobility and instill prophylactic principles, and gymnasium and general exercise programs to provide functional and physical reactivation.

Preliminary findings from an ongoing study by Williams[82] show significant benefits for patients with chronic low back pain.

Williams studied patients with chronic (> 3 months) mechanical spinal pain who were off work and had been on earnings-related compensation for 3 months or longer and who were referred to the center by general practitioners throughout New Zealand. Patients initially completed a battery of questionnaires collecting data relating to demographics, clinical history, pain, functional status (Dallas Pain Questionnaire), depression (Zung), somatic perceptions (Modified Somatic Perceptions Questionnaire), fear avoidance beliefs (Fear Avoidance Beliefs Questionnaire), and pain locus of control (modified Multidimensional Health Locus of Control). Physical examination followed assessment of spinal mobility, straight-leg raise, neurologic deficit, and signs and symptoms of nonorganic illness. Patients were then assessed according to the standard McKenzie protocol including repeated end-range spinal movements and static loading tests to determine the direction of therapeutic spinal movement and appropriate resting positions. Patients were prescribed individualized exercise programs involving patient-generated repeated end-range passive exercise and repeated end-range passive exercise on REPEX equipment. Patients also undertook active strengthening exercises and reactivation. Individualized home exercise and gymnasium programs were prescribed for self-management following discharge. Patients were reassessed at exit and followups undertaken at 3 months and 1 year.

Of 79 patients referred to the center, 15 were excluded, 64 entered the program, and 3 dropped out. Patients entering had a mean age of 37 years, a mean current episode duration of 3.1 years, and had been off work an average of 1.9 years. At discharge, 62 percent reported a "marked improvement" or better in their pain level, and overall the group yielded a median value of 70 percent relief on a pain relief analog scale. At entry, the numbers of patients reporting most distal pain location as the leg, the thigh, or the low back were 35, 16, and 10, respectively. At discharge the corresponding values were 21, 15, and 25 ($P < 0.001$). Pre- and posttreatment mean values for pain impact on the Dallas Pain Questionnaire were 57 and 33 percent, respectively ($P < 0.001$) with each of the four subscales yielding significant changes ($P < 0.001$). Significant improvements in spinal mobility (21 percent, $P < 0.001$) and straight-leg raise ($P < 0.001$) were also obtained. At entry, 7 patients were classified as "normal," 33 as "risk," and 21 as "distressed" according to the Distress and Risk Assessment Method. Corresponding figures at discharge were 28, 22, and 11. Patients exhibited significant mean reductions in fears regarding the effect of activity on their pain ($P < 0.001$), a decreased chance locus of pain control ($P < 0.01$), and an increased internal locus of pain control ($P < 0.001$).

Williams concluded that although the uncontrolled nature of this study precluded conclusions as to the cause(s) of these changes, the length of time these patients had had their symptoms and been off work suggested their conditions were likely to have reached relatively stable states. Although other causes could not be ruled out, the marked changes in pain location and intensity, function, and psychological status over the 2-week period were consistent with McKenzie's claim that repeated end-range spinal movements were able to rapidly reverse underlying pathology. Follow-up assessments were being undertaken to determine the stability of these findings.

## CONCLUSIONS

The McKenzie approach to the diagnosis of spinal pain is often misunderstood. It does not treat all patients with extension as though it were the opposite of Williams' flexion exercises. It is also a much more complex discipline to carry out than this brief description can convey.

The McKenzie system is based primarily on pain and its behavior, as well as the presence of acute spinal deformity, as the only direct links we have with the unknown underlying pathology. Meanwhile, the large majority of acute and chronic patients can be effectively treated and recurrences can be prevented or quickly resolved simply by monitoring the pain and its behavior during a comprehensive mechanical assessment that identifies and uses self-treatment principles to the fullest extent for a wide range of patients.

To impact the low-back population and its high cost to our society, we cannot remain content with letting patients spontaneously recover as we dispense unproven, passive modalities while at the same time claiming credit. We also cannot justify performing invasive injection procedures, prescribing medications and bed rest, or applying manual therapy to a population of patients who can effectively treat themselves.

The success of the McKenzie system is dependent on the training and expertise of the physician and therapist especially. Typically, 2 years of clinical experience with assessment and treatment of mechanical spinal disorders, coupled with appropriate education and certification, is a minimum requirement for effective education in this method.

Progressive repeated end-range passive exercise offers an exciting tool for the treatment of low back pain in the future. Much research is required to validate its value and identify its most useful role. Early findings, however, and my own experience allow me to speculate that this "device" will alter the course of conservative therapy of the lower back. Only time will tell.

## REFERENCES

1. McKenzie RA: Mechanical diagnosis and therapy for low back pain: toward a better understanding. p. 157. In Twomey LT, Taylor JR (eds): Clinics in Physical Therapy. Physical Therapy of the Low Back. Churchill Livingstone, New York, 1987
2. Landen BR: Heat and cold for the relief of low back pain? Phys Ther 47:1126, 1967
3. Klein RG, Eek BC: Low energy laser and exercise for chronic low back pain: double-blind controlled trial. Arch Phys Med Rehabil 71:34, 1990
4. Deyo RA, Walsh N, Martin D et al: A controlled trial of transcutaneous electronic nerve stimulation (TENS) and exercise for chronic low back pain. N Engl J Med 322:1627, 1990
5. Spitzer WO, LeBlanc FE, Dupuis M et al: Scientific approach to the assessment and management of activity-related spinal disorders. A monograph for clinicians. Report of the Quebec Task Force on spinal disorders. Spine 12:75, 1987
6. Nwuga VCB: Ultrasound in treatment of back pain resulting from prolapsed intervertebral disc. Arch Phys Med Rehabil 64:88, 1989
7. Gnatz SM: Increased radicular pain due to therapeutic ultrasound applied to the back. Arch Phys Med Rehabil 70:493, 1989
8. Nachemson A: Clin Orthop Relat Res 279:8, 1992
9. Meade TW, Dyer S, Browne W et al: Low back pain of mechanical origin: randomised comparison of chiropractic and hospital outpatient treatment. Br Med J 300: 1431, 1990
10. Vanharanta H, Sachs BL, Spivey MA et al: The relationship of pain provocation to lumbar disc deterioration as seen by CT/discography study. Spine 12:295, 1987
11. Vanharanta H, Guyer RD, Ohnmeiss DD et al: Disc deterioration in low back syndromes: a prospective, multicenter CT/discography study. Spine 13:1345, 1988
12. Zucherman J, Derby R, Hsu K et al: Normal magnetic resonance imaging with abnormal discography. Spine 13:1355, 1988
13. Kornberg M: Discography and magnetic resonance imaging in the diagnosis of lumbar disc disruption. Spine 14:1368, 1989
14. Butler D, Trafimow JH, Anderson GBJ et al: Discs degenerate before facets. Spine 15:111, 1990

15. Kuslich SD, Ulstrom RN, Michael CJ: The tissue origin of low back pain and sciatica: a report of pain response to tissue stimulation during operations on the lumbar spine using local anesthesia. Orthop Clin North Am 22:181, 1991
16. Smyth MJ, Wright V: Sciatica and the intervertebral disc. An experimental study. J Bone Joint Surg 40A:1401, 1958
17. Hirsch C: The anatomical basis for low back pain. Acta Orthop Scand 33:1, 1963
18. Mooney V: University of Arizona Symposium on Back Pain: The present and the future, Tucson, Arizona, March 11–14, 1992
19. Jackson RP, Jacobs RR, Montesano PX: 1988 Volvo Award in Clinical Sciences. Facet joint injection in low-back pain. A prospective statistical study. Spine 13:966, 1988
20. Luilius G, Laasoner EM, Myllynen P et al: Lumbar facet joint syndrome. A randomized clinical trial. J Bone Joint Surg 77B:1108, 1989
21. Dixon A: Diagnosis of low back pain. In Jayson M (ed): The Lumbar Spine and Back Pain. Pitman Medical, Tunbridge Wells, England, 1980
22. Potter NA, Rothstein JM: Intertester reliability for selected clinical tests of the sacroiliac joint. Phys Ther 65:1671, 1985
23. Cyriax J: Textbook of Orthopaedic Medicine. 5th Ed. Vol. 1. Baillière Tindall, London, 1980
24. Bogduk N: The causes of low back pain. Med J Aust 156:151, 1992
25. Bogduk N: The sources of low back pain. In Jayson MIV (ed): The Lumbar Spine and Back Pain. 4th Ed. Churchill Livingstone, Edinburgh, 1992
26. Suzuki N, Seiichi E: A quantitative study of trunk muscle strength and fatigability in the low back pain syndrome. Spine 8:1, 1983
27. Twomey L, Taylor J: Age changes in the lumbar intervertebral discs. Acta Orthop Scand 56:496, 1985
28. Coventry MB, Ghormley RK, Kernohan JW: The intervertebral disc: part II. Changes in the intervertebral disc concomitant with age. J Bone Joint Surg 27:233, 1945
29. Coventry MB, Ghormley RK, Kernohan JW: The intervertebral disc: part III. Pathological changes in the intervertebral disc. J Bone Joint Surg 27:460, 1945
30. Vernon-Roberts B: The pathology and interrelation of intervertebral disc lesions. In Jayson M (ed): The Lumbar Spine and Back Pain. 2nd Ed. Pitman Medical, Tunbridge Wells, England, 1980
31. Schiotz EH, Cyriax J: Manipulation past and present. Heinemann, London, 1975
32. Brunarski DJ: Clinical trials of spinal manipulation. J Manip Phys Ther 7:4, 1984
33. Doran DML, Newell DJ: Manipulation in treatment of low back pain: a multicenter study. Br Med J 2:161, 1975
34. Farrell JB, Twomey LT: Acute low back pain. Comparison of two conservative treatment approaches. p. 162. Proceedings of Manipulative Therapists Association of Australia, Perth, Western Australia, 1983
35. Hadler NM, Curtis P, Gillings DB, Stinnett S: A benefit of spinal manipulation as adjunctive therapy for acute low back pain: a stratified, controlled trial. Spine 12: 7, 1987
36. Hoehler FK, Tobis JS, Buerger AA: Spinal manipulation for low back pain. JAMA 245:1835, 1981
37. Sims-Williams H, Jayson MIV, Young SMS: Controlled trial of mobilisation and manipulation for patients with low back pain in general practice. Br Med J 2:1338, 1978
38. Assendelft WJJ, Bouter LM, Kessels AGH: Effectiveness of chiropractic and phys-

iotherapy in the treatment of low back pain: a critical discussion of the British randomized clinical trial. J Manip Phys Ther 14:281, 1991

39. Nachemson A: Conservative treatment of low back pain. In Jayson M (ed): The Lumbar Spine and Back Pain. 2nd Ed. Pitman Medical, Tunbridge Wells, England, 1980

40. McKenzie RA: The Lumbar Spine. Mechanical Diagnosis and Therapy. Spinal Publications Limited, Waikanae, New Zealand, 1981

41. McKenzie RA: The Cervical and Thoracic Spine. Mechanical Diagnosis and Therapy. 1st Ed. Spinal Publications (N.Z.) Limited, Waikanae, New Zealand, 1990

42. Donelson R, Murphy K, Silva G: Centralization phenomenon: its usefulness in evaluating and treating referred pain. Spine 15:3, 1990

43. DiMaggio A, Mooney V: Conservative care for low back pain; what works? J Musculoskel Med 4:27, 1987

44. DiMaggio A, Mooney V: The McKenzie program: exercise effective against back pain. J Musculoskel Med 4:63, 1987

45. Van Wijmen PM: Lumbar pain syndromes. p. 442. In Grieve GP (ed): Modern manual therapy of the vertebral column. Churchill Livingstone, New York, 1986

46. McKenzie RA: Treat Your Own Back. Spinal Publications, Lower Hutt, New Zealand, 1981

47. McKenzie RA: Treat Your Own Neck. Spinal Publications, Lower Hutt, New Zealand, 1983

48. McKenzie RA: A physical therapy perspective on acute spinal disorders. p. 211. In Mayer TG, Mooney V, and Gatchel RJ (eds): Contemporary Conservative Care for Painful Spinal Disorders: Concepts, Diagnosis and Treatment. Lea & Febiger, Malvern, PA, 1991

49. Stevens BJ, McKenzie RA: Mechanical diagnosis and self treatment of the cervical spine. In Grant R (ed): Physical Therapy of the Cervical and Thoracic Spine. Churchill Livingstone, New York, 1988

50. Donelson R: The McKenzie approach to evaluating and treating low back pain. Orthop Rev XIX:681, 1990

51. Donelson RG, McKenzie R: Mechanical assessment and treatment of spinal pain. p. 1627. In Frymoyer JW (edf): The Adult Spine: Principles and Practice. Vol. 2. Raven Press, New York, 1991

52. Donelson RG: Identifying appropriate exercises for your low back pain patient. J Musculoskel Med 8:14, 1991

53. Nelson MA, Allen P, Clamp S et al: Reliability and reproducibility of clinical findings in low-back pain. Spine 4:2, 1979

54. Matyas TA, Bach TM: The reliability of selected techniques in clinical arthrometrics. Aust J Physiother 31:175, 1985

55. Gonnella C, Paris S, Kutner M: Reliability in evaluating passive intervertebral motion. Phys Ther 62:437, 1982

56. Shepperd JAN: Patterns of internal disc dynamics, cadaver motion studies. Video presented at the International Society for the Study of the Lumbar Spine Meeting, Boston, June 13–14, 1990

57. Cloward RB: Cervical diskography: a contribution to the etiology and mechanism of neck, shoulder and arm pain. Ann Surg 150:1052, 1959

58. Murphey F: Sources and patterns of pain in disc disease. Clin Neurosurg 15:343, 1968

59. Adams MA, Hutton WC: Prolapsed intervertebral disc: a hyperflexion injury. Spine 7:3, 1982

60. Adams MA, Hutton WC: Gradual disc prolapse. Spine 10:6, 1985
61. Taylor JR, Twomey LT: The lumbar spine from infancy to old age. p. 1. In Twomey LT and Taylor JR (eds): Clinics in Physical Therapy. Physical Therapy of the Low Back. Churchill Livingstone, New York, 1987
62. Farfan HF: Mechanical Disorders of the Low Back. Lea & Febiger, Philadelphia, 1973
63. Panjabi M, Krag MH, Chung TQ: Effects of disc injury on mechanical behaviour of the human spine. Spine 9:7, 1984
64. McKenzie RA: Prophylaxis in recurrent low back pain. NZ Med J 89:627, 1979
65. McKenzie RA: Manual correction of sciatic scoliosis. NZ Med J 76:484, 1972
66. Cherkin D: Pilot randomized trials of physical and educational interventions for low back pain. p. 2. BOAT Newsletter. Vol. 2. University of Washington, Seattle, Washington, June 1992
67. The Backletter 7:7, 1992, Skol Publishing, Madison, New Hampshire
68. Ponte DJ, Jensen GJ, Kent BE: A preliminary report on the use of the McKenzie protocol versus Williams protocol in the treatment of low back pain. J Orthop Sports Phys Ther 6:130, 1984
69. Nwuga G, Nwuga V: Relative therapeutic efficacy of the Williams and McKenzie protocols in back pain management. Physiother Pract 1:99, 1985
70. Kopp JR, Alexander AH, Turocy RH et al: The use of lumbar extension in the evaluation and treatment of patients with acute herniated nucleus pulposus. A preliminary report. Clin Orthop 202:211, 1986
71. Williams MM, Hawley JA, McKenzie RA, Van Wijmen PM: A comparison of the effects of two sitting postures on back and referred pain. Spine 16:1185, 1991
72. Alexander AH, Jones AM, Rosenbaum Jr DH: Nonoperative management of herniated nucleus pulposus: patient selection by the extension sign—long term follow-up. Presented to North American Spine Society Annual Meeting, Monterey, California, August 8–11, 1990
73. Stankovic R, Johnell O: Conservative treatment of acute low-back pain. A prospective randomized trial: McKenzie method of treatment versus patient education in "Mini Back School." Spine 15:2, 1990
74. Spratt KF, Lehmann TR, Weinstein JN, Sayre HA: A new approach to the low-back physical examination. Behavioral assessment of mechanical signs. Spine 15: 2, 1990
75. Roberts AP: The conservative treatment of low back pain. Thesis, Nottingham, 1990
76. McKinney LA: Early mobilisation and outcome in acute sprains of the neck. Br Med J 299:1006, 1989
77. Elnaggar IM, Nordin M, Sheikhzadeh A et al: Effects of spinal flexion and extension exercises on low-back pain and spinal mobility in chronic mechanical low-back pain patients. Spine 16:967, 1991
78. Vanharanta H, Videman T, Mooney V: Comparison of McKenzie exercises, back trac and back school in lumbar syndrome; preliminary results. Annual Meeting of International Society for the Study of the Lumbar Spine, Dallas, Texas, May 28–June 9, 1986
79. Donelson RG, Grant WD, Kamps C, Medcalf R: Low back and referred pain response to mechanical lumbar movements in the frontal plane. Presented at International Society for the Study of the Lumbar Spine Meeting, Heidelberg, May 12–16, 1991
80. Rath WW, Rath JND, Duffy CG: A comparison of pain location and duration with

treatment outcome and frequency. Presented at First International McKenzie Conference, Newport Beach, California, July 20–21, 1989

81. Riddle DL, Rothstein JM: Intertester reliability of McKenzie's classifications of the syndrome types present in patients with low back pain. Spine 18:1333, 1993

82. Williams M, Grant R: Effects of a McKenzie spinal therapy and rehabilitation programme: preliminary findings (abstract). Presented at The Society for Back Pain Research, Annual Scientific Meeting, London, October 30, 1992

83. Anderson J, Boumphrey F, Bell G: Early decompression in cauda equina syndrome. Presented at the International Society for the Study of the Lumbar Spine Meeting, Chicago, May 20–24, 1992

84. McIlwain WA: A technique for improving results of soft tissue repair in low back patients utilising the LPM 100. 1991 (in press)

# 7 | Clinical Assessment: The Use of Combined Movements in Assessment and Treatment

*Brian C. Edwards*

The physical examination of the lumbar spine requires a high degree of skill combined with a thorough knowledge of structure and function, particularly when the treatment to be prescribed is manipulative therapy. This is because very close attention needs to be paid to the way in which the patient's signs and symptoms react to relatively small changes in posture and movement. If movement is the preferred method of treatment, the more precise the information on the reaction of signs and symptoms to movement the more specific and effective the passive movement (manipulative procedure) will be.

However, it is important to expand the usual orthopedic examination by including movements that will highlight signs and symptoms that might normally be masked. This involves combining movements, which will increase or decrease the stretch and compressive effects on structures associated with the joint (e.g., the capsule, ligaments, and muscle attachments). This enables the therapist to establish movement patterns that assist not only in the choice of the movement techniques to be used but also in the progression of treatment and prognosis.

## HISTORY TAKING AND SUBJECTIVE EXAMINATION

A standard orthopedic examination of the lumbar spine initially involves history taking. At the outset an accurate account of the symptoms and their distribution must be obtained. This can be achieved in a number of ways. The patient can be given a simple body chart (Fig. 7-1) and asked to draw in the areas of pain or discomfort. However, such a method usually requires the therapist to repeat the examination in more detail, which can be very time consuming. A useful compromise is to ask the patient to map out on the body chart using one finger the areas of paresthesia and anesthesia, including a description of the type and depth of pain. In the case of the lumbar spine particularly, specific questions need to be asked related to perineal anesthesia or paresthesia alteration in micturition or bowel habit (particularly if associated with severe pain) and the responses require careful assessment. Care must be taken at this point to explain to the patient that it is important and necessary to describe the symptoms experienced at the time of assessment. If the distribution of symptoms has changed, the change can be superimposed on the same diagram or a separate diagram can be used. This is an important aspect of the examination since a clear understanding of those symptoms that are currently experienced as compared to those originally experienced can have an important bearing on both the diagnosis of the condition and selection of the treatment techniques.

Once descriptions of the symptoms and their distribution have been established, the patient should be questioned about how symptoms in different areas

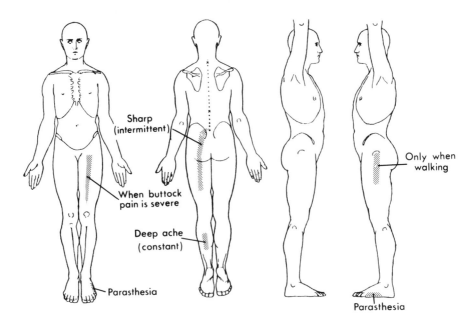

**Fig. 7-1.**  A body chart used to show distribution of symptoms in a patient.

are related to each other (e.g., has there been an increase in pain in one area with a corresponding change in another area? In what sequence did the symptoms originally appear?). Such questioning is often omitted in history taking. However, the answers provided by the patient highlight and implicate the anatomic structures likely to be affected, which may be the cause of the patient's symptoms. They can also help in identifying the level of involvement of referred symptoms when it comes to the objective examination.

The constancy of a patient's symptoms and the variability in the intensity of pain are also important aspects of the history taking and must be established. Following this, activities that cause any change in symptoms should be noted (i.e., the ease with which symptoms are aggravated; the activities that cause this aggravation; the relation between the type of activity and the duration and intensity of the symptoms produced, sometimes called irritability). These are often a useful guide to the amount of physical examination or treatment that may be carried out on the first day.

Activities that aggravate, relieve, or do not affect the symptoms need to be carefully described and analyzed in relation to the anatomy and biomechanics of the vertebral column, and to the distribution of the patient's symptoms. The simple activity of digging in the garden may be performed quite differently by two patients.

Once aggravating and easing factors have been identified, it is useful to evaluate which particular combined movements are being performed during the activity. This is especially important in the case of a patient with a severe or irritable condition, when it is important to identify a pain-easing position. If sitting, standing, or lying positions aggravate or relieve the symptoms, this should be carefully noted. Particular attention should be paid to the positions adopted by the patient at the time of examination and treatment.

## 24-Hour Variation

The history of present and past attacks of low back pain in terms of the type of activity responsible (if any) and the mode of onset of the symptoms needs to be clearly described by the patient and noted by the physical therapist. The onset of the symptoms is frequently related to and may have resulted from a particular incident or activity. However, it is not unusual for patients to have difficulty in remembering the particular incident, as they may regard it as trivial or it may have occurred some time before the onset of the symptoms.[1]

The need for accurate questioning and skill in the interpretation of answers cannot be overemphasized. It is essential to have this information as a sound base before proceeding to the next step of the objective examination. The interpretation of the subjective examination also requires considerable patience and skill on the part of the therapist.

# OBJECTIVE EXAMINATION OF THE LUMBAR SPINE

## Definition

The term *objective examination* is something of a misnomer. Objectivity in its pure form is difficult to achieve when the physical therapist includes in such examination not only movements but also the patient's description of the symptoms reproduced by the movements. The objective examination therefore contains some elements that are subjective in the sense that patient response requires interpretation by the therapist. It is important that reference is constantly made to the specific areas of pain and the symptoms for which the patient has come seeking treatment. It must be emphasized that attention to small details of a patient's answers and to individual movements is essential if the objective examination is to help identify particular structures as likely sources of the patient's symptoms.

The principal aim of the objective examination is to establish the effect of movement of the lumbar spine on those symptoms that have already been described by the patient. In doing this the identification of the muscles, joints, and ligaments involved in the patient's disorder is of primary importance. Careful observation of the way the vertebral column moves areas of hyper- and hypomobility, and areas of relative muscle hypertrophy or atrophy are assessed.

## Observation

The first part of the examination consists of observation. Three important aspects of observation are general movement, posture and shape of joints, and gait.

### General Movement

Observation of the care with which a patient moves while adopting the sitting position or moves out of such a position, and how the patient moves while disrobing, with any changes in facial expression, assists the interpretation of the patient's symptoms. A pertinent question to be asked when a particular posture produces pain is "Is it 'the' pain or is it different from the pain for which you are seeking treatment?" Such observations may suggest to the therapist the movements that are likely to reproduce the symptoms.

### Posture and Shape of Joints

Alteration in posture and joint outline may be of recent or long-standing duration and include many so-called postural deformities that may well be perfectly normal for a particular individual. It should be emphasized that some fairly obvious deformities (e.g., marked kyphosis, lordosis, or scoliosis) may be of no significance in the patient's current problem.

### Gait

Obvious gait alterations can be observed initially. Changes such as altered weight distribution and lack of mobility in hips, knees, or ankles, or a positive Trendelenburg sign may be noted. With the exception of the latter, lack of mobility may be inhibition of movement due to pain originating in the lumbar spine, or due to a previous unrelated peripheral joint involvement.

## SPECIFIC MOVEMENT AND OBSERVATION

At this time, it is important to compare the symptoms and signs produced on movement to the answers given to the related subjective questions. Thus links may be established between the symptoms described by the patient and those elicited by the movement. The patient needs to be undressed sufficiently to observe the whole of the spine as well as the lower limbs.

### Observation from Behind

When observing from behind the following may be observed and variation noted:

1. Altered leg length
2. Altered shoulder height
3. Position of head on neck and neck on shoulders
4. Kyphosis or lordosis (exaggerated or diminished)
5. Position of scapulae
6. Valgus or varus deformity of knees and feet
7. Scoliosis (postural or structural)
8. Position of sacrum and iliac crests
9. Prominence or depression of vertebral spinous processes
10. Skin contour and color

### Observation from the Front

When observing from the front, a clinician should take note of the following features:

1. Height or level of iliac crests
2. Position or level of the knees

3. Shape of trunk
4. Relative position of shoulders, head, and feet
5. Skin contour

## Observation from the Side

When observing from the side, a clinician should be aware of the following:

1. Position of head
2. Shape of cervical, thoracic, and lumbar spinal curves (any increased or decreased kyphosis or lordosis)
3. Skin contour

## Movements

The lumbar spine is most easily examined from behind.

### Flexion

When suitably undressed the patient is asked first to describe exactly where the symptoms are at present. The patient is then asked to bend forward to where there is any increase in any part of the symptom complex. This flexion range is usually recorded by measuring the distance from the outstretched fingertips to the floor or in relation to the position of the fingertips on the legs (e.g., patella, midthigh). The patient is then asked to move in a controlled manner further into the painful range (Fig. 7-2). This range and any alteration in the symptoms are noted.

In addition to noting the full range of movement, considerable attention is paid to the way in which the individual vertebrae move during flexion. Areas of hyper- and hypomobility, as well as any deviation from the median sagittal plane, are recorded. Surface contour should be carefully considered, particularly noting areas of prominence or depression. At this time it is important to compare those symptoms and signs produced on flexion to those answers given to the related subjective questions. Thus any links may be established between the symptoms described by the patient and those elicited by the movement. The distribution of the symptoms and the range of movement needs to be very carefully recorded. In one patient buttock pain may be produced during the first 10° of flexion, but the patient may also be able to continue to full range without any alteration in the distribution of the pain. In another patient, buttock pain may be produced in the first 10° of flexion but on continuing the movement toward full range, the pain may progress to the calf. *Both patients have the same range of forward flexion but they produce quite different symptoms, which need to be treated quite differently.*

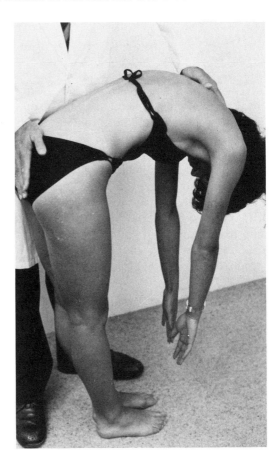

**Fig. 7-2.** Part 1 of the general examination: flexion.

The effect of a controlled amount of overpressure (i.e., gentle passive forcing of the movement from the patient's end range further into range) is also necessary under certain circumstances, not only to observe the way the symptoms react but also to test the *end feel* of the physiologic movement. The end feel of a movement is the relationship between the pain experienced and the resistance to movement. Such resistance may be due to intrinsic muscle spasm or tightness of the ligaments and capsule of the joint.

The end feel of the physiologic movement, mentioned above, may be different from the end feel with localized passive movement procedures (described later). However, quite distinct solid, springy, soft, or hard end feelings may be distinguished. The end feel needs to be noted because if there is a difference between what is found with localized procedures compared to the more general movement procedures, then an attempt needs to be made to define those differences and the possible reasons for them.

On occasion it is important to hold the full range position of flexion for a period of time. This becomes a necessary part of the examination, especially if during the subjective examination and activity involving sustained flexion is reported by the patient as a position where symptoms are eased. Such a procedure is valuable because if the symptoms are not eased, more detailed questioning and examination is necessary.

The return from the flexed to the upright position is also an important movement to monitor, both in terms of the way the vertebral column moves and the production of symptoms. A postural scoliosis or tilt may become on adoption of the erect position, which is not evident on bending forward. Another important aspect of assessment of flexion and the return to the upright position is the reproduction of a painful arc; that is, pain that is produced through a part of the range and then is eased as the movement continues. This can happen either during the flexion movement or during the return to the upright position. The range within which such symptoms are produced as well as the distribution of the symptoms should be carefully recorded and related if possible to the subjective findings. Often those patients with painful arcs are slower to respond to treatment, particularly if the painful arc is variable in its position in the range.

On occasion, symptoms may be produced some time after the movement has been completed (i.e., latent pain). This latent pain possibly may have a large chemical/inflammatory component in its production or etiology. Occasionally repeated flexion movements or varying the speed of the movement may be necessary to reproduce this symptom.

In addition to the general observation of changes in signs and symptoms on full range flexion, particular consideration needs to be given to the way in which motion segments are moving on flexion. There is a cephalad movement of the inferior zygapophyseal facets at one level in relation to the superior facets of the level below. This is accompanied by a stretching of the soft tissues of the posterior elements of the motion segment, including the posterior parts of the disc and the canal structures, as well as the posterior ligaments, capsules, and muscles. There is an accompanying compression of the anterior parts of the disc (nucleus and anterior annulus including the anterior longitudinal ligament).

**Lateral Flexion**

The patient stands in the same position as for flexion and is asked to slide the hand down the lateral aspect of the leg. Measurement is usually taken of the distance from the fingertips to the head of the fibula. Areas of hypo- and hypermobility can be observed at segmental levels by closely matching the movement behavior of the vertebrae, comparing the relative movement of the motion segment(s) with those above and below, and their sideways movement behavior compared one to the other. As with flexion, the use of overpressure and repeated and sustained movements may be necessary, in addition to the observance of deformity and presence or absence of a painful arc.

The effect of lateral flexion on that part of the motion segment on the contralateral extended side (away from that which the movement is performed on) is similar to that observed with sagittal plane flexion. There is a cephalad movement of the inferior zygapophyseal facet of the superior vertebra on the

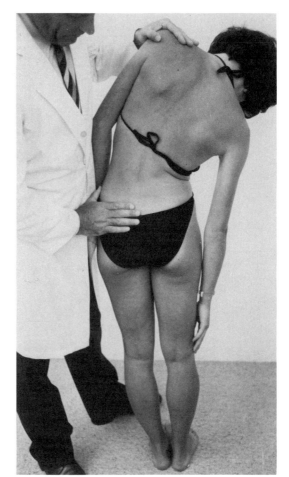

**Fig. 7-3.** Part I of the general examination: right lateral flexion.

superior zygapophyseal facet of the vertebra below. This stretches the soft-tissue structures (e.g., discs, joint capsules,) on the side opposite the direction of lateral flexion. On the side toward which the lateral flexion is performed these structures are compressed (Fig. 7-3).

## Extension

The therapist stands behind the patient, who is asked to bend backward. Measurement can be made of the distance the fingertips pass down the posterior aspect of the thigh. Areas of hypo- and hypermobility are observed as well as the distribution of symptoms at the end of range and through range. Overpressure and repeated and sustained movements are used as necessary.

The effect of extension on the motion segment is such that there is a caudal movement of the inferior zygapophyseal facets of a vertebra on the facets of

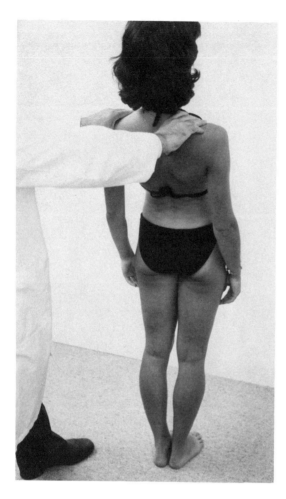

**Fig. 7-4.** Part 3 of the general examination: thoracolumbar extension.

the vertebra below. There is also a compression of the posterior parts and a stretching of the anterior parts of the intervertebral disc (Fig. 7-4).

### Axial Rotation

Rotation as a testing procedure in the lumbar spine is not a movement that often produces significant alteration in signs and symptoms. Strangely enough, it is a movement often preferred as a passive movement treatment technique by therapists. One method of testing rotation is for the therapist to stand on the left side of the patient and take hold of the patient's right ileum with the right hand and the patient's right shoulder with the left. The patient's pelvis is then rotated to the right while applying counterresistance to the shoulder (Fig. 7-5).

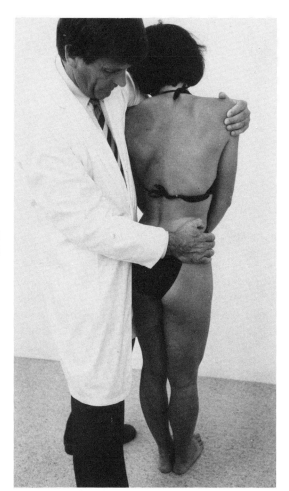

**Fig. 7-5.** Part 4 of the general examination: lumbar rotation to the left.

## General Assessment of Standard Active Physiologic Movements

In addition to recording the ranges of movements that are available and the way in which the vertebral segments move, detailed attention must also be given to the distribution of the symptoms and the type of symptoms involved with each movement. The importance of the patient's descriptions of these symptoms cannot be overemphasized. Comparison needs to be made between the way the patient describes the symptoms produced with various activities as elicited during the subjective questioning to those produced and observed in the objective testing of lumbar movements mentioned above. Similar descriptions of type of symptoms as well as distribution are important (i.e., the pain may be described as diffuse, lancinating, or referred to a limb, etc.). At this stage, the therapist should look for similarities between the movements of general daily activities that bring on the symptoms and the active movements that elicit the pain. For example, a patient may report that bending activity in the garden for about 1 hour brings on back pain, while on subsequent examination one repetition of forward flexion is shown to produce the same pain. Careful questioning is required to define the type and distribution of the symptoms, because sustained flexion (if that is the movement adopted while gardening) is unlikely to produce the same quality and quantity of pain as would be produced by one movement of flexion. Such careful questioning can help both in diagnosis as well as the selection of a treatment technique.

## Combined Movements

Habitually, movements of the vertebral column occur in combination across planes rather than as pure movements in one plane only. Many aspects of this phenomenon have been investigated.[2–6] Gregerson and Lucas[7] found that axial rotation of the lumbar spine to the left accompanied lateral flexion to the left and rotation to the right accompanied lateral flexion to the right. However, in one case they found the reverse combination occurred. Stoddard[5] stated that the direction of this conjoined rotation varied, depending on whether the lateral flexion was performed with the lumbar spine in flexion or extension. He suggested that the conjoined rotation is to the same side when the movement of lateral flexion is performed in flexion and to the opposite side when the movement of lateral flexion is performed in extension. Kapandji[8] also stated that lateral rotation occurs in conjunction with lateral flexion. Personal laboratory observation on fresh human cadaveric specimens seems to indicate that the direction of axial rotation is in the opposite direction to that to which the lumbar spine is laterally flexed, regardless of whether the spine is in flexion or extension. The presence of degenerative processes within the disc or zygapophyseal joints affects the amount of rotation, and occasionally there is an unexplained apparent reversal of the axial rotation.

Because of this, the usual objective examination of the lumbar spine should be expanded to incorporate combined movements. This is because symptoms and signs produced by lateral flexion, flexion, extension, and rotation as pure movements may alter when these movements are performed in a combined manner.[1]

### Lateral Flexion in Flexion

The therapist stands on the right-hand side of the patient so that the therapist's right anterosuperior iliac spine is in contact with the lateral aspect of the patient's right hip. The therapist's right hand is placed over the posterior aspect of the patient's left shoulder. The therapist's left hand grips the patient's left ilium. The patient is asked to bend forward: the range at which the symptoms

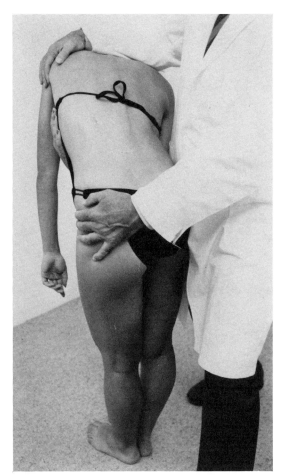

**Fig. 7-6.** Part 1 of the combined movements examination: lateral flexion in flexion.

are reproduced is noted and while this position is maintained, lateral flexion to the right is included as part of the total pattern (Fig. 7-6).

## Lateral Flexion in Extension

The therapist stands on the right-hand side of the patient, with the right arm placed around the patient's chest so that the therapist's right hand grips the patient's left shoulder. The thumbs and index finger of the therapist's left hand are placed over the transverse process of the vertebral level to be examined. The patient is then bent backward and laterally flexed to the right (Fig. 7-7).

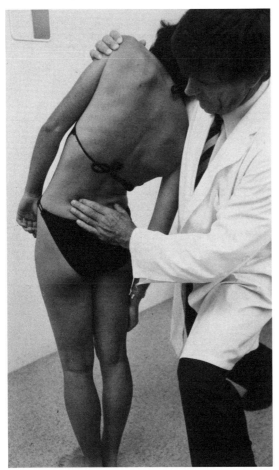

**Fig. 7-7.** Part 2 of the combined movements examination: lateral flexion in extension.

### Flexion and Rotation

The therapist stands on the right-hand side of the patient and places the hands posteriorly on the patient's shoulder. The patient then bends forward and rotates to the right (Fig. 7-8).

### Extension and Rotation

The same hand positions are adopted as with extension and lateral flexion. The patient's lumbar spine is extended and rotated to the right as well (Fig. 7-9).

## Passive Accessory Movements in Combined Positions

The usual accessory movements of transverse, central, and unilateral pressure[9,10] may also be carried out in combined positions. The lumbar spine is placed in the combined positions described above and the appropriate accessory movements are performed.

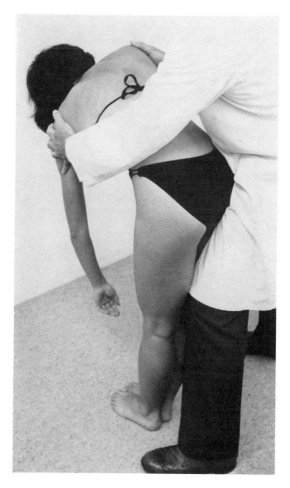

**Fig. 7-8.** Part 3 of the combined movements examination: flexion and rotation.

## Central Vertebral Pressure in Extension and Right Lateral Flexion

The patient lies prone in a position of extension and right lateral flexion. Central vertebral pressure is applied over the spinous process. Then the pressure is directed caudad on the spinous process of L4; the compressive effect particularly on the right-hand side will be increased on the right between L4–L5 but decreased between L3–L4 (Fig. 7-10).

## Transverse Pressure to the Left in Flexion and Left Lateral Flexion

With the patient prone and in a position of flexion and left lateral flexion, transverse pressure over the right side of the spinous process is applied. This will tend to increase the stretching effect on the right (Fig. 7-11).

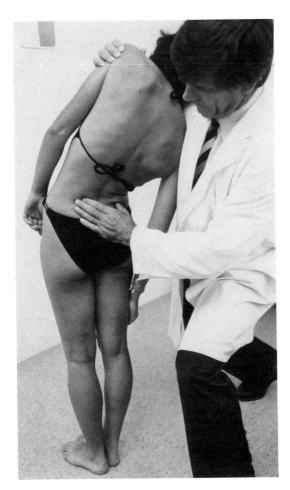

**Fig. 7-9.** Part 4 of the combined movements examination: extension and rotation.

## Unilateral Pressure on the Right in Flexion and Left Lateral Flexion

With the patient positioned in flexion and right lateral flexion, unilateral pressure on the right over the transverse process of the vertebrae is applied. If this pressure is directed cephalad on the transverse process of L4 there will be an increase in the stretching effect on the right between L4–L5 and a decrease between L3–L4 (Fig. 7-12).

## Passive Testing of Physiologic Movements

Standard passive physiologic tests of the movements of flexion, extension, lateral flexion, and axial rotation can also be carried out and are a useful adjunct to the examination procedures.

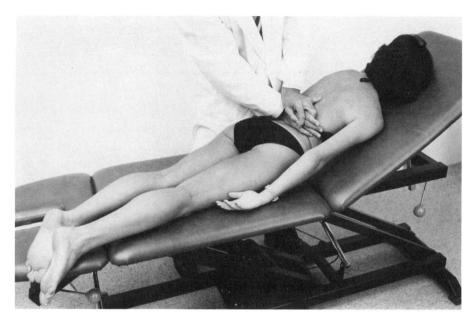

**Fig. 7-10.** Passive accessory movements in part 1 of the combined positions examination: central vertebral pressure in extension and right lateral flexion.

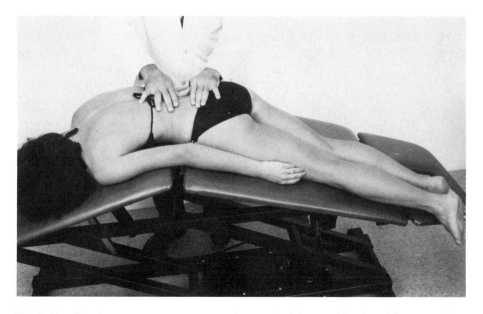

**Fig. 7-11.** Passive accessory movements in part 2 of the combined positions examination: transverse pressure to the left in flexion and left lateral flexion.

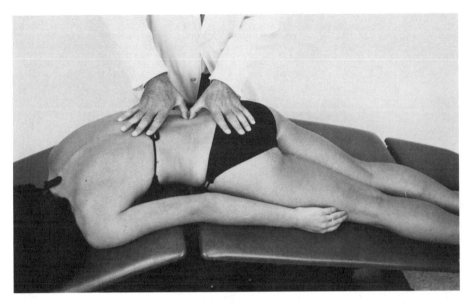

**Fig. 7-12.** Passive accessory movements in part 3 of the combined positions examination: unilateral pressure on the right in flexion and left lateral flexion.

## Assessment of Combined Movements

The movements of flexion, extension, lateral flexion, and rotation performed in the neutral position are termed *primary movements*. On the initial examination it is usual for one of these primary movements to reproduce part or all of the symptoms of which the patient is complaining. It is to this primary movement that the other movements are added. It is essential when performing the primary movement that the movement is taken to the point where the symptoms begin, and then taken in a controlled manner further into the painful range of the movement. At this stage the movement of lateral flexion or rotation or both is added.

Care must be taken when adding other movements that the starting position into the range of the primary movement is not altered. The basic principle is to combine movements that have similar mechanical effects on the motion segment and to observe if symptoms are increased or decreased by such maneuvers. On flexion there is a cephalad movement of the inferior zygapophyseal facet, for instance of L4 on the superior zygapophyseal facet of L5. The posterior elements are stretched: the posterior part of the intervertebral disc, the posterior longitudinal ligament, the ligamentum flavum, and capsules of the zygapophyseal joints. The anterior structures are compressed.

With right lateral flexion, for example, the left interior zygapophyseal facet of L4 moves upward on the left superior zygapophyseal facet of L5. This movement produces a stretching of the elements on the left side of the motion segment with completion of the right side of the motion segment. When flexion and right lateral flexion are combined, the stretching effects on the left are increased and slight stretching effects are produced on the right.

With extension there is a downward movement of the inferior zygapophyseal facet (e.g., of the L4 vertebrae on the superior zygapophyseal facet of L5). This is accompanied by compression of the posterior elements of the motion segment. When the movement of right lateral flexion is combined with extension, there is an increase on the compressive effects on the right and a decrease on the left.

### Regular and Irregular Patterns

The combination of these movements can, under many circumstances, produce recognizable symptom patterns, which may be described as regular or irregular.[1] Regular patterns are those in which similar movements at the intervertebral joint produce the same symptoms whenever the movements are performed. The symptoms, however, may differ in quality or severity. The regular pattern may be divided further: (1) regular patterns: stretch and compressive; (2) irregular patterns: those that show no recognizable pattern.

**Regular Compressive Pattern.** Right lateral flexion increases right buttock pain. This pain is made worse when right lateral flexion is performed in extension, and eased when right lateral flexion is performed in flexion. Therefore, if the patient's symptoms are produced on the side to which the movement is directed, then the pattern is a compressing pattern.

**Regular Stretch Pattern.** Right lateral flexion increases left buttock pain. This pain is made worse when right lateral flexion is performed in flexion and eased when right lateral flexion is performed in extension. Therefore, if the symptoms are present on the opposite side from that to which the movement is directed, then the pattern can be considered a stretching pattern.

**Irregular Pattern.** All of those patients who do not fit into the regular category are classified as irregular. There are many of these (e.g., when right lateral flexion reproduces right buttock pain, which is made worse when right lateral flexion is combined with flexion on the right. In this movement, the right compression of right lateral flexion is counteracted by the stretching of flexion). Another example is left lateral flexion producing right buttock pain (a stretching movement). This pain is made worse when the same movement is performed in extension (a compressing movement) and eased when the movement of left lateral flexion is performed in flexion (another stretching movement).

The irregular pattern may indicate that there is more than one component to the joint disorder (e.g., zygapophyseal joint and intervertebral disc, canal and foranimal structures). Generally traumatic injuries (e.g., whiplash and early disc lesions) have irregular patterns, whereas chronic disc lesions or zygapophyseal joint lesions with no history of trauma leave regular patterns.

Contained within one type of pattern there may be elements of other patterns. These should be recognized, and time provided so as to decide whether any irregular patterns have some recognizable, regular components.

The recognition of different patterns can assist in choosing the direction of technique, allowing a combined movement end-of-range (CME), procedure to be used, and assessing the manner in which the signs and symptoms may improve.

When choosing the direction of the technique in the case of regular patterns (either stretch or compressive), the first choice of movement is in the direction that is away from the movement that reproduces the symptom. For example, if right lateral flexion reproduces the right buttock pain and this pain is made worse when the right lateral flexion is performed in extension (that is, a regular compressive pattern), the first choice would be to carry out the opposite movement (i.e., left lateral flexion in flexion). As the symptoms improve, the technique of left lateral flexion in flexion is changed to right lateral flexion in flexion and progresses to right lateral flexion in extension as symptoms improve further.

If the patient presents with a regular stretch pattern (e.g., right lateral flexion reproduces left buttock pain and this pain is made worse when right lateral flexion is performed in flexion and eased when right lateral flexion is performed in extension), the first choice technique would be the opposite movement (i.e., left lateral flexion in extension). This technique can then progress to performing right lateral flexion in flexion as the symptoms improve.

The use of the box diagram is a simple way to show this:

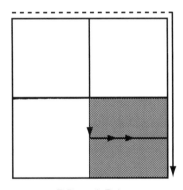

**R** Buttock Pain

Progression: (1) left lateral flexion in flexion, (2) right lateral flexion in flexion, (3) right lateral flexion in extension.

Or, for example 2:

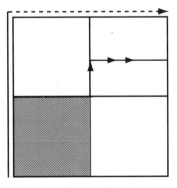

**L** Buttock Pain

Progression: (1) left lateral flexion in extension, (2) left lateral flexion in flexion, (3) right lateral flexion in flexion.

These procedures are described in greater detail elsewhere.[1]

CME procedures should be used. There is evidence that end-of-range procedures (i.e., passive movements performed at the limit of a range of movement) are more effective in reducing pain perception and improving the range of movement.[10-13] By combining movements, it is possible to use end-of-range movements in a relatively painless way. The most painful movement for the patient can be used as a treatment technique in its least painful combined position. The movement technique can be carried out in a manner that causes the least pain but is performed at the end of the available range. This position is progressed to what was the most painful position for the patient as the symptoms improve.

Assessing the improvement in a patient's condition means recognizing the patterns, regular or irregular, that can help in predicting the way in which the symptoms will improve. In the case of a regular compressive pattern where, for example, right lateral flexion produces right buttock pain and this pain is worse when the movement is performed in extension, then right lateral flexion in neutral will improve before right lateral flexion in extension. With a regular stretch pattern, for example, of right lateral flexion causing left buttock pain, this pain being worse when right lateral flexion is performed in flexion, then right lateral flexion in neutral will improve before right lateral flexion in flexion. The response in the case of irregular patterns is not as predictable and the improvement in the signs and symptoms may appear in an apparently random fashion.

## TREATMENT TECHNIQUE

### Right Lateral Flexion in Neutral

The treatment table is adjusted so as to have the thoracic spine at the desired position of lateral flexion. This position will correspond to that found on examination. The lumbar spine is placed in a neutral position. The therapist's right hand is placed at the level at which the lateral flexion is to be centered, with the therapist's left hand placed over the patient's right greater trochanter. The moment of lateral flexion is performed by moving the left hand in a cephalad direction so as to laterally flex the pelvis to the right (Fig. 7-13).

### Right Lateral Flexion in Flexion

The treatment table is adjusted and the therapist's hands are placed in a manner as described above. The patient's hips and knees are flexed so as to flex the lumbar spine to the required position. The patient's feet are placed over the therapist's flexed left thigh. This maintains the angle of lumbar flexion.

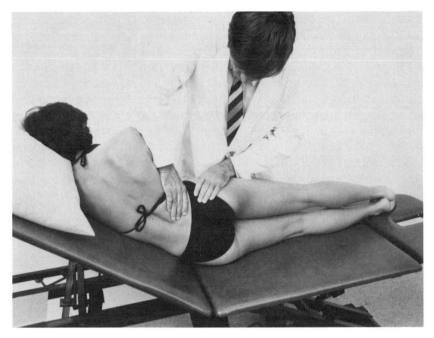

**Fig. 7-13.**   Part 1 of the technique examination: right lateral flexion in neutral.

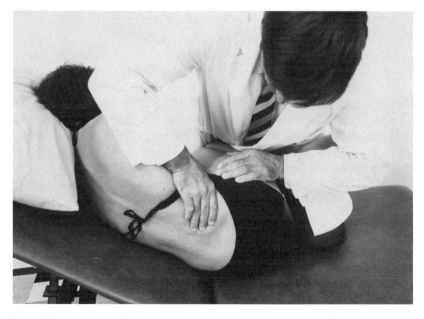

**Fig. 7-14.**   Part 2 of the technique examination: right lateral flexion in flexion.

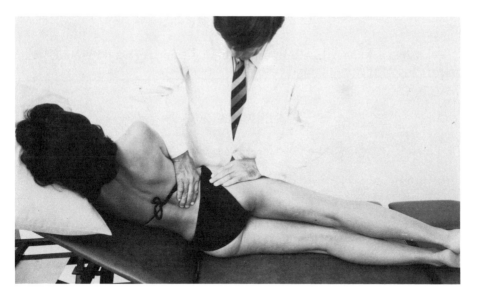

**Fig. 7-15.** Part 3 of the technique examination: right lateral flexion in extension.

The movement of lateral flexion is carried out by moving the left hand cephalad while maintaining the flexion of the lumbar spine (Fig. 7-14).

## Right Lateral Flexion in Extension

The table and hand position are placed in a manner as described above. The lumbar spine is placed in a position of extension. Lateral flexion is carried out by moving the left hand in a cephalad direction while maintaining the position of extension (Fig. 7-15).

## SUMMARY

The examination of the lumbar spine requires considerable patience and skill. The principle of combining movements provides an addition to the standard examination and a means by which changes in signs and symptoms can be readily assessed and specific symptom patterns observed. These symptom patterns are of assistance in the selection of passive movement treatment technique, because the ability to predict the likely result enables the therapist to use the CME technique, even in acutely painful conditions.

## ACKNOWLEDGMENTS

I wish to acknowledge the considerable assistance of David Watkins in the preparation of the photographs used in this chapter.

## REFERENCES

1. Edwards BC: Manual of Combined Movement. Churchill Livingstone, London, 1992
2. Farfan HF: Muscular mechanics of the lumbar spine and the position of power and efficiency. Orthop Clin N Am 6:135, 1975
3. Loehl WY: Regional rotation of the spine. Rheumatol Rehabil 12:223, 1973
4. Rolander SD: Motion of the lumbar spine with special reference to the stabilising effect of posterior fusion—an experimental study of autopsy specimens. Acta Orthop Scand, suppl 90, 1966
5. Stoddard AC: Manual of Osteopathic Technique. Hutchison, London, 1959
6. Troup JDG, Hood CA, Chapman AE: Measurements of the sagittal mobility of the lumbar spine and hips. Am Phys Med 9:308,1968
7. Gregerson GC, Lucas DB: An in vivo study of the axial rotation of the human thoracolumbar spine. J Bone Joint Surg 49A:247, 1967
8. Kapandji IA: Physiology of Joints. Vol. 3. Churchill Livingstone, London, 1974
9. Maitland GD: Vertebral Manipulation. Butterworths, London, 1985
10. Nade S, Newbold PJ: Factors determining the level and changes in intra-articular pressure in the knee joint of the dog. J Physiol 338:21, 1983
11. Baxendale RH, Ferrell WR: The effect of knee joint afferent discharge on transmission in flexion reflex pathways in decerebrate cats. J Physiol 315:231, 1981
12. Grigg P, Greenspan BJ: Response of primate joint afferent neurons to mechanical stimulation of the knee joint. J Neurophys 40:1, 1977
13. Lundberg A, Malmgren K, Schomburg ED: Role of joint afferents in motor control exemplified by effects on reflex pathways from ib afferents. J Physiol 284:327, 1978

# 8 | Manipulative Physical Therapy in the Management of Selected Low Lumbar Syndromes

Patricia H. Trott
Ruth Grant
Geoffrey D. Maitland

Patients referred for manipulative physical therapy can be divided into two groups according to the history. Patients in the first group have a *history of injury,* such as a fall or direct blow, or are referred following surgery. The tissues that are injured depend on the direction and force of the injury, and thus the therapist cannot predict the pattern of the symptoms and signs or the response to treatment. The second group includes patients who have a *history of symptoms occurring spontaneously* or following some trivial incident such as sneezing or bending to pick up a light object. Patients in this second group have symptoms, signs, and histories that are easily recognized, and these conditions respond in a predictable way to manipulative physical therapy.

This chapter is predicated on a recognition and understanding of the pathology and patterns of pain presentation given in previous chapters, and is therefore specifically directed to technique selection and application in the management of some common syndromes (clinical presentations) of the low lumbar spine (L4–S1) seen in physical therapy practice. Although discussion is restricted to the use of passive movement techniques, the need for a detailed assessment of the soft-tissue components and the muscular control of the spine and pelvis is stressed, and these aspects together with ergonomic advice are included in the overall management of low lumbar problems (these aspects are covered in other chapters of this book).

Before describing such lumbar conditions, discussion of the factors that govern the selection of passive movement techniques is necessary.

## SELECTION OF TECHNIQUES

### Diagnosis

In the clinical setting, reaching a definitive diagnosis is not always possible. This is particularly the case for low lumbar disorders, and relates to the following factors.

1. In many cases the etiology is multifactorial and includes both an inflammatory and a mechanical cause.
2. Pain arising from certain tissues does not follow a specific anatomic pattern.
3. A particular pathologic process can give differing patterns of symptoms and signs.

For example, patients with a diagnosis of disc herniation with nerve-root irritation can exhibit differing clinical presentations; that is, the symptoms may be acute and severe, or chronic. The distribution of pain may vary, being worse either proximally or distally, with or without neurologic changes. The pattern of limitation of movements may vary from gross restriction of flexion and straight-leg raising (SLR) due to pain, to full range and pain-free flexion but with marked restriction of extension.

Clearly, a diagnostic label on its own is of limited assistance when choosing physical treatment modalities, and in particular when selecting passive movement techniques. Rather, treatment selection is based on the way the condition presents in terms of the patient's symptoms, abnormalities of movement, and the history of the disorder. Knowing which structures can cause pain and the different patterns of pain response that can occur during test movements is fundamental to the selection of passive movement techniques.

Physical therapists, and in particular manipulative physical therapists, are skilled in the diagnosis of mechanical disorders of the neuromusculoskeletal system. They are also trained to recognize when symptoms do not have a mechanical basis and when to suspect an inflammatory component. In many cases radiologic and hematologic tests are required to exclude other pathologies.

# Pain-Sensitive Structures and Their Pain Patterns

In the lumbar spine the common structures that cause symptoms are the joints[1,2] and their supportive tissues,[2] and the pain-sensitive structures in the vertebral and foraminal canals.[3–7]

## Intervertebral Joints

**Intervertebral Disc.** Pain from disorders of the intervertebral disc is commonly deep and ill defined, presenting as a wide area across the low back or as a vague buttock pain. This pain may spread to the upper posterior thigh or lower abdomen, but pain originating in the disc itself is not referred into the lower leg.[8] The pain may be central, to one side, or bilateral (symmetric or asymmetric).

A damaged disc may impinge against the posterior longitudinal ligament or the dura or, as it herniates, disc material can impinge on or irritate the nerve-root sleeve or the nerve root causing referred pain.[2,9]

Discogenic pain behaves differently from pain arising from other structures, in that (1) following a sustained posture, rapid reversal of that posture is both painful and stiff (e.g., standing up quickly after prolonged sitting), and (2) speed of movement will vary the position in range at which pain is experienced (i.e., with increased speed, pain is experienced earlier in the range). Discogenic pain may be aggravated by either compressive or stretching movements.[10]

**Zygapophyseal Joint.** Like other synovial joints, the zygapophyseal joint may present with an intraarticular disorder (which is made worse, that is, more painful, when the articular surfaces are compressed) or a periarticular disorder (which is worsened by movements that place stress on the capsule).

Commonly, zygapophyseal joint pain is felt locally as a unilateral back pain, which when severe can spread down the entire limb.[2,11] The site of pain is not exclusive to one zygapophyseal joint; therefore, the source of pain must be confirmed by clinical examination. In its chronic form, there may be no local pain over the affected joint, but a distal localized patch of pain. This is a common phenomenon in the thoracolumbar region; similar clinical findings for the lower lumbar area have not been substantiated by research.

**Ligamentous and Capsular Structures.** Referred pain from specific spinal ligamentous structures follows no known neurologic pattern.[2,12] Based on clinical experience, Maitland[10] reported that ligamentous and capsular pain is felt maximally over the ligament and that the pain may spread into the lower limb. Movements that stretch the ligament/capsule may produce sharp local pain or a stretched sensation at the symptomatic site.

## Structures in the Vertebral and Foraminal Canals

The pain-sensitive structures in the vertebral and foraminal canals are the dura anteriorly,[5,6] the nerve-root sleeves, the ventral nerve roots, and the blood vessels of the epidural space.[7,13]

The structures comprising the vertebral canal that are pain sensitive are the posterior longitudinal ligament, posterior portions of the annuli fibrosi, and the anterior aspect of the laminae.[1] The pain-sensitive components of the foraminal canals are the posterolateral aspect of the intervertebral discs and the zygapophyseal joints.[1]

Passive-movement tests will implicate a loss of mobility and/or increase in tension of the neuromeningeal tissues.

**Dura and Nerve-Root Sleeve.** Dural pain does not have a segmental pattern of reference.[3] However, stimulation of the nerve-root sleeve gives rise to symptoms of similar distribution to those arising from stimulation of that nerve root. The only reported difference is that the nerve root frequently gives rise to symptoms that are more severe distally and the pain is often associated with paresthesia. These phenomena are not seen with irritation of the nerve-root sleeve.[14]

**Radicular Pain.** Mechanical or chemical irritation of the sensory nerve root causes pain and/or paresthesia to be experienced in the distal part of a dermatome, or if felt throughout a dermatome, these symptoms are often worse distally.[15] Movements that narrow the intervertebral canal and foramen (extension, rotation, and lateral flexion to the affected side) are likely to reproduce or aggravate the nerve-root pain/paresthesia. Clinically, pain can be conclusively attributed to the nerve root only if there are neurologic changes indicating a loss of conduction along that nerve root.

Passive movement tests that specifically test the neuromeningeal structures are SLR, prone knee flexion (PKF), passive neck flexion (PNF), and the slump test. These tests are described in major textbooks on manipulative therapy.[9,10,16,17] They are used not only as examination techniques but also in treatment.

## Range/Pain Response to Movement

Test movements of the low lumbar intervertebral joints and the neuromeningeal tissues produce common patterns.

### Stretching or Compressing Pain

Unilateral back pain may be reproduced by either stretching (e.g., lateral flexion away from the painful side)or by compressing the faulty tissues (e.g., lateral flexion toward the painful side).

### End-of-Range or Through Range Pain

Pain may be reproduced at the limit of a particular movement (i.e., when the soft-tissue restraints are put on stretch) or during the performance of a movement, increasing near the limit of the movement. Through range pain is common in joints in which there is a constant ache.

## Local and Referred Pain

In patients who have referred pain, the pain response to test movements influences the selection of passive movement techniques. For example, test movements even when firmly applied may elicit only local back pain. In these patients the movement may be applied firmly without risk of exacerbation of symptoms. In cases where the test movement has to be sustained at end of range in order to reproduce the referred pain, a treatment technique that is sustained will be required. In contrast to this, test movements that immediately cause distal leg symptoms require very gentle treatment in a manner that does not reproduce the distal symptoms. Test movements that cause latent referred pain or that cause the referred pain to linger also indicate caution in treatment.

## History

Any history taken should include the onset and progression of the disorder. Conditions that have a spontaneous (nontraumatic) onset have a characteristic progressive history; that is, there is a pattern that is typical of a degenerating disc or of postural ligamentous pain. Knowing the history that is typical for these conditions helps the clinician to recognize the present stage of the disorder and to match this with the symptoms and signs to form a syndrome. Typical histories are presented in the case studies at the end of this chapter.

A detailed history gives information as to the stability or progressive nature of the disorder. This will guide the extent and strength of techniques used and may contraindicate certain techniques. This is particularly important in cases of a progressive disc disorder when injudicious treatment may convert a potential disc protrusion into a herniated disc with neurologic changes.

The progression of the disorder allows prediction of the outcome of treatment, number of treatment sessions needed, and long-term prognosis.

The following case history illustrates these aspects of history taking.

A 25-year-old gardener presented with a 10-year history of low back pain, which started one school vacation when he worked as a builder's laborer. He then remained symptom free until he began work as a gardener 7 years ago. Prolonged digging caused low back pain, which initially would be gone by the next morning, but this slowly worsened to the extent that the pain spread to his left buttock and posterior thigh and took longer to settle. In the last 6 months he has required treatment; two or three treatments of heat and extension exercises have completely relieved his symptoms. Two weeks ago, he tripped over a stone and experienced sharp pain in his left calf and paresthesia of his left fifth toe. This has not responded to heat and exercises, but he has been able to continue his gardening.

This history is typical of a progressive and worsening disc disorder and the patient is now at a stage where he has nerve-root irritation. Although a trivial incident provoked this episode, the disorder is relatively stable in that he can continue gardening without worsening his symptoms.

More specific treatment will be required and can be performed firmly without risk of exacerbation of his symptoms. The expectation of treatment is to make him symptom free while anticipating that there may be further episodes due to the progressive nature of his disorder.

## Symptoms

The area in which a patient feels the symptoms and the manner in which they vary in relation to posture and movement assist in the recognition of syndromes, and if they match the response to physical examination, can assist in the selection of passive movement techniques. A movement or combination of movements that simulate a position or movement described by the patient as one that causes the pain, can be used as the treatment technique. The following case history illustrates this.

> A right-handed tennis player complains of chronic right-side low back pain as he commences serving. In this position his low lumbar spine is extended, laterally flexed, and rotated to the right. Examination confirms that this combined position reproduces his pain and testing of intervertebral movement reveals hypomobility at the L5–S1 joint.

An effective treatment would consist of placing his low lumbar spine into this combined position and then passively stretching one of these movements, carefully localizing the movement to the L5–S1 joint.

Two other important aspects of the patient's symptoms are the *severity* of the pain and the *irritability* of the disorder. Severity relates to the examiner's interpretation of the severity of the pain based on the patient's description and functional limitations due to the pain. Irritability (or touchiness) of the disorder is based on three things: (1) how much activity the patient can perform before being stopped by pain; (2) the degree and distribution of pain provoked by that activity; and (3) how long the pain takes to subside to its original level. (This is the most informative part and serves as a guide to the probable response of the symptoms to examination and treatment.)

In the previous example of the tennis player, a nonirritable disorder would be one in which he experiences momentary pain each time he serves (in this case the treatment described previously would be applicable). In contrast to this, an irritable disorder would be one in which his back pain lasts for several minutes after serving a ball, and this pain increases to the extent that after serving one game his back is so painful that he cannot continue to play and has to rest for 1 hour to ease his pain. In this example, a technique that reproduced his symptoms would not be the initial choice of treatment, but rather his lumbar spine would be positioned in the most comfortable position and a technique performed that was pain free.

## Signs

*Signs* refer to physical examination findings. Physical examination tests are used to incriminate or exclude certain structures as the source of a patient's symptoms. In particular, the tests determine the involvement of the intervertebral joints and neuromeningeal tissues and whether conduction of the spinal cord and cauda equina is altered. They help indicate the degree of irritability of the disorder and demonstrate whether symptoms have a stretch or compression component.

The physical examination of movements includes three sections. These are examination of

1. The gross physiologic movements of the lumbar spine (flexion, extension, lateral flexion; and rotation). It may be necessary to examine these movements in different combinations and in varied sequences, to sustain these positions or to perform them with distraction or compression
2. Passive physiologic and accessory movements at each intervertebral segment
3. The neuromeningeal tissues in the vertebral and foraminal canals (using SLR, PNF, PKF, and the slump test)

Reaching a diagnosis of a mechanical disorder of the neuromusculoskeletal tissues is important, to isolate the structures at fault by knowing the symptom distribution and the response to physical tests. Knowledge of the movements that increase or decrease the symptom response are the main determinants of how to apply passive movement in treatment (not the diagnostic title per se).

## Selection of Technique Based on Effect

### Mobilization/Manipulation

Passive movement as a treatment technique can be broadly divided into its use as mobilization (passive oscillatory movements) or manipulation (small amplitude thrust/stretch performed at speed at the limit of a range of movement).

Mobilization is the method of choice for most lumbar disorders because it can be used as a treatment for pain or for restoring movement in a hypomobile joint. It can be adapted to suit the severity of the pain, the irritability of the disorder, and the stages and stability of the pathology.

Manipulation is the treatment of choice when an intervertebral joint is locked. To regain mobility in cases of an irritable joint condition, a single localized manipulation may be less aggravating than repeated stretching by mobilization.

## Position of the Intervertebral Joint and Direction of the Movement Technique

Treatment by passive movement involves careful positioning of the particular intervertebral segment and the selection of the most effective direction of movement. These are based on a knowledge of spinal biomechanics and the desired symptom response.

**Manipulation.** Manipulation is applied in the direction of limitation in order to stretch the tissues in that particular direction. For example, using biomechanical principles, the lumbar spine can be positioned (in lateral flexion and contralateral rotation) to isolate movement to the desired intervertebral segment and a rotary thrust applied in the appropriate direction.

**Passive Mobilization.** When using passive mobilization both the position of the intervertebral joint and the direction of movement are varied according to the desired effect of the technique. Some examples are:

1. *To avoid any discomfort or pain:* In cases where the pain is severe or the disorder is irritable, the symptoms should not be provoked or aggravated. The lumbar spine would be positioned so that the painful intervertebral segment was pain free and the movement technique performed must also be pain free.

2. *To cause or to avoid reproduction of referred pain:* Provocation of referred pain is safe when the pain is chronic and nonirritable, and when it is not an acute radicular pain. In these cases it may be necessary to cause some leg pain to gain improvement; thus the spine is positioned to either provoke some symptoms or to enable the treatment technique to provoke the referred symptoms. Findings indicating radicular pain (i.e., pain worse distally and the presence of neurologic changes), when the examination of movements reproduces the distal pain, should warn the clinician against using a technique that provoked the referred pain.

3. *To open one side of the intervertebral joint* (i.e., to stretch the disc, distract the zygapophyseal joint, and widen the foraminal canal on one side): This would be the choice in cases of nerve-root irritation/compression or in cases of a progressive unilateral disc disorder. For example, to widen the right side of the L4 to L5 intervertebral space, the spine would be positioned in the combined position of flexion, lateral flexion, and rotation to the left. Which of these movements would be emphasized as the treatment technique would depend on the pain response.

4. *To stretch tissues that are contracted:* Joints that are both painful and hypomobile can respond differently to passive mobilization depending to a large extent on the irritability. The pain response during the performance of a technique and its effect over a 24-hour period will guide the clinician in the choice of which direction to move the joint and how firmly to stretch the contracted tissues. A favorable response to gentle oscillatory stretches is that the pain experienced during the technique decreases, thus allowing the movement to be performed more strongly. A worsening of the pain response indicates that this direction of movement is aggravating the condition.

5. *To move the intervertebral joints or the canal structures:* During the physical examination, if movements of the intervertebral joints and of the neuro-meningeal structures in the canal both reproduce the patient's leg symptoms, a technique directed at altering the intervertebral joint movements should be the first choice of treatment. The effect on the intervertebral joint signs and the canal signs is noted and if the latter are not improving, movement of the neuromeningeal tissues is added or substituted. In cases of only back and/or buttock pain and where the canal tests more effectively reproduce this pain, then the first choice would be to use movement of the canal structures (e.g., PNF, SLR, PKF, or the slump test).

## Manner of Movement Technique Performance

Selection of a treatment technique does not merely relate to the direction of movement but also to the manner in which it is applied. The amplitude can be varied from a barely perceptible movement to one that makes use of the total available range. The rhythm can be varied from a smooth, evenly applied movement to one that is staccato. Similarly, the speed and the position in range in which the movement is performed can be altered.

Passive movement techniques must be modified according to the intention of the technique, and this is based on the symptoms experienced by the patient during the technique, the quality of the movement, the presence of spasm, and the end feel. It is not possible to discuss these details in any depth in this chapter, but only to present the two ends of the symptom spectrum that ranges from a constant ache with pain experienced through range, to stiffness with mild discomfort felt only at the end of range of certain movements as presented below. For a full description, see Maitland.[10]

**Constant Aching with Pain Through Range.** The lumbar spine must be placed in a position of maximal comfort (usually one of slight flexion and mid-position for the other movements). The treatment technique will be of small amplitude, performed slowly and smoothly (so that there is no discomfort produced or where discomfort is constant, with no increase in the level of the aching). The movement technique may be a physiologic or an accessory movement, and its performance should result in an immediate lessening of the level of aching. In some patients there may be an immediate effect, but in others the effect should be noted over a 24-hour period.

**Stiffness with Mild Discomfort Felt Only at the End of Range of Certain Movements.** The lumbar spine is carefully positioned at or near the limit of the stiff directions of movement (i.e., in the position that best reproduces the stiffness and discomfort). The treatment technique will be one that places maximal stretch on the hypomobile intervertebral segment. The technique should be firmly applied, of small amplitude, and either sustained or staccato in rhythm. If the level of discomfort increases with the firm stretching, large amplitude movements can be interspersed every 40 to 60 seconds.

# CASE STUDIES

In this section some of the common syndromes with a history of spontaneous onset of symptoms are presented. Management is restricted to treatment by passive movement. The syndromes are presented as case histories; however, the reader is encouraged to read Grant et al.[18]

## Acute Back Pain (Discogenic)

### History

A 35-year-old man experienced a mild central low backache after pushing a car one morning. This ache intensified during a 40-minute drive to work, and he was unable to get out of the car unaided due to severe low back pain. He had no previous history of backache and radiographs of his lumbosacral region were reported as being normal. After 2 days in bed without any improvement in his symptoms, physical therapy was requested by his doctor.

### Symptoms

There was a constant dull backache centered over the L4 to L5 region. The patient was unable to move in bed due to sharp jabs of pain. His most comfortable position was supine with his hips and knees flexed over two pillows in crook lying or side lying with his legs (and lumbar spine) flexed.

### Signs

The patient was examined supine. SLR was almost full range as was PNF, but both tests slightly increased his back pain. Spreading and compression of the ilia were pain free and there was no abnormality in lower limb reflexes or sensation (testing muscle strength was not undertaken due to back pain). In crook lying, lumbar rotation to each side was reduced to half range due to pain.

### Interpretation

The history suggests discogenic pain—pushing a heavy car would raise intradiscal pressure—with pain worsened by sitting followed by inability to extend the spine. The physical examination was too restricted by pain to be helpful in confirming the source of his symptoms.

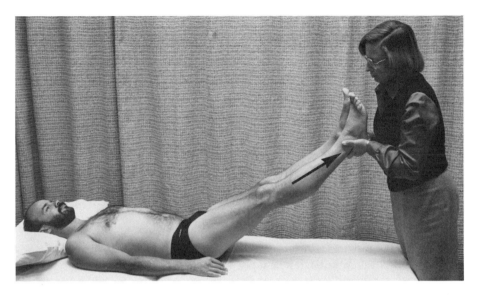

**Fig. 8-1.** Longitudinal caudad mobilization of the lower lumbar spine, produced by manual traction to the lower limbs.

## Management

**Day 1 (Treatment 1).** Because SLR was of good range, both legs were comfortably flexed at the hips to 50° and gentle manual traction was applied by pulling on his legs (Fig. 8-1). During traction his backache decreased. A series of four gentle but sharp tugs were applied to his legs. With each tug, a jab of back pain was experienced but there was no increase in his constant backache. On reassessment, PNF was full and painless but SLR remained unchanged. The treatment was repeated resulting in a slight improvement in his SLR on both sides and in his range of lumbar rotations performed in supine.

**Day 2 (Treatment 2).** The patient reported greater freedom of movements in bed and had been out of bed twice for a hot shower. Examination of his lumbar mobility in standing showed marked limitation of flexion by pain centered over L5 and there was obvious spasm in his erector spinae. Extension was half range and he had a full range of lateral flexion to each side. Bilateral SLR was full and painless. Manual traction effected no change in his mobility so he was placed in a prone position with two pillows under his abdomen. From this position of comfort, he was asked to gently passively extend his spine using a modified push-up technique.[19] This technique was repeated 10 times, sustaining the position for 5 seconds. The patient was encouraged to extend his lumbar spine to his comfortable limit. However, particular care was taken to avoid development of a backache. On reassessment in standing, flexion had improved so that he could reach fingertips to his patellae and extension was three-quarters of usual range.

The technique was repeated but this time lying over only one pillow. Following two more applications the patient could lie comfortably prone without a pillow, and in weightbearing there was a further slight increase in his ranges of flexion and extension.

The patient was asked to repeat this technique hourly (three sets of 10 push-ups, at the end of which he allowed his back to sag into sustained extension for 1 minute, providing that there was no reproduction of backache). He was allowed out of bed for short periods but was to avoid sitting.

**Day 3 (Treatment 3).** The patient was pain free when moving in bed and could be ambulant for more than 1 hour before his ache returned. His range of flexion was such that he was able to reach his fingertips to midshin level (normally he could reach his ankles) and to fully extend his lumbar spine with only a mild ache.

The extension push-ups were repeated with the manipulative therapist stabilizing the patients' pelvis flat on the floor. As this was pain free, the patient was asked to sustain the position allowing his lumbar spine to sag fully into extension. In this extended position, gentle posteroanterior pressures were applied to L5, taking care to cause only mild discomfort. On resuming the flat prone position, sharp deep pain was felt over L5 but this quickly subsided with repeated gentle extension.

The above regimen was repeated prior to reassessing his mobility in standing. Flexion and extension were now full range. Gentle overpressure to extension reproduced the same deep, sharp pain.

**Days 4, 6, and 10 (Treatments 4, 5, and 6).** Subsequent treatments were conducted at the manipulative therapist's clinic and consisted of restoration of full pain-free range of lumbar extension using posteroanterior pressures on L5 with the patient's lumbar spine in extension. By day 6 the patient was symptom free, but experienced a deep ache with firm sustained posteroanterior pressure on L5. When seen 4 days later, no pain could be elicited by sustained or staccato posteroanterior oscillatory movement.

The patient was discharged with advice regarding lifting and care of his back during sustained postures (especially flexion).

## Severe Nerve-Root (Radicular) Pain

### History

A 35-year-old man had suffered from recurrent attacks of low back pain over the last 5 years. These were associated with lifting strains. This present episode commenced 4 days ago when he bent to move the garden hose. He experienced only mild aching in his low back, but over the next few hours his back pain disappeared and he felt strong pain in his left buttock and calf. His calf pain had worsened in the last 24 hours and spread into his left foot.

## Symptoms

The patient had constant severe pain in the lateral aspect of his left calf and foot and numbness of the lateral aspect of his left foot. Less severe aching was experienced in his left buttock. Weight bearing and sitting aggravated his back and calf pain, and coughing aggravated his back pain. He could gain some relief of symptoms by lying on his right side with his legs (and lumbar spine) flexed.

## Signs

The following movements aggravated his buttock and calf/foot pain: flexion to touch his patellae, extension and left lateral flexion half range, and left SLR limited to 25°. Neurologic examination revealed a reduced left ankle jerk, reduced sensation over the lateral border of the foot, and weak toe flexors (calf power could not be tested due to pain on weightbearing).

## Interpretation

There was evidence of S1 nerve-root compression. The history of a trivial incident causing this episode and the presence of worsening symptoms indicated that the disorder is both unstable and progressive, requiring care with treatment so as not to worsen the condition.

## Management

**Day 1 (Treatment 1).** In position of ease (i.e., lying on right side with lumbar spine comfortably flexed), the pelvis was gently rotated to the right taking care not to aggravate calf/foot or buttock pain. The technique was performed as far as possible into range without aggravating symptoms; SLR was used as reassessment. After two applications of rotation, flexion was also reassessed. The patient reported easing of his calf symptoms and both flexion and left SLR had minimally improved; however, extension range remained unaltered.

The patient was advised to rest in bed as much as possible and to avoid sitting.

**Day 2 (Treatment 2).** The patient reported that his symptoms were unchanged, and his physical signs and neurologic status were found to be unaltered. Rotary mobilization was repeated (as on day 1) with a similar response.

**Day 3 (Treatment 3).** No alteration in symptoms or signs. As his symptoms were aggravated by weightbearing, lumbar traction was given (15 lb for 10 minutes). During traction his calf/foot pain was eased and afterward his SLR improved by 10°.

**Day 4 (Treatment 4).** Definite reduction in calf/foot pain and improvement in all physical signs. Traction was repeated (15 lb for 20 minutes). At subsequent treatments both the time and the strength of the traction were increased.

**Day 10 (Treatment 8).** There were no leg symptoms, but buttock pain was experienced with prolonged sitting. Physical examination revealed full recovery of neurologic function. The extreme range of flexion, with the addition of neck flexion, reproduced buttock pain; the other spinal movements were full range and pain free. On passive overpressure, left SLR lacked 20° and also reproduced left buttock pain.

### Interpretation

At this stage, spinal mobility was full and painless but movement of the neuromeningeal tissues was restricted and reproduced the patient's only remaining symptom. A gentle technique to stretch the neuromeningeal tissues should be used, but if reproduction of nerve-root symptoms occurred it would contraindicate its use at this stage.

**Treatment 8 (Continued).** A gentle stretch was applied to left SLR, causing only buttock pain. Following this, flexion plus neck flexion were pain free.

**Day 12 (Treatment 9).** The patient was now symptom free, but left SLR still caused buttock pain at 75°.

### Interpretation

Despite an excellent response to treatment, in view of the progressive disorder, a decision not to stretch his SLR more firmly was taken. It was decided to review his progress in 2 weeks.

When seen 2 weeks later he had remained symptom free but his left SLR had not improved. Now that his disorder had stabilized, his SLR was strongly stretched, restoring full range with no return of symptoms.

## Chronic Nerve-Root (Radicular) Aching

This may present as either (1) residual symptoms from an acute episode of nerve-root pain; or (2) chronic aching (not pain) with signs of nerve-root compression.

In both cases, the disorder is nonirritable and does not restrict the patients' activities; however, because most low lumbar nerve-root problems are of discogenic origin, sitting causes an increase in leg symptoms. The disorder is stable and permits stronger techniques to be applied safely. The following case history illustrates the second type.

### History

A 40-year-old housewife presented with a past history of recurrent low back pain for 7 years. One year ago she noticed a dull ache in her left leg. At that time, two or three treatments of passive mobilization completely relieved her symptoms. The current episode began 3 weeks ago following paving of the garden path with bricks. While stooping to lay the bricks she was conscious of aching in her buttock and down the posterior aspect of her left leg. Rotary mobilization had not helped.

### Symptoms

A constant dull ache spread from her left sacroiliac area, down the posterior aspect of her buttock to the heel, together with paresthesia of the lateral aspect of her foot. The ache in her calf and the paresthesia were worsened if she sustained a flexed posture (e.g., vacuuming carpets) for more than 30 minutes or sat for more than 60 minutes.

### Signs

There was a full range of pain-free spinal movements, even when these were sustained. Poor intervertebral movement was noted below L3 on extension and on left lateral flexion. By adding left lateral flexion to the fully extended position, buttock aching was reproduced. The addition of left and right rotation made no change in the symptoms. Testing of intervertebral movement confirmed hypomobility at both L4–L5 and L5–S1 motion segments and posteroanterior pressure over L5 (performed with her spine in extension/left lateral flexion) caused buttock pain.

Tests for the neuromeningeal tissues revealed full SLR but the left leg had a tighter end feel; the slump test was positive (i.e., left knee extension lacked 30° and caused calf pain, which was eased by releasing cervical flexion). She had slight weakness of her left calf, but otherwise showed no neurologic deficit.

### Interpretation

The history implicated a disc disorder that was slowly progressing to interfere with nerve-root function. The disorder was stable in that the patient could continue with her daily activities as a housewife. Treatment to change both her intervertebral joint signs and neuromeningeal signs was necessary, using techniques that would temporarily aggravate her leg ache. Treating the intervertebral joint hypomobility first was safer, while observing its effect on both the joint and neuromeningeal signs.

## Management

**Day 1 (Treatment 1).** With the patient's low lumbar spine positioned in extension/left lateral flexion, firm posteroanterior pressures were applied to L4 and L5 spinous processes for 60 to 90 seconds, causing local pain and a mild increase in left buttock aching (Fig. 8-2). On reassessment, lumbar extension/left lateral flexion no longer reproduced an increase in buttock ache and low lumbar mobility had improved. The slump test had improved (left knee extension improved by 10°). Treatment was repeated with no further gain in mobility; neurologic function was unchanged.

**Day 3 (Treatment 2).** The patient reported no ill effects from treatment, and a lessening of her left leg aching. Physical examination showed that she had maintained the improvement gained on day 1. Neurologic function was unchanged. The above treatment was repeated even more strongly and sustained to stretch the tight tissues. The reproduction of only local pain (no referred buttock pain) supported the safety of using a strong stretch. The result of this stretch was that extension/left lateral flexion was painful only when sustained, and in the slump position, knee extension

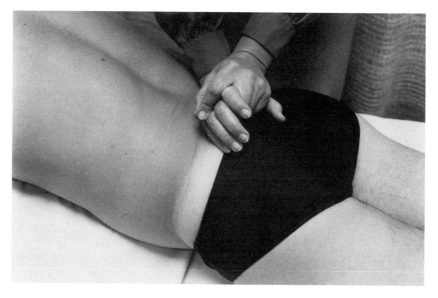

**Fig. 8-2.** Posteroanterior pressures on L5 with the lumbar spine positioned in extension/left lateral flexion.

improved by another 10°. Repeating the technique twice gained no further change to the slump test.

**Day 5 (Treatment 3).** The patient was delighted with her progress. She no longer had a constant ache down her left leg. The ache and paresthesia returned only if she sat for more than 1 hour. On examination, her left calf had regained full strength. Left SLR was no longer tighter than on the right; however, in the slump position, left knee extension still lacked 10° and caused buttock pain.

Treatment was changed to restore mobility in the neuromeningeal tissues. In the slump position, her left knee was stretched into full extension, causing sharp buttock pain (Fig. 8-3). This technique was not repeated until its effect on nerve-root conduction was known. This can only be assessed over 24 to 48 hours.

**Day 7 (Treatment 4).** There was no return of symptoms following the last treatment. Her calf strength and ankle reflex were normal. In the slump position, knee extension still reproduced sharp buttock pain. The stretch to the neuromeningeal tissues was increased by stretching the knee into

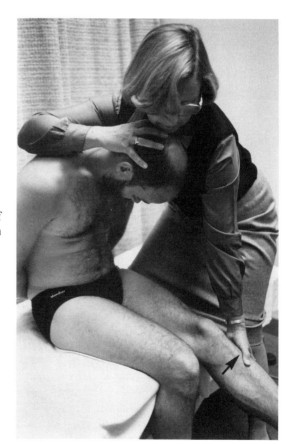

**Fig. 8-3.** Passive extension of the left knee performed while in the slump position.

full extension and stretching the ankle into full dorsiflexion in the slump position. This again caused sharp buttock pain. Reassessment of knee extension in the slump position showed it to be full range with minimal buttock pain. The technique was repeated once more. The patient was asked to experiment with activities such as sustained flexion and sitting for long periods during the next week.

**Day 14 (Treatment 5).** The patient reported that she experienced no leg symptoms but that her back ached after activities involving sustained flexion for more than 45 minutes and after sitting more than 90 minutes. She considered that this was better than she had been for several years. Examination of the slump test revealed full mobility, but caused slight buttock pain. The patient was discharged with a home exercise program to maintain the mobility of both her lower lumbar spine and her neuromeningeal tissues.

## Mechanical Locking

### History

A 20-year-old man complained of a sudden onset of unilateral back pain, which prevented him from standing upright. He had bent forward quickly to catch a ball near his left foot and was unable to straighten because of sharp back pain. He had no past history of back pain and no spinal radiographs had been taken.

### Symptoms

There was no pain when his back was held in slight flexion, but on standing upright pain was experienced to the right of the L5 spinous process.

### Signs

The patient was prevented by pain from extending, laterally flexing, or rotating his low lumbar spine to the right. The other movements were full and painless. Passive testing of intersegmental movement revealed an inability to produce the above painful movements at L4–L5 with marked spasm on attempting to do so. Unilateral posteroanterior pressures over the right L4–L5 zygapophyseal joint produced marked pain and spasm.

### Interpretation

A rapid unguarded movement in flexion/left lateral flexion gapped the right lumbar zygapophyseal joints, following which there was mechanical blocking of the movements that normally appose the articular surfaces (extension, lateral flexion, and rotation of the trunk to the right). The mechanism of mechanical locking remains a contentious issue.[20–22]

A manipulation, localized to the affected intervertebral level, to gap in this case the right L4–L5 zygapophyseal joint, will restore normal joint function.

### Management

A rotary manipulation was performed to gap the right L4–L5 zygapophyseal joint. The patient was positioned on his left side with his low lumbar spine flexed and laterally flexed to the right until movement could be palpated at the L4–L5 intervertebral level (Fig. 8-4). In this position, with thumb pressure against the right side of the spinous process of L4 (to stabilize L4), a quick left rotary thrust was applied through the pelvis and to L5 by finger pressure against the left side of L5 spinous process (to pull L5 into left rotation).

Immediately afterward the patient could fully extend, laterally flex,

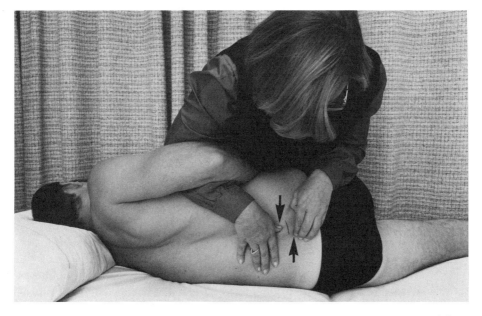

**Fig. 8-4.** Rotary manipulation is used to open the right L4–L5 zygapophyseal joint.

and rotate his trunk to the right with only soreness experienced at the extreme of these movements. This soreness was lessened by gentle large amplitude posteroanterior pressures performed unilaterally over the right L4–L5 zygapophyseal joint. The next day the patient reported by telephone that he was symptom free.

## Zygapophyseal Joint Arthropathy (Causing Only Referred Symptoms)

### History

A 50-year-old man described a gradual onset, over 3 days, of aching in the right trochanteric area. This had been present for 1 month. He could not recall any injury to his back, hip, or leg, and he had not experienced pain in any other area. He had no past history of back or lower extremity symptoms.

Radiographs of the lumbar spine and hip were reported to be normal. He was diagnosed by the referring doctor as suffering from trochanteric bursitis.

### Symptoms

The patient experienced a constant deep ache over his right greater trochanter, which was unaltered by posture or activity.

### Signs

Lumbar movements were full and pain free with overpressure. Tests for the neuromeningeal tissues, hip, and trochanteric bursitis were negative.

Deep palpation (through the erector spinae) over the right L4–L5 zygapophyseal joint revealed stiffness, local spasm, and tenderness, and there was an area of thickening at the right side of the interspinous space between L4 and L5. These signs were absent on the left side. Reproduction of referred pain was not possible.

### Interpretation

Anatomically, pathology of the L4–L5 zygapophyseal joint could give rise to referred pain at the trochanteric area. In the absence of other physical signs, it would be appropriate to mobilize the hypomobile L4–L5 zygapophyseal joint and note any effect on his trochanteric aching. An association between the hypomobile L4–L5 zygapophyseal joint and the trochanteric pain can be made only in retrospect.

## Management

The hypomobility was localized to the L4–L5 right zygapophyseal joint; therefore, passive stretching should be localized to this joint.

**Day 1 (Treatment 1).** Posteroanterior oscillatory pressures were applied firmly for 60 seconds to the spinous processes of L4 and L5, and unilaterally over the painful joint. On being questioned, the patient reported no change in his constant trochanteric ache.

**Day 2 (Treatment 2).** The patient reported that his right trochanteric pain was now intermittent (and continued unrelated to movement or to changes of posture of his trunk). The treatment was repeated giving three applications of posteroanterior pressures lasting 60 seconds each. These were interspersed with gentle large amplitude oscillations to ease the local soreness.

**Days 4, 6, and 8 (Treatments 3, 4, and 5).** The patient reported continued improvement of his symptoms and the mobilization of L4–L5 was progressed in strength and sustained for longer periods to achieve a better stretch on the tight soft tissues (capsule and ligaments). At the last visit, it was necessary to place his lower lumbar spine into full extension and direct the posteroanterior pressures more caudally in order to detect any residual hypomobility. By this stage, he experienced only occasional transient aching in his thigh, so treatment was stopped, with a review in 2 weeks.

**Day 22 (Treatment 6).** When reassessed 2 weeks later the patient reported that he was symptom free. Passive mobility tests showed no hypomobility or thickening of soft tissues on the right of the L4–L5 joint.

## Zygapophyseal Joint Arthropathy (Intra-articular Problem)

### History

A 75-year-old woman complained of a sharp pain to the right of L5 following stepping awkwardly with her right foot into a shallow depression in the pavement 1 week previously. She had become aware of aching in her back and this worsened with each step until it became constant. Because her back was both painful and stiff the following morning, she consulted her doctor. He ordered radiographs to be taken, which revealed narrowing of her lumbosacral disc space and osteoarthritic changes in her lumbosacral zygapophyseal joints. She was given anti-inflammatory medication and advised to rest as much as possible. Five days later her pain was no longer constant but certain spinal movements still caused considerable pain and she was referred for physical therapy. She had a past history of low backache for many years if she stood for long periods.

### Symptoms

Sharp pain just lateral to the spinous process of L5 on the right was provoked by turning in bed from a supine position onto her right side, and on bending to the right when standing.

### Signs

All movements of her low lumbar spine were hypomobile. Lumbar extension and lateral flexion to the right reproduced her pain. Pain was experienced at half range, increasing at the limit of these movements.

Palpation of passive accessory movements revealed marked hypomobility of L4–L5 and L5–S1 segments and posteroanterior pressure and transverse pressure to the left reproduced her back pain. Tests for neural mobility and conduction were negative.

### Interpretation

This was an elderly woman with a degenerative, stiff lower lumbar spine. A trivial injury (i.e., a jar up through her right leg) caused the hypomobile joint to become painful.

This was thought to be an intraarticular problem because pain was experienced with movements that closed the right side of the intervertebral joint and because pain was felt early and throughout these movements. Such articular problems respond well to large amplitude passive mobilization, performed carefully to avoid compression of the articular surfaces. Later, when pain is minimal, one may progress to mobilization with the surfaces compressed.

### Management

**Day 1 (Treatment 1).** With the patient lying comfortably on her right side in slight flexion, gentle large amplitude left lateral flexion oscillations were produced by moving the pelvis (Fig. 8-5). Care was taken not to cause any discomfort. Following this, extension and right lateral flexion were reassessed. A favorable response was noted in that pain started later in

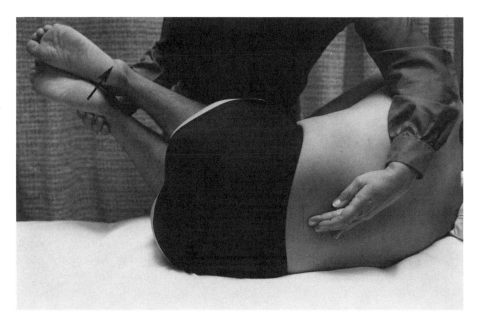

**Fig. 8-5.** Passive left lateral flexion mobilization of the lower lumbar spine, produced by moving the lower limbs and pelvis.

the range of both of these movements. The technique was repeated but no further improvement was noted.

**Day 3 (Treatment 2).** The patient reported no change in her symptoms but the improvement in the signs gained with the first treatment had been maintained. The day 1 treatment was repeated twice, following which the pain response to right lateral flexion improved, but extension was unchanged. The technique was changed to accessory posteroanterior central pressures to L4 and L5, again employing large amplitude movements. This achieved an immediate improvement in the range of extension and a reduction in the pain response.

**Day 5 (Treatment 3).** The patient was delighted with her progress in that she had no pain turning in bed and her daily movements were painless. Mild pain was experienced at the limit of both extension and right lateral flexion. By adding extension to right lateral flexion, sharp pain was produced. For treatment, her lumbar spine was placed in the position of slight right lateral flexion combined with extension. In this position, posteroanterior pressures were performed for 30 seconds as a large amplitude movement, causing slight pain at first. During performance of the technique, the pain disappeared, so the spine was placed further into extension and right lateral flexion. Slight pain was again experienced and again this disappeared with another application of the mobilization. On reassessment, combined right lateral flexion with extension was pain free. Slight pain was experienced only on overpressure.

**Day 7 (Treatment 4).** The patient was still symptom free and right lateral flexion with extension was no longer painful when performed with overpressure. However, when right lateral flexion was added to extension, slight pain was experienced.

The spine was placed in this combined position in the same order (full extension and then full right lateral flexion) and posteroanterior central pressures performed as a strong stretching technique. This caused marked pain and required gentle large amplitude posteroanterior pressures to ease the soreness. Following this the patient complained of aching across her lower lumbar area. Pulsed short-wave diathermy for 15 minutes (on a low frequency and low dosage) eased her ache.

**Days 10 and 24 (Treatments 5 and 6).** The patient remained symptom free but extension plus right lateral flexion still reproduced slight pain to the right of L5. By combining these movements on the left side, a similar pain was produced. This was considered likely to be her normal response and no further treatment was given. This was verified by finding the same signs 2 weeks later, during which time she had remained symptom free.

## Postural Pain

### History

A 28-year-old mother of three children presented with a 6-month history of gradual onset of low back pain. She could not recall an incident that had caused her symptoms. During her third pregnancy 2 years ago, she had experienced the same pain but this had settled after the birth. There was no history of trauma and her radiographs were reported to be normal.

### Symptoms

The patient was asymptomatic in the morning but by midafternoon her low back began to ache. This ache worsened as the day progressed, especially during activities requiring her lumbar spine to be held in sustained flexion (bathing the children, making beds, sweeping, vacuuming) and when lifting the children. Sitting and lying eased the pain.

### Signs

The patient stood with an increased lumbar lordosis; she had a full range of pain-free movements. Overpressure into full extension was painful and by combining this with lateral flexion to either side the pain was made worse on that side. Testing of intervertebral movements revealed excellent mobility with the exception of posteroanterior gliding of L5 on the sacrum, which was slightly hypomobile. Tests for the neuromeningeal tissues were normal. Her lower abdominal and gluteal muscles muscles were slack and weak.

### Interpretation

This was a patient with a young, mobile spine that became painful when the tissues restraining flexion were stressed (posterior ligamentous structures and zygapophyseal joints). There was poor support by the abdominal muscles, which co-contract with the erector spinae and gluteals to stabilize the spine during flexion. Pain was relieved by rest (when stress was taken off the painful tissues).

### Management

**Day 1 (Treatment 1).** An explanation of the cause of the symptoms was given, the need to strengthen the lower abdominals, gluteals, and erector spinae was stressed. Large amplitude accessory posteroanterior mobilization of her L5–S1 joint to restore her normal mobility at this segment will help this joint to become pain free, but the primary objective is to strengthen abdominal, gluteal, and erector spinae muscle groups. This was complemented by postural correction (pelvic tilting) and by giving advice on correct lifting techniques and how to restore the lumbar lordosis after periods of sustained flexion (discussed in more detail in other chapters).

**Day 5 (Treatment 2).** The patient was seen again to check that she was performing her exercises correctly and regularly. As her strength improved the exercises were progressively increased in difficulty. Her lumbosacral joint was again mobilized. She reported no change in her symptoms. She was urged to continue her exercises regularly.

**Day 21 (Treatment 3).** The patient reported that she was virtually symptom free, experiencing slight aching if she was excessively busy and tired. On examination, lumbar extension combined with lateral flexion to each side was full and painless, as was posteroanterior accessory gliding of L5. The patient was discharged with the advice to maintain good muscle support of her spine by regular exercise.

## Coccygeal Pain

### History

A 22-year-old female bank clerk complained of a gradual onset over 3 days of localized coccygeal pain. There was no history of lumbar or pelvic symptoms, trauma, or childbirth.

## Symptoms

The patient's coccygeal pain was present only in sitting and worsened if she slouched. Standing eased her pain almost immediately. Her pain was unaltered by sitting on a hard surface, defecation, or squatting.

## Signs

The patient's sitting posture was poor and passive overpressure to the slouched sitting posture reproduced her coccygeal pain. The addition of cervical flexion and knee extension did not alter her pain. Also the addition of posteroanterior pressure to the coccyx (flexion of the sacrococcygeal joint) did not alter her pain, although the coccyx was very tender.

Lumbar movements were full and pain free to overpressure; however, there was a loss of intersegmental mobility below L3 on both flexion and extension. Testing of intervertebral mobility revealed hypomobility, pain, and spasm on central posteroanterior pressure over L5, but the coccygeal pain was not reproduced. Pain associated with pressure on L5 was unaltered by the addition of posteroanterior pressure on L4. There was no thickening on careful palpation of the sacrococcygeal joint and the ligaments attaching to the coccyx.

## Interpretation

Coccygeal pain of musculoskeletal origin can arise from the sacrococcygeal joint or ligamentous attachments to the coccyx, secondary to direct trauma such as sitting heavily on the buttocks, or childbirth, or be referred from the low lumbar spine. In this case, the lack of coccygeal trauma, pain on passive movement of the coccyx, and thickening of the sacrococcygeal joint or coccygeal ligamentous attachments negated a local source of pain. Local joint signs at L5–S1 incriminated this joint as the source of symptoms. This could be verified by treating the L5–S1 joint and reassessing symptom production by sitting.

## Management

**Day 1 (Treatment 1).** The explanation was given that the likely source of symptoms was the lumbar spine and that treatment would entail correction of sitting posture and restoration of low lumbar joint mobility. Large amplitude accessory posteroanterior mobilization was applied for 60 seconds to L5 to restore normal pain-free mobility. This effected an immediate lessening of the degree of pain on retesting of overpressure to slouched sitting. The technique was repeated with further improvement. The session ended with postural correction of the patient's sitting posture and she was asked to set up a protocol by which she could monitor her sitting posture at work.

**Day 4 (Treatment 2).** The patient reported increased pain associated with sitting, for 2 days following her examination and first treatment; since then her symptoms had greatly improved. On questioning, she reported that she monitored her posture at the completion of each customer transaction. On reassessment, slouched sitting with overpressure was symptom free but her L5–S1 joint remained hypomobile and painful to posteroanterior pressure testing. Day 1 treatment was repeated.

**Day 7 (Treatment 3).** The patient reported that she was symptom free. Since her second treatment she had experienced coccygeal aching only twice, associated with periods of prolonged sitting. Posture correction immediately abolished the aching. The L5–S1 joint was firmly mobilized and home exercises checked and progressed.

## Spinal Stenosis

### History

A 60-year-old ex-nurse complained of a 20-year history of low back pain for which she had never sought treatment. In the last 6 months she had experienced vague aching in both lower limbs, which had become progressively worse to the stage where it now severely interfered with walking. She found that she could still ride her bicycle without pain. Having been a nurse she suspected peripheral vascular disease, possibly secondary to diabetes mellitus. Tests for these were negative. Plain radiographs of her lumbar spine showed narrowing of the L4–L5 disc space and marked bilateral osteoarthrosis of the zygapophyseal joints at L4–L5 and L5–S1. No spondylolisthesis was present.

### Symptoms

Symptoms included deep aching and pain in both calves and the dorsal and lateral aspects of both feet, worse on the left side. Symptoms were provoked by standing for more than 15 minutes or walking for more than 3 to 4 minutes. They were eased only by sitting.

### Signs

Signs included excessive lumbar lordotic curve with adaptive shortening of erector spinae muscles. Extension of the lumbar spine reproduced low back pain and if sustained with passive overpressure for 20 seconds, bilateral calf aching developed. Other lumbar movements were hypomobile below L3, but pain free. SLR was equal on both sides, but there was an increased feeling of posterior thigh tightness on the left. There was no neurologic deficit, and peripheral pulses were normal. Deep palpation (through the erector spinae) revealed bilateral thickening, hypomobility, local spasm, and tenderness over the L4–L5 and L5–S1 zygapophyseal joints. Firm pressure did not reproduce referred leg symptoms.

### Interpretation

Gradual onset of bilateral extrasegmental lower extremity pain associated with walking suggested vascular or neurogenic (cauda equina) etiology. A neurogenic source was supported by the easing of symptoms with sitting, which widens the spinal canal, and by reproduction of both back and bilateral leg pains with lumbar extension. A vascular source was unlikely because leg symptoms were not eased by standing still and her peripheral pulses were normal.

In consultation with her medical practitioner, a computed tomography (CT) scan of her low lumbar spine was taken. This confirmed the presence of spinal canal stenosis at L5–S1 with indentation of the thecal sack.

### Management

**Day 1 (Treatment 1).** Management consisted of an explanation to the patient of the likely etiology of her symptoms and for the need to widen her spinal canal by flattening her lumbar lordosis. Passive mobilization of her lower lumbar zygapophyseal joints would help to ease her back symptoms, possibly by lessening joint effusion.

In crook lying the patient was unable to actively flatten her lumbar curve; therefore, the tight erector spinae were lengthened using a combination of reciprocal relaxation and passive stretching techniques performed at the limit of lumbar flexion in the sitting posture. This resulted in the patient being able to achieve some flattening of her lumbar spine and she was instructed to repeat this 10 times at home, four times daily.

**Day 3 (Treatment 2).** Symptoms were unchanged. Review of active posterior pelvic tilting revealed an improved range of lumbar flexion but poor movement below L3. Lengthening techniques for erector spinae were repeated, but this effected no palpable improvement in low lumbar flexion. In crook lying with the abdominal wall relaxed, anteroposterior mobilization was applied by slowly depressing the abdomen with the thumb pads until the anterior aspect of the vertebral bodies were palpated. Following this, there was improvement in the passive range of low lumbar flexion. This was followed by refining the active posterior tilting exercise to encourage recruitment of the low abdominals. The patient was then asked to gently (submaximal effort) flatten her lumbar spine by hollowing her abdomen.[23] The same regimen of home exercises was prescribed.

**Day 5 (Treatment 3).** Symptoms were unchanged. Treatment 2 was repeated with emphasis on re-education of low abdominal control of low lumbar/pelvic flexion. This included being able to hold the flattened lumbar position while flexing alternate hips.

**Day 8 (Treatment 4).** Symptoms were unchanged and lumbar extension was the same as on day 1. Treatment 2 was repeated with the addition of unilateral posteroanterior mobilization, performed bilaterally L3 to L5. Lumbar extension caused less back pain and, after a second application, extension had to be sustained for 5 seconds before producing back pain. Abdominal hollowing was progressed to standing and maintenance during walking.

**Day 14 (Treatment 5).** The patient was now able to stand for 20 minutes before leg symptoms developed, and walking was unaltered. The improvement gained in lumbar extension from unilateral posteroanterior mobilization had been maintained, so this was repeated. Following this only a vague ache was experienced in the calves after sustaining full extension for 40 seconds. The avoidance of lumbar lordosis when walking was emphasized.

**Day 21 (Treatment 6).** The patient was now able to walk for 6 minutes before needing to sit to relieve her leg symptoms. Treatment 5 was repeated with most time spent on maintenance of a flattened lumbar spine during walking and climbing stairs.

**Day 28 (Treatment 7).** The patient was able to walk 10 to 15 minutes before needing to sit. Treatment 6 was repeated.

**Day 56 (Treatment 8).** When reviewed 1 month later patient reported that she could walk for 20 minutes and that standing to do household duties was symptom free as long as she remembered to maintain her slightly flexed lumbar posture. Her lumbar extension and passive intersegmental mobility L3 to L5 were reassessed and found to have been maintained. The need for ongoing abdominal exercises and lumbar posture correction was emphasized.

## CONCLUSIONS

Most lumbar dysfunctions have a mechanical component that responds well to carefully applied manipulative physical therapy. Manipulative physical therapy is safe, effective, and an important part in the overall management of patients with these conditions. However, the decision to apply manipulative therapy must be based on a thorough examination, sound judgment of which techniques to select, and repeated reassessment of the effects of these techniques if the optimal results are to be achieved.

# REFERENCES

1. Bogduk N, Tynan W, Wilson AS: The nerve supply to the human lumbar intervertebral discs. J Anat 132:39, 1981
2. Bogduk N: The innervation of the lumbar spine. Spine 8:286, 1983
3. Cyriax J: Dural pain. Lancet 1:919, 1978
4. Wyke B: Neurological aspects of low back pain. p. 189. In Jayson MIV (ed): The Lumbar Spine and Back Pain. Sector, New York, 1976
5. Kimmel D: Innervation of the spinal dural mater and dura mater of the posterior cranial fossa. Neurology 10:800, 1961
6. El Mahdi MA, Latif FYA, Janko M: The spinal nerve root innervation and a new concept of the clinicopathological interrelations in back pain and sciatica. Neurochirurgia 24:137, 1981
7. Pedersen HE, Blunck CFJ, Gardner E: The anatomy of lumbo-sacral posterior rami and meningeal branches of spinal nerves (sinu-vertebral nerves). J Bone Joint Surg 38A:377, 1956
8. Simmons FH, Segil CM: An evaluation of discography in the localization of symptomatic levels in discogenic disease of the spine. Clin Orthop 108:57, 1975
9. Grieve GP: Common Vertebral Joint Problems. 2nd Ed. p. 144. Churchill Livingstone, London, 1981
10. Maitland GD: Vertebral Manipulation. 5th Ed. Butterworths, London, 1986
11. Mooney V, Robertson J: The facet syndrome. Clin Orthop 115:149, 1976
12. McCall IW, Park WM, O'Brien JP: Induced pain referral from posterior lumbar elements in normal subjects. Spine 4:441, 1979
13. Edgar MA, Nundy S: Innervation of the spinal dura mater. J Neurol Neurosurg Psychiatry 29:530, 1966
14. Edgar MA, Park WM: Induced pain patterns on passive straight-leg-raising in lower lumbar disc protrusion. J Bone Joint Surg 56B:658, 1974
15. Austen R: The distribution and characteristics of lumbar-lower limb symptoms in subjects with and without a neurological deficit. p. 252. In Proceedings 7th Biennial Conference, Manipulative Physiotherapists Association of Australia, North Fitzroy, Australia, 1991
16. Cyriax J: Textbook of Orthopaedic Medicine. 7th Ed. Vol 1. Baillière Tindall, London, 1978
17. Butler DS: Mobilisation of the Nervous System. Churchill Livingstone, Melbourne, 1991
18. Grant R, Jones M, Maitland GD: Clinical decision making in upper quadrant dysfunction. p. 51. In Grant R (ed): Physical Therapy of the Cervical and Thoracic Spine. Churchill Livingstone, New York, 1988
19. McKenzie RA: The Lumbar Spine. Mechanical Diagnosis and Therapy. Spinal Publications, Waikanae, New Zealand, 1981
20. Kos J, Wolf J: Les menisques intervertebraux et leur role possible dans les blocages vertebraux. Ann Med Phys 15:203, 1972
21. Bogduk N, Jull G: The theoretical pathology of acute locked back: a basis for manipulative therapy. Man Med 1:78, 1985
22. Bogduk N, Twomey LT: Clinical anatomy of the lumbar spine. 2nd Ed. Churchill Livingstone, Melbourne, 1991
23. Richardson C, Jull G, Toppenburg R, Comerford M: Technique for active lumbar stabilisation for spinal protection: a pilot study. Aust J Physiother 38:105, 1992

# 9 | Rehabilitation of Active Stabilization of the Lumbar Spine

*Gwendolen A. Jull*
*Carolyn A. Richardson*

Rehabilitation of the trunk muscle system is one of the most important aspects of treatment undertaken by physical therapists to help patients regain function and to prevent recurring episodes of back pain. A vital function of the muscle system is to support and control the back in posture, movement, and its load-bearing activities. Not surprisingly, current exercise programs emphasize the aim of enhancing active trunk muscle stabilization.[1-3]

## SUPPORT AND CONTROL FOR THE LUMBAR SPINE

The provision of support and control for the lumbar spine involves a complex interaction between many muscles of the trunk and girdles. While some muscles perform and control the primary action, other muscles must work automatically in synergy to balance any asymmetrical forces, control unwanted movement, and offer support to articular structures. The positional and directional requirements of the task dictate the combination of muscles used and the nature of their work.[4-7] The rehabilitation of active trunk stabilization is concerned not only with torque-producing capabilities of muscles in each plane of motion, but more pertinently with a person's ability to automatically coordinate an optimal pattern of muscle activity to control postures and functions safely and effectively.

## Supporting Role of Muscles of the Lumbopelvic Area

All muscles of the trunk and pelvis contribute to trunk control. However, clinicians and researchers recognize that trunk muscles such as the oblique abdominals and the deep transversus abdominis have key roles in spinal support and control.[2,3,8–14] Their anatomic design and location provide a dynamic corsetlike structure suitable for fixation and support. The transversus abdominis, and to a variable extent the internal obliques, further contribute to lumbar noncontractile supportive mechanisms through their attachments to the thoracolumbar fascia.[10,12,15] Here they augment sagittal and coronal plane control. The internal and external oblique abdominals act in synergy with the multifidus to provide rotatory control of the trunk.[16] However, within this synergy, it is primarily the obliques that have the torque-producing capacity to provide the torsional stability in sagittal plane function,[17] whereas rectus abdominis and the erector spinae produce and control the primary movement. As a group, these lateral abdominal muscles have the anatomic design to provide and augment control in all three planes of motion. Optimal and safe function, especially in the sagittal plane, is commensurate with their automatic recruitment to a level sufficient to support the trunk when it is required to carry load and to perform common daily activities. These muscles must be also capable of offering this supporting activity over time.

The short one-joint muscles in the pelvic region also have the anatomic design and alignment to provide major support to the lumbar region. For example, of the hip extensors, gluteus maximus would have the prime supporting role. Of the many, often long fusiform muscles that can perform hip flexion, the deep iliopsoas would be more suited to the supporting role.

In summary, all muscles associated with the lumbar region must contribute in some way to its stabilization. It is argued that the function of some specific muscles is more aligned to a supporting role.

## Dysfunction in Muscles in Their Supporting Role

Studies comparing back pain patients and normal controls, although plagued with variables, have shown that the back muscles and the abdominals become weaker with chronic back pain, and more conclusively, that they lose endurance capacity (see Beimborn and Morrissey[18] for review). Although these studies provide data on gross muscle function, more specific information is required on the pattern and degree to which individual muscles contribute to the dysfunction. This is necessary because clinical evidence suggests that dysfunction may be disproportionate between muscles.[19–21]

Although all abdominal muscles can become weak, the lateral abdominal muscles (i.e., oblique abdominals and transversus abdominis) appear to be particularly vulnerable to loss of their trunk-supporting role.[22,23] There is also some suggestion that lack of control and fatigability of these particular muscles may predispose to back strain. Parnianpour et al[24] required subjects to repeat 15 cycles of full trunk flexion and extension as quickly and as accurately as they could at 70 percent of their maximum extension torque. They found a loss of precision and control, measured particularly as an increase in movement in the transverse and coronal planes with the onset of fatigue. These authors considered that this loss of active control may deny protection to the lumbar structures and could be a mechanism for industrial and recreational injury.

Our own initial investigation of a method to measure the stability capacity of these lateral abdominal muscles found that 8 of 20 asymptomatic subjects demonstrated poor automatic rotatory control of their trunks when required to take the weight of one leg. This was improved when subjects consciously contracted their obliques and transversus abdominis prior to holding their leg weight.[25] Such findings are in accordance with the clinical practice of focusing on activating these muscles.[1-3,8]

Other muscles involved in the control of the lumbopelvic area also appear to be vulnerable to loss of their supporting function. Gluteus maximus (compared to other hip extensors), gluteus medius (compared to other hip abductors), and iliopsoas (compared to other hip flexors) are recognized as muscles that often show signs of dysfunction. Dysfunction in these muscles together with the abdominals could contribute significantly to the onset of back pain.[9,19-21,26]

The conclusion that dysfunction occurs specifically in the supporting muscles has been deduced through clinical observation and laboratory research. There is a need for physical therapists and their patients to have an objective, practical assessment of the specific muscle dysfunction that can be used easily in the clinical situation. Such a measurement would also allow patients to monitor their own improvement with home exercises.

## Clinical Assessment of Specific Supporting Muscle Dysfunction

Recognition of specific deficits in these muscles has led to various indirect methods of clinically assessing the muscles' supporting dysfunction. These include postural analysis and assessment of muscle lengths. Such assessments are based on the premise that a muscle that loses its supporting role usually lengthens due to the effect of gravity. This will indirectly affect various body postures.[9,26,27] Movement patterns are also used to detect dysfunction through a change in muscle recruitment patterns. Muscles such as gluteus maximus may either not be recruited at all or display delayed recruitment in movements such as hip extension.[28]

These assessment procedures, when performed in the clinic, rely on the observational skills of the physical therapist and lack objectivity. It was therefore considered important to develop additional specific tests for these muscles that could illustrate a well-defined deficit in muscle function and that could be easily and objectively measured in the clinic.

The test advocated is one that examines the muscle's ability to activate in isolation under low-load conditions and further tests its ability to hold an isometric contraction. The basis for this test evolved from studying the possible mechanisms that could have caused the loss of support and control in these muscles. Insight into the physiologic changes that occur in antigravity muscles when subjected to disuse could explain clinical findings and rationalize this objective test.

Richardson[29] proposed that patterns of normal use as well as changes that occur due to pain and reflex inhibition lead to a progressive lack of use in such muscles as the oblique abdominals and gluteals. Such supporting, antigravity muscles when subject to disuse are likely to undergo some physiologic changes. Reduced neural input (neural traffic) seems to affect the slow twitch fibers within the muscle to a greater extent than the fast twitch fibers.[30] Many research studies both on animals and humans suggest that the slow-twitch fibers of a disused antigravity muscle take on more of the characteristics and functional role of fast-twitch fibers.[31–40]

Because it is the slow twitch fibers within a muscle that are primarily concerned with postural support,[22] their changing function would affect the support and control offered by the whole muscle. Therefore, when an antigravity muscle is not used over a period of time, it would be reasonable to suggest that it would have particular difficulty sustaining and controlling a low-load isometric contraction (i.e., 30 to 40 percent maximum) without phasic, erratic contractions occurring.

The test advocated requires that the target muscle is assessed in relative isolation so that its functional status is not masked by substitution by other neighboring muscles. Body positioning and limb load is used to help isolate the muscle but no added weight is applied. The patient is asked to hold an isometric contraction with good control. The length of time this contraction is held while maintaining the limb in a steady position provides an objective measure of any dysfunction of the slow twitch fibers within a muscle.

This clinical test has proved very useful for depicting a functional deficit in the supporting muscles. The pelvic–hip muscles such as the gluteals can be tested in some degree of isolation with a carefully applied grade 3 classical muscle test.[9] More sensitivity seems to be obtained if the physical therapist passively lifts the limb into the inner range, then requiring the patient to hold the position. The patient's ability to activate the muscle and maintain the contraction without losing control of limb position can then be assessed.

In relation to the obliques/transversus group, a special low-load test had to be devised that would test their capacity selectively without contribution from rectus abdominis. This was a challenging task, because the classical tests for the oblique abdominals involve a significant contribution by often more active muscles. For example, the external oblique abdominals are usually tested with a trunk curl-up with rotation action.[41] This would necessarily involve rectus abdominis contraction. The internal obliques are tested by ipsilateral pelvic tilting and rotation toward the contralateral side.[41] The oblique abdominal activation would be difficult to differentiate from the contraction of rectus abdominis and quadratus lumborum in such a test. It was the muscle test for transversus abdominis that provided the possible answer. Lacote et al[41] used the action of sucking in the stomach and depressing the abdominal wall to test transversus abdominis function. This is a similar action to drawing in the stomach suggested by Kendall and McCreary[9] as a method of activating an oblique abdominal contraction. It was proposed that such a test may activate both the oblique abdominals and transversus and separate their action from rectus abdominis.

Studies were undertaken to test this assumption. Multichannel electromyography (EMG) was used to investigate this and other methods of activating the supporting muscles of the trunk.[25,42] The results revealed that setting the abdominals by drawing in the stomach and tightening the waist[9] activated the obliques/transversus abdominis muscles and most importantly dissociated their activity from that of rectus abdominis. A similar pattern of activity was demonstrated with an abdominal bracing action.[8] These techniques fulfilled the requirements of the test in that they separated the lateral abdominals from rectus abdominis, but objective methods of quantification were lacking as well as a method of assessing the holding capacity or fatigability of these muscles. A new assessment tool had to be devised to allow these two parameters to be easily quantified in the clinical situation.

This need led to the development of a simple pressure sensor (Stabilizer, Chattanooga, Australia). It consists of a trisectional, single-cell unit made of a nonelastic material. The sensor is inserted between the low back and exercise surface and is inflated to fill the irregularly shaped space. It operates on the principle that body movement or change of position in any plane causes volume changes in the cell, which are measured as pressure changes.

Out studies[42] in the supine crook lying and reclined sitting positions demonstrated that the pressure sensor can be used as a clinical measure to indicate the successful, or not, activation of the lateral abdominal musculature or to detect if incorrect substitution strategies are used (Fig. 9-1). From a baseline pressure of 40 mmHg (i.e., the pressure in the cell that fills the space behind the back giving the patient an awareness only of its presence), the correct abdominal setting or bracing actions cause a slight flattening of the lumbar spine, which registers as a pressure increase of approximately 10 mmHg. Inability to activate the muscles registers as a nil increase in pressure. Inappropriate recruitment of rectus abdominis, to substitute for the correct muscle contraction, causes posterior pelvic tilt and lumbar flexion and this results in a more marked increase in pressure (e.g., up to 20 mmHg).[42] The pressure sensor can be used in conjunction with multichannel EMG to check the correct activation of the abdominal muscles.

The holding capacity or fatigability of these muscles is judged by the time that the correct activation is held. There will be a slight fluctuation ($\pm 2$ mmHg) registered by the pressure sensor with the movement associated with breathing, but fatigue in the muscles can be instantly detected by either a gradual or often quite rapid loss in pressure. A gradual switch to rectus abdominis activity is discernible by a subtle, gradually increasing pressure over time. In this way, the pressure sensor provides both a measure and feedback system for the patient.

This test of abdominal setting by drawing in the stomach and tightening

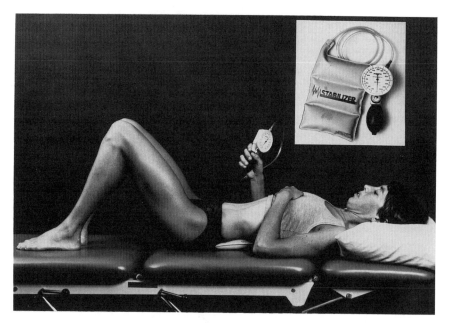

**Fig. 9-1.**   The pressure sensor (inserted) used in the test of the abdominal setting action.

the waist or by a bracing action, as a test of the activation of the lateral abdominals and their holding capacity, appears to be very relevant to these muscles' functional supporting and postural role. It is proving useful as a clinical test. However, further refinement of the technique is needed for its validation as a research tool.

When the dysfunctions in the ability to consciously activate and statically hold and control a muscle contraction are detected in muscles such as the lateral abdominals and key girdle muscles, it provides a specific focus for the initial stages of the stabilization program. We believe that these muscles require specific training in isolation in the first instance, to enhance their activation and to train their supportive role. This initial step is necessary to ensure their appropriate participation in higher levels of function where they are required to coactivate with all trunk and girdle muscle to support and protect the spine.

## A REHABILITATION APPROACH FOR ACTIVE STABILIZATION

The aim of this stabilization program is to re-activate the stabilizing muscles, retrain their holding capacity, and retrain their ability to automatically contract appropriately with other synergists to support and protect the spine under various functional loads and skills. Based on our research and clinical observations, a four-stage progressive approach to stabilization training has been developed. Rehabilitation is commenced at the level appropriate to the patient and progressed sequentially through higher degrees of loaded control and skill. Progression is guided by continuous reassessment.

In focusing on a particular aspect of rehabilitation, it is easy to detract attention from the often complex nature of the physical dysfunction that may be present in the back pain patient. The articular, neural, and muscle systems and their central nervous control are interdependent in function and dysfunction.

In the first instance, pain, swelling, and pathology have powerful influences on the muscle system and muscles quickly react by either inhibition or spasm.[43] Lumbar osseoligamentous stability is aided by an optimal return of movement to the lumbar joints so that the joints can share the load created in normal functional activities. The most obvious illustration of this necessity is demonstrated in the instability that can occur in the segment adjacent to fusion sites in the lumbar spine.[44] Likewise, the range of movement of the joints and tightness in the muscles of the pelvic girdle, hips, and lower limbs can exert substantial influences on lumbar spine posture and movement. Problems in these structures are often present in the back pain patient and are part of the total problem.[9,26,45–49] Movement and muscle control of these regions are closely related. Therefore, any rehabilitation program must evaluate and address the total problem, and emphasis must be placed on the component of rehabilitation of active trunk stabilization.

## Stage 1: Isolation and Facilitation of Target Muscles

In the initial assessment of the oblique abdominals and transversus abdominis, it is found that many back pain patients have an inability to isolate, activate, hold, and control a setting contraction. This constitutes a problem at a very basic level and these dysfunctions must be addressed and abilities restored before the patient can progress further into the program. The patient trains to gain conscious control of these muscles at submaximal levels in this stage.

It is not uncommon to find that patients often experience initial difficulty in re-activating the muscle pattern of the obliques and transversus abdominis voluntarily. There does not seem to be a similar problem in activating rectus abdominis,[3] and patients will readily substitute with this muscle action. It is therefore important from the outset that the patient has a conscious awareness and perception of the correct activation in the setting contraction and can themselves detect when their performance is incorrect or ineffective. The emphasis in this stage is on accuracy. There is not an emphasis on effort, because this will encourage recruitment of inappropriate muscles near and far.

The first essential step in retraining is good demonstration and verbal instruction, because different patients respond to different verbal cues. Varying instructions such as drawing in and hollowing the lower abdomen, drawing the navel up and in toward the spine,[11] or feeling the muscles tighten at the waist[8] may variously cue the patient. When the patient uses substitution strategies

258 *Physical Therapy of the Low Back*

for the correct muscle action, these must be identified and explained to the patient. As previously mentioned, the most common is the often subtle substitution with rectus abdominis that is observed by a posterior pelvic tilt action, a depression in the anterior rib cage, and a tendency for a rounding of anterior abdominal wall rather than a hollowing. Alternatively, patients may effectively mimic the setting action by inhaling and merely elevating their rib cage, which makes their abdomen look flat. From the beginning, the patient must be taught to dissociate breathing from the setting action and learn to breathe normally while activating and holding the abdominal set.

As the patient trains to improve the holding capacity of these muscles, it is not always easy to know whether the abdominal setting action is being performed correctly or when muscle fatigue is occurring. The visual feedback provided by the pressure sensor is proving to be a very potent monitoring and feedback system. It is used in both the teaching and practice of the setting action, providing feedback to the patient, through the pressure readings, of their successful or unsuccessful performance. An inability or poor ability to activate the muscles registers as a nil or minimal increase in pressure, whereas substitution with rectus abdominis will cause pressure changes greater than those associated with the isolated contraction of the obliques and transversus abdominis. In this way, the pressure sensor assists the patient in the motor learning process for acquiring this abdominal setting skill and for training the holding capacity of these muscles. This quantification of performance thus helps in the teaching process and also enhances compliance, especially when practicing at home.

Motor learning abilities and the level of dysfunction in the lateral abdominal muscles will vary between patients, and physical therapists will use the various facilitation techniques at their disposal to encourage conscious activation of the muscles. When patients are having difficulties initially, the easiest positions to teach conscious muscle activation is in four-point kneel or prone lying (Fig. 9-2). These positions use the forward drift of the abdominal contents as a stretch facilitation to the setting action. In the prone position, visual feedback can augment the facilitation. The pressure sensor is placed under the abdomen and inflated to a baseline pressure of approximately 70 mmHg. Instead of trying to increase pressure, as required when the sensor is behind the back, the patient sets the lateral abdominals and draws the stomach off the pad, aiming for a decrease in pressure of at least 10 mmHg.

Manual guidance subtly directed through multifidus in the prone, standing, and sitting positions can also assist activation of the muscle pattern and can be applied by either the therapist or patient. This action directly guides the very subtle lumbar flexion that occurs with the abdominal setting action and also directly facilitates the multifidus, which cocontracts with the obliques to support the spine.

The abdominal setting action is also taught and practiced in the supported standing and sitting positions as well as in supine crook lying. This is a necessary component for postural retraining and for future exercise. Facilitation techniques such as sweep tapping in conjunction with visual feedback can be helpful

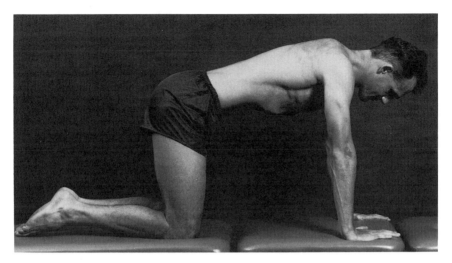

**Fig. 9-2.** Abdominal setting in four-point kneeling position.

here. Although a 10-mmHg increase in the pressure sensor is sought with correct activation in these positions, patients may achieve lesser increases in the preliminary stages. These readings will gradually improve as patients enhance their skills. While the ability to activate the lateral abdominal muscles is required in all the positions mentioned, patients must start training in those where they can more easily achieve the isolated contraction. The emphasis is on attainable goals, because unachievable tasks will encourage substitution strategies.

If patients cannot consciously activate the lateral abdominal muscles and when marked weakness is considered to be a major problem, it may be necessary to begin retraining by using direct resistance to the trunk to encourage activation. It has been shown that a rotatory resistance applied to the trunk via the pelvis or shoulders will directly activate the supporting muscles with little contribution from rectus abdominis.[14] It is also very appropriate to use a technique that emphasizes facilitation of the multifidus within the cocontraction pattern because localized dysfunction in this muscle has been identified. Using diagnostic ultrasound and imaging, a study of patients with their first episode of acute unilateral back pain revealed that there is unilateral inhibition within this multifascicle muscle, primarily at the lumbar level of dysfunction.[50] Providing a reason for this selective segmental inhibition is challenging and it may represent pain inhibition mediated via a long loop reflex pathway.[51] Nevertheless, these findings do provide a basis for including exercise techniques that aim to facilitate multifidus at the dysfunctional segmental level (Fig. 9-3).

The resistance applied in any of these exercises should be low load and facilitatory, with the patient encouraged to sustain the submaximal contraction. Rhythmic stabilizations and alternating isometrics are also suitable techniques to employ to activate particular supporting muscles.[52] While exercises using direct resistance proceed, the patient continues to work to achieve a conscious isolated activation of these muscles.

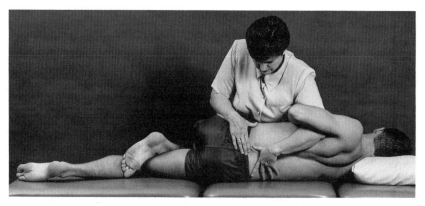

**Fig. 9-3.** The multifidus is facilitated via a gentle rotatory resistance applied to the dysfunctional segment.

The second phase of this initial stage of rehabilitation is directed toward improving the holding capacity of these muscles. Once the patient can consciously activate the abdominal set, they practice to increase the holding time of this contraction. Preference is given to practicing repeated holding contractions short of muscle fatigue. This is to ensure accuracy of training to the lateral abdominal muscles and to prevent the recruitment of unwanted synergists that fatigue may provoke. For example, the patient may practice to hold for 5 seconds, rest 5 seconds, repeating the sequence 10 times and building up the sequence to 10-second intervals. Whenever possible they monitor their performance with the pressure sensor and cease the instant loss of control or substitution is detected.

The holding capacity of these muscles can also be trained by monitoring the control of the abdominal setting action under very low loads provided by unilateral leg movement. A leg movement such as abduction/external rotation (Fig. 9-4) provides a low force that tends to rotate the pelvis and trunk. This addition of a low facilitatory eccentric load is a good method for measurement of holding ability. A loss of control during a continuous abdominal setting contraction while performing repetitions of this leg movement results in rotatory movement of the pelvis and lumbar spine. This movement can be easily detected either through observation or use of feedback from the pressure sensor.

Repetition is essential to this retraining process. Formal practice of these types of exercises should be undertaken at least twice a day to monitor and reinforce effective performance. This is augmented by incorporating regular repetitions of the holding contraction into daily activities. This helps the regimen to not be too invasive on a patient's time. The repeated activation and endurance training of the lateral abdominal supporting muscles is also intimately related to the re-education of static and dynamic postural control and form.

A similar dysfunction to that found in the lateral abdominal muscles is often detected in pelvic girdle muscles such as the gluteals and iliopsoas. It is treated with the same approach of facilitating the muscle in isolation at low

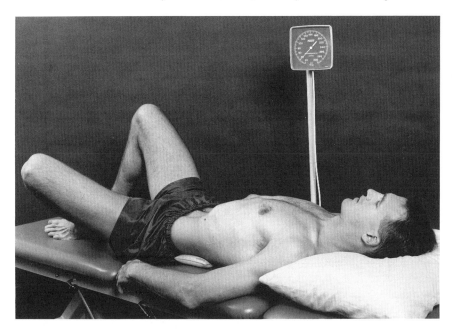

**Fig. 9-4.** Monitoring the ability to sustain an abdominal set with low levels of leg load. Leg rotation in the prone position is also used.

loads and training its holding capacity. Stability of the whole lumbopelvic area is dependent on the support of these muscles, and their rehabilitation is in tandem with that of the lateral abdominals.

This first stage of conscious activation and control of key muscles of the trunk and girdle at low levels of effort must be achieved before the trunk stabilization program can be progressed. The stage can be frustrating for the patient but if these muscles are not capable of functioning at the low levels, their appropriate contribution to more complex motor behaviors and loads is unlikely. The muscle activation is commenced immediately in the rehabilitation program even in the treatment of many acute back pain patients. The minimal loads involved in the exercise techniques do not overload injured structures. The added benefit is that control of pain is often commensurate with the reactivation of the muscle support system.

## Stage 2: Training of Trunk Stabilization Under Static Conditions of Increasing Load

Following their activation in isolation, the lateral abdominal muscles are now trained in their stability role under more functional conditions. This involves retraining the total motor program used for trunk stabilization, which requires a balanced interaction between the lateral abdominals, rectus abdominis, and the back muscles.

The aim of this stage is to enhance muscle control for trunk stabilization by gradually adding load both directly to the trunk and indirectly with the use of limb load. This second stage of stabilization training requires the trunk to be held and controlled in a midposition and continues to train the static capacity of the trunk muscles.

The static mode of training as the initial functional level has several advantages. From a pathoanatomic viewpoint, the lumbar spine is maintained in a more mid- or neutral position. This lessens the risks of adverse stress on the injured or pathologically compromised lumbar articular structures that may be provoked by through range or end-of-range exercises. Training can be progressed to this level even in the early stages of a treatment program.

The level and effectiveness of a patient's muscle control of trunk position for stabilization can be monitored objectively with the pressure sensor in this static method of training. It is placed behind the back to ensure that stabilization of the lumbopelvic region is maintained during the progressively loaded exercise. The principle employed for the use of such a device is that if the trunk muscle control is at an appropriate level and balanced between muscles for the load applied, no movement in the lumbopelvic region will occur and hence there will be no pressure variation during the exercise. In dynamic trunk exercise, it is very difficult if not impossible to quantitatively evaluate if this balance of activity is occurring between the muscles producing and controlling the primary movement and those having a supportive function in that plane.

Another important consideration when training an interaction of muscle activity under conditions of increasing loads is that too much resistance on a weakened muscle can be inhibitory.[19] As already discussed, it is often found clinically that the oblique abdominals and transversus abdominis are often either not automatically recruited appropriately or demonstrate weakness in the back pain patient. With too much load, the patient can easily lose control of trunk stability or substitute with inappropriate muscles and lose the correct synergistic interaction of the trunk muscles. Having the accuracy provided by the pressure sensor in the clinic, it has clearly emphasized that back pain patients often have to start training at very low loads, because it is only at these levels that they can maintain trunk control initially. The objective monitoring system also helps the physical therapist and the patient resist the temptation to add too much load too quickly, but rather concentrate on precision and control. By accurately monitoring the level of control of the coactivation of the trunk muscles, the pressure sensor is used to direct progression of the load safely and appropriately during this stage of stabilization training.

A great deal of emphasis is given to training active trunk stabilization with leg load resistance, because this allows monitoring of control, the feedback helping the patient to focus on the concept of muscle coordination and control rather than the more familiar strengthening types of exercise.

### Static Training with Leg Loading

In the low-load leg exercises, patients continue to consciously set their abdominals prior to and during the exercise to ensure activation of the obliques and transversus abdominis in the total trunk motor program. They monitor their

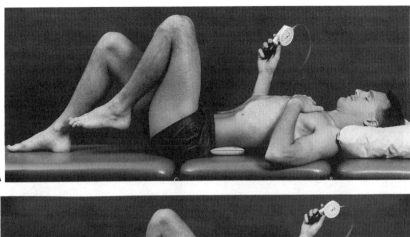

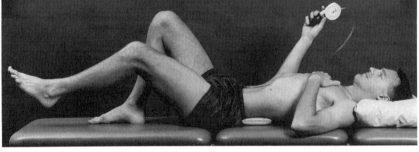

**Fig. 9-5.** Crook lying, low-level unilateral leg loads using straight or diagonal lifts. Arms should not provide trunk support. (**A**) Single leg lift to 90° hip flexion and lowering. (**B**) Single leg extension and flexion movement.

performance with the pressure sensor and cease the exercise if control is lost or with the onset of fatigue. It should be noted that preference is given to exercises involving unilateral leg-loading activities. The leg movement can be in the sagittal plane or the leg placed in some degree of abduction to allow diagonal movement. Such unilateral exercises highlight the demand for rotatory control by the lateral abdominal muscles to complement the activity of rectus abdominis and the back extensors (Fig. 9-5).

Progression of leg loading can be given in a variety of starting positions (Fig. 9-6). Attention is simultaneously given to correct activation and control of the girdle muscles during these exercises. For example, both trunk control and appropriate gluteus maximus activity should be monitored in prone, leg extension exercises. Load is gradually and carefully increased to both the trunk and girdle muscles by methods such as increasing limb lever length or by adding resistance to the limbs with elastic straps or light weights.

Once the patient has progressed through the program to the higher leg load exercises (Fig. 9-7), automatic activation of the lateral abdominal muscles in balance with rectus abdominis should now be occurring. To reinforce this balance, the patient aims to maintain a steady reading on the pressure sensor as well as maintaining a flattish abdominal wall during the exercise.[11]

Additional types of exercises are given in this stage in conjunction with

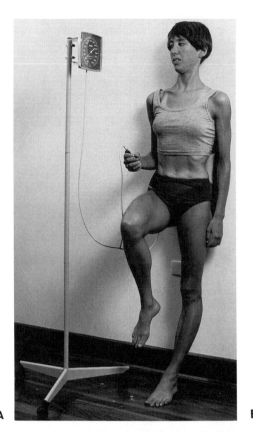
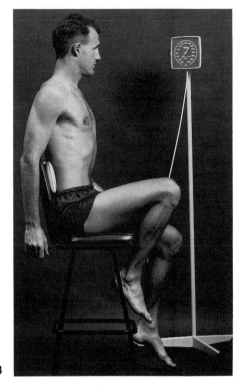

**Fig. 9-6.** Examples of leg loading activities in the sagittal plane: **(A)** standing unilateral hip flexion, **(B)** sitting unilateral hip flexion, **(C)** prone lying unilateral hip extension.

leg-loading activities. This is necessary so that the patient learns muscle control in a variety of situations.

### Static Training with Direct Resistance to the Trunk

Isometric trunk exercises using such techniques as rhythmic stabilizations in a variety of starting positions are useful exercises for the clinic.[52] Control of the lumbar spine in a neutral or midposition continues to be emphasized.

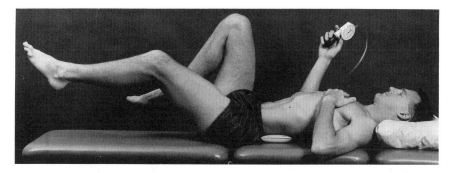

**Fig. 9-7.**   An example of higher level of unilateral leg loading.

This type of exercise can be adapted for self-application at home (Fig. 9-8). The manual resistance applied by either the therapist or the patient at home should be well controlled, the magnitude of resistance aimed at working the trunk muscles at approximately 30 percent of their maximum in line with their holding and controlling role. At later stages, the speed of change of application of resistance can be increased to facilitate automatic postural responses.

### Static Training Using Different Body Positions

Trunk muscle control in the neutral position of the lumbar spine is trained in a variety of body positions, with the four-point kneeling and bridging positions being especially useful. Exercises are progressed through increasing degrees of difficulty, introducing more unstable bases and making more strength and endurance demands on the trunk stabilizers (Fig. 9-9).

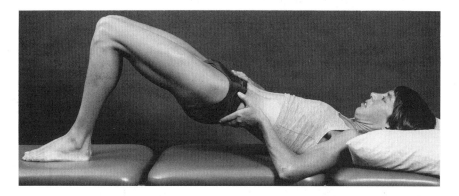

**Fig. 9-8.**   Self-applied rotatory resistance in the bridge position while the patient consciously sets the abdomen.

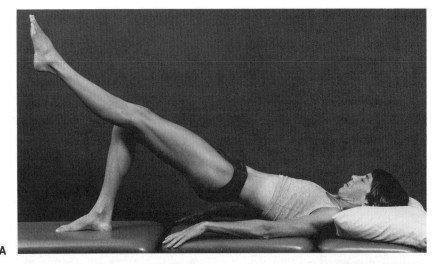

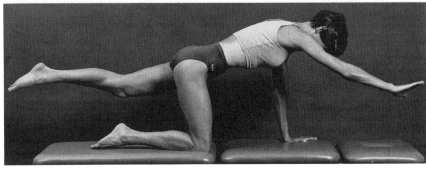

**Fig. 9-9(A&B).**    Static training in different positions. The patient must control the trunk in a neutral position.

### Static Trunk Control in Conjunction with Other Treatment Techniques

Trunk control is emphasized and monitored in other components of the total management program of the back pain patient. This is particularly relevant to muscle-lengthening techniques where the shortened muscle has attachments to either the lumbar spine or pelvic girdle. Such muscles include the hamstrings, tensor fascia lata and iliotibial band, rectus femoris, the iliopsoas (when tight) and upper limb muscles such as latissimus dorsi (Fig. 9-10). Substitute movement or loss of control of the neutral position of the lumbar spine can mimic apparent muscle length gains. This not only reduces the effectiveness of muscle lengthening techniques, but more importantly can make the lumbar joints vulnerable to strain. Likewise, trunk control is emphasized in exercise used to strengthen the lower or upper limb musculature.

Throughout all exercises in this second stage of trunk stabilization training,

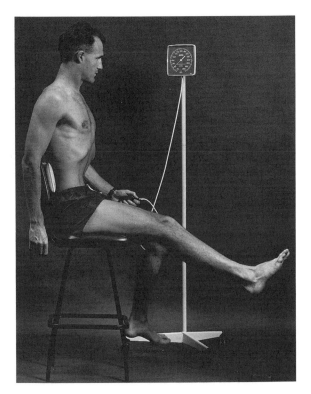

**Fig. 9-10.**   Lengthening of hamstrings in sitting combined with training for active trunk control.

the patient works to control a mid- or neutral position of the lumbopelvic complex and attention is simultaneously directed toward the correct activation of the girdle muscles. Substitution strategies that the patient may attempt to adopt to control the trunk position need to be carefully monitored, explained to the patient, and corrected.

## Stage 3: Development of Trunk Stabilization During Slow Controlled Movement of the Lumbar Spine

Once stability has been trained through static stabilization procedures, the program is progressed to introduce controlled trunk movement (i.e., movement of the trunk with appropriate activation of the supporting muscles). If progressive training has been followed, automatic protective muscle stabilization should now begin to occur during movement. If necessary, the patient can still voluntarily activate the supporting muscles, because movement is slow enough to gain conscious feedback for activation.

Trunk movement is resisted in each plane of motion. Resistance or load

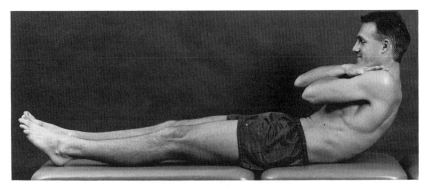

**Fig. 9-11.** Slow controlled curl-up with emphasis on the correct abdominal interaction.

can be applied to the trunk muscles using body weight and exercise apparatus, and through functional retraining. Exercises such as curl-ups and curl-ups with rotation are appropriate at this stage, provided that they are undertaken at a slow speed and the lateral abdominal muscles are active with rectus abdominis (Fig. 9-11). A flattish abdominal wall during the curl-up is indicative of a more balanced activity.[11] Trunk control during back extension exercises can be enhanced by incorporating activation of the lower scapular stabilizers and lateral abdominal muscles.

Isokinetic apparatus can be used in this stage to provide accommodating resistance to through range trunk movements. Exercise can be conducted in each of the sagittal, coronal, and importantly, transverse planes. Programs can be instituted for both concentric and eccentric work.

This stage also introduces the more advanced functional retraining or work hardening. Emphasis is on quality of movement and muscle control. Lifting, carrying, pushing, or other activities as required by the patient's occupation are gradually progressed to heavier loads.

Physical therapists are familiar with the types of exercise and functional retraining that are performed in this third stage of stabilization training. The important issue is that with movement, there are difficulties in objectively monitoring if the appropriate levels of activation are occurring in the trunk muscles in their stability role. For this reason it is prudent not to progress to this stage until the patient can demonstrate trunk muscle control under the measurable static positions of stage 2.

## Stage 4: Lumbar Stabilization During High-Speed and Skilled Movement

When the patient's sport or occupation involves high-speed or skilled movements, it is necessary to ensure that there is adequate stabilization and muscle control for these activities. These high-speed activities should not be introduced too early into a treatment program, and indeed more ballistic-type exercises should not form part of a program to enhance stabilization. High-speed phasic activity is the antithesis of the tonic continuous activity required for joint support.

This delay in introducing high-speed movement is in response to several factors. Our approach to the retraining of stabilization has been essentially based on the ability to monitor if the supporting muscles are capable of controlling the lumbopelvic area, and secondly on the patient's ability to consciously correct and retrain the muscles in order to gain automatic activation in the supporting muscles. Both these elements become very difficult to achieve when the patient is performing fast, highly skilled activities and exercises. For this reason the first three stages of the program are more suited to the training of dysfunction in the supporting muscles.

In addition, the action of the muscles aligned with stability may be adversely affected by a person performing a predominance of fast repetitive movements. This may even be a factor in the development of poor postural control and supporting ability. It is pertinent to briefly review some studies on the effects of fast movements on the muscle system, because their results explain why an emphasis on this stage of rehabilitation is unwise and why those engaging in various training and fitness programs involving a predominance of such activities need to be closely monitored.

Research has been directed to muscles of the knee, ankle, hip, and more recently the trunk. Richardson and Bullock[53] studied the effect of increasing speeds of ballistic knee flexion–extension movements on the quadriceps musculature. They found that within the knee extensor muscle group, increasing speeds of movement were associated with increasingly higher levels of rectus femoris activity. The vastus medialis and vastus lateralis, in contrast, demonstrated no increase in activity levels with increasing speeds of knee movement. These results highlight a possible relationship between rapid knee joint movement and reduced activity in the surrounding one-joint supporting muscles.

Similar findings have been described for the ankle plantarflexors with the two-joint gastrocnemius more activated in fast repetitive plantar flexion than the antigravity, stabilizing muscle, soleus. Smith et al[54] found that the gastrocnemius of the cat performed the very rapid movements of paw shaking while soleus was inhibited. A study on humans confirmed this pattern of muscle activation.[55] Subjects were trained over a 4-week period in rapid plantar flexion, heel-raising movements in standing. Significant increases in jumping height abilities were found but these were accompanied by a significant loss of static function of the soleus muscle. Repeating rapid plantar flexion movements could reduce the stability role of the soleus.

It appears that gluteus maximus may react in a similar way when exposed to repetitive, fast hip extension activities. A study of elite track cyclists determined that these subjects had a significantly reduced ability to hold an inner range gluteus maximus contraction when compared to a noncycling control population.[56] In fact, most cyclist subjects could not hold the position at all.

There is also evidence that repetition of fast trunk movements may be related to reduced trunk stabilization. Thortensson et al[57] reported that increasing the speed of trunk flexion movement resulted in increased rectus abdominis activity, which was not accompanied by similar increases in the oblique abdominal muscle activity. A recent study investigated the effect of speed of performance of curl-up exercises on subjects' ability to actively stabilize their lumbar spine.[58] This was measured by the ability to hold the lumbar spine steady during leg extension movements in supine while load was increased by increments of leg weight. It was shown that subjects who regularly performed curl-ups at high speeds demonstrated lower levels of active stabilization, whereas higher levels were demonstrated by those subjects who regularly performed curl-ups in a slow and controlled fashion.

The results of these studies of the effects of high-speed movement on the nature of muscle activity highlight the importance in stabilization training of progressing the patient slowly and methodically through the earlier stages of the program. This is to ensure that automatic and appropriate levels of stabilization can be achieved before this more advanced final stage. This fourth stage of training is principally required for those patients whose life-style demands include fast and skilled movements (e.g., sports persons or those involved in high levels of physical activity). It is not routinely given to all patients. When required, retraining is approached by first progressively increasing the speed at which various formal exercises for the trunk or limbs are performed. This can then be transferred to increasing the rate at which functional activities are attempted. In this way the rehabilitation of trunk stabilization can be progressed to this highest level of speed and skill.

## CONCLUSIONS

Physical therapists worldwide recognize the importance of retraining active trunk stabilization within the total management program of the back pain patient, as well as in preventative programs. This is reflected both in the literature and in current instructional programs. This type of training, which initially emphasizes control in a midtrunk position, has the advantage of allowing exercise to be introduced early in the treatment program.

The key factors that have influenced the development of the program presented here are evolving from our research. This has been concerned with methods of identifying and measuring the nature of dysfunction of muscles, in their supporting role, through an isolated test of their activation and holding capacity. Additionally a pressure sensor has been developed as a simple clinical method to measure the complex interaction of all trunk muscles to provide support for the trunk by monitoring a steady trunk position when distal load is applied.

Providing methods by which both the physical therapist and patient can appreciate the muscle dysfunction, in objective terms, has given a positive step forward in enhancing the effectiveness and efficiency of stabilization exercises. Physical therapists are able to quantify the dysfunction, and therefore plan a suitable level of exercise for the patient. In addition, patients are most compliant when they can understand the dysfunction in their muscles and can monitor their own progress during rehabilitation. This is vital because the relearning and retraining of the ability of the trunk muscles to optimally support the spine may take some patients several weeks and may also require long-term exercise training to prevent the recurrence of their pain.

There are multiple causes of muscle dysfunction and the loss of optimal control for trunk stabilization. This program is presented as a step forward in the gradual understanding of a complex problem. It is one that blends clinical effectiveness with a rationale based on current research. It is hoped that it stimulates further research initiatives into the effectiveness of physical therapy exercise programs for the rehabilitation and prevention of back pain.

## REFERENCES

1. Saal JA, Saal JS: Nonoperative treatment of herniated lumbar intervertebral disc with radiculopathy. An outcome study. Spine 14:431, 1989
2. Liemohn W: Exercise and the back. Rheum Dis Clin North Am 16:945, 1990
3. Robison R: The new back school prescription: stabilization training part I. Occup Med 7:17, 1992
4. Farfan H: Muscular mechanism of the lumbar spine and the position of power and efficiency. Orthop Clin North Am 6:135, 1975
5. Kumar S: Physiological responses to weight lifting in different planes. Ergonomics 23:987, 1980
6. Pope MH, Anderson GBJ, Broman et al: Electromyographic studies of lumbar trunk musculature during the development of axial torques. J Orthop Res 4:288, 1986
7. Oddson L, Thorstensson A: Task specificity in the control of intrinsic trunk muscles in man. Acta Physiol Scand 139:123, 1990
8. Kennedy B: An Australian program for management of back problems. Physiotherapy 66:108, 1980
9. Kendall FP, McCreary EK: Muscles. Testing and Function. 3rd Ed. Williams & Wilkins, Baltimore, 1983
10. Gracovetsky S, Farfan H, Helleur C: The abdominal mechanism. Spine 10:317, 1985
11. Miller MI, Medeiros JM: Recruitment of internal oblique and transversus abdominis muscles during the eccentric phase of the curl-up exercise. Phys Ther 67:1213, 1987
12. Tesh KM, Dunn JS, Evans JH: The abdominal muscles and vertebral stability. Spine 12:501, 1987
13. Zetterberg C, Anderson GBJ, Schultz AB: The activity of individual trunk muscles during heavy physical loading. Spine 12:1035, 1987
14. Richardson C, Toppenberg R, Jull G: An initial evaluation of eight abdominal exercises for their ability to provide stabilisation for the lumbar spine. Aust J Physiother 36:6, 1990
15. Macintosh JE, Bogduk N, Gracovetsky S: The biomechanics of the thoracolumbar fascia. Clin Biomech 2:78, 1987
16. Macintosh JE, Bogduk N: The detailed biomechanics of the lumbar multifidus. Clin Biomech 1:196, 1986
17. Bogduk N, Twomey LT: Clinical Anatomy of the Lumbar Spine. 2nd Ed. Churchill Livingstone, Melbourne, 1991

18. Beimborn DS, Morrissey MC: A review of the literature related to trunk muscle performance. Spine 13:655, 1988
19. Janda V: Muscles, motor regulation and back problems. p. 27. In Korr IM (ed): The Neurologic Mechanisms in Manipulative Therapy. Plenum, New York, 1978
20. Janda V, Schmid HJA: Muscles as a pathogenic factor in back pain. p. 1. In Proceedings 4th International Conference of the International Federation of Orthopaedic Manipulative Therapists. Christchurch, New Zealand, 1980
21. Sahrmann SA: Muscle imbalances in the orthopaedic and neurological patient. p. 836. In Proceedings 10th International Congress of the World Confederation for Physical Therapy. Sydney, Australia, 1987
22. Caix M, Outrequin G, Descottes B et al: The muscles of the abdominal wall: a new functional approach with anatomical deductions. Anat Clin 6:101, 1984
23. Nouwen A, Van Akkerveeken PF, Versloot JM: Patterns of muscular activity during movement in patients with chronic low back pain. Spine 12:777, 1987
24. Parnianpour M, Nordin M, Kahanovitz N, Frankel V: The triaxial coupling of torque generation of trunk muscles during isometric exertions and the effect of fatiguing isoinertial movements on the motor output and movement patterns. Spine 13:982, 1988
25. Jull G, Richardson C, Toppenberg R et al: Towards a measurement of active muscle control for lumbar stabilisation. Aust J Physiother 39:187, 1993
26. Jull GA, Janda V: Muscles and motor control in low back pain: assessment and management. p. 253. In Twomey LT, Taylor JR (eds): Physical Therapy of the Low Back. Churchill Livingstone, New York, 1987
27. Sahrmann S: Postural applications in the child and adult. Neurodevelopmental aspects. Adult posturing. p. 295. In Kraus S (ed): TMJ Disorders. Management of the Craniomandibular Complex. Churchill Livingstone, New York, 1988
28. Bullock-Saxton J: Changes in muscle function at hip and low back following chronic ankle sprain. p. 1470. In Proceedings 11th International Congress of the World Confederation for Physical Therapy. London, 1991
29. Richardson CA: The need for more precise methods of testing and exercising stability muscle function. (Submitted for publication)
30. Kuno M: An hypothesis for neural control of the speed of muscle contraction in the mammal. Adv Biophys 17:69, 1984
31. Fischbach GD, Robbins N: Changes in contractile properties of disused soleus muscle. J Physiol 201:305, 1969
32. Edstrom L: Selective atrophy of red muscle fibres in the quadriceps in long standing knee joint dysfunction: injuries to the anterior cruciate ligament. J Neurol Sci 11:551, 1970
33. Ianuzzo CD: The cellular composition of human skeletal muscle. p. 31. In Knuttgren HG (ed): Neuromuscular Mechanisms for Therapeutic and Conditioning Exercise. University Park Press, Baltimore, 1976
34. Oganov V, Skuratova S, Potapov N, Shirvindkaye M: Physiological mechanisms of adaptation of skeletal muscles of mammals to the weightless state. p. 17. In Cuba F, Maredal G, Takacs O (eds): Advances in Physiological Science. Pergamon Press, Hungary, 1980
35. Zetterberg C, Aniansson A, Grimby G: Morphology of the paravertebral muscles in adolescent idiopathic scoliosis. Spine 8:457, 1983
36. White MJ, Davies CTM: The effects of immobilisation, after lower leg fractures, on the contractile properties of human triceps surae. Clin Sci 66:277, 1984
37. Fitts RH, Brimmer CJ: Recovery in skeletal muscle contractile function after prolonged hindlimb immobilization. J Appl Physiol 59:916, 1985

38. Richardson CA: Atrophy of vastus medialis in patellofemoral pain syndrome. p. 400. In Proceedings 10th International Congress of the World Confederation for Physical Therapy. Sydney, Australia, 1987
39. Templeton GH, Sweeney HL, Himson BF et al: Changes in fibre composition of soleus muscle during hind limb suspension. J Appl Physiol 65:1191, 1988
40. Appell HJ: Muscular atrophy following immobilisation: a review. Sports Med 10: 42, 1990
41. Lacote M, Chevalier AM, Miranda A et al: Clinical Evaluation of Muscle Function. Churchill Livingstone, London, 1987
42. Richardson CA, Jull GA, Toppenberg R, Comerford M: Techniques for active lumbar stabilisation for spinal protection: a pilot study. Aust J Physiother 38:105, 1992
43. Ekholm J, Eklund G, Skoglund S: On the reflex effects from the knee joint of the cat. Acta Physiol Scand 50:167, 1960
44. Froning EC, Frohman B: Motion of the lumbosacral spine after laminectomy and spine fusion. Correlation of motion with the result. J Bone Joint Surg 50A:897, 1968
45. Pope MH, Bevins T, Wilder DG, Frymoyer W: The relationship between anthropometric, postural, muscular and mobility characteristics of males aged 18–55. Spine 10:644, 1985
46. Mellin G: Correlations of hip mobility with degree of back pain and lumbar spine mobility in chronic low back pain patients. Spine 13:668, 1988
47. Mierau D, Cassidy JD, Yong-Hing K: Low-back pain and straight leg raising in children and adolescents. Spine 14:526, 1989
48. Sward L, Erikssen B, Peterson L: Anthropometric characteristics, passive hip flexion and spinal mobility in relation to back pain in athletes. Spine 15:376, 1990
49. Waddell G, Somerville D, Henderson I, Newton M: Objective clinical evaluation of physical impairment in chronic low back pain. Spine 17:617, 1992
50. Hides JA, Stokes MJ, Saide M et al: Asymmetry of lumbar multifidus muscle size measured by real-time ultrasound imaging in patients with acute back pain. Spine (in press)
51. Stokes MJ, Hides JA, Jull GA, Cooper DH: Mechanism of human paraspinal muscle wasting with acute low back pain, abstracted. J Physiol 452:280p, 1992
52. Sullivan PE, Markos PD: Clinical Procedures in Therapeutic Exercise. Reston Publishing, Reston, VA, 1987
53. Richardson CA, Bullock MI: Changes in muscle activity during fast, alternating flexion-extension movements of the knee. Scand J Rehabil Med 18:51, 1986
54. Smith JO, Betts B, Ederton VR, Zernicke RF: Rapid ankle extension during paw shakes: selective recruitment of fast ankle extensors. J Neurophysiol 43:612, 1980
55. Ng G, Richardson CA: The effects of training triceps surae using progressive speed loading. Physiother Theory Pract 6:77, 1990
56. Richardson CA, Sims K: An inner range holding contraction. An objective measure of stabilising function of an antigravity muscle. p. 829. In Proceedings 11th International Congress of the World Confederation for Physical Therapy, London, 1991
57. Thortensson A, Oddsson L, Carlson H: Motor control of voluntary trunk movements in standing. Acta Physiol Scand 125:309, 1985
58. Wohlfahrt DA, Jull GA, Richardson CA: The relationship between the dynamic and static function of the abdominal muscles. Aust J Physiother 39:9, 1993

# 10 Intensive Physical Rehabilitation for Back Pain

Lance T. Twomey
James R. Taylor

The current epidemic of low back pain and spinal dysfunction in Western society, with its consequent huge costs to the individual and to the communities concerned, has demanded increasing attention in recent years. It is suggested that contemporary health science is currently unable to contain the ever-increasing costs of treatment,[1] and is failing to provide definitive answers to the multifaceted problem. However, closer analysis and investigation reveals that in some areas there have been significant recent advances, particularly in our ability to rehabilitate those with chronic back pain.[2,3]

Few people escape back problems and associated pain during their lives and all vertebral columns show changes with age that make them potentially less able to cope with the variety of physical stresses of daily life. It is now generally considered that 80 percent of adults in Western industrialized societies suffer low back pain during their lifetime. In terms of work loss and treatment costs, back pain is the single most expensive musculoskeletal ailment in Western society.[1,4,5] At any time, about 40 percent of any large gathering will indicate that they currently have low back pain, while as many as 60 percent of the population will have experienced some degree of low back pain in the past year.[6] For many years it has been assumed that low back pain is an epidemic only in industrialized societies, but is not a significant problem in less "developed" countries. However, recent research indicates that when back pain clinics are opened in less industrialized societies, people flock there for treatment.[7]

It is unlikely that the prevalence of back pain has significantly altered in recent years, but the cost to the community is now much better understood.

In the absence of a complete knowledge of the pathogenesis of back pain, and because of the inadequacy of some diagnostic procedures, many of the diagnostic labels attached to patients are uncertain and treatment is often empirical.[2,4] However, recent biologic and epidemiologic studies continue to fill in the gaps in our knowledge of normal spinal structure and function, and of the patterns of age changes and related pathology in the spine.[5] Low back pain and low-back dysfunction or disability need to be carefully distinguished.[1] While both may reflect pathology and structural change, soft-tissue or biochemical pathology are not readily diagnosed by current investigative methods and the assessment of pain and dysfunction still rests primarily on the individual's subjective history. This is influenced by the patient's beliefs and attitudes,[8] and the subjective report of the severity of back pain may reflect a host of other influences. These influences include concepts as diverse as a person's learned response to pain, their interpretation of the meaning of their back pain, and avoidance behavior associated with unpleasant aspects of the patient's lifestyle or occupation.

## EXERCISE AND BACK PAIN

This chapter does not consider the treatment of acute low back pain, since this is covered elsewhere in this volume and because there are so many treatment methodologies used by orthodox and alternative medicine that appear to be effective. The reader is referred to Grieve[9] and to Corrigan and Maitland[10] for excellent descriptions of many of the methods used. This chapter does consider the treatment of chronic low back pain, since it is this disorder that is most prevalent in all Western societies and has been the focus of considerable research effort with some important progress made during the last decade.

In recent years, it has become abundantly clear that physical activity is beneficial and necessary to patients with back pain; active rehabilitation not only restores function, but is also strongly associated with a reduction in pain.[1,3,5,8,11–13] There is no evidence that prolonged rest, or the avoidance of exercise/activity brings about a reduction in chronic back pain; indeed the evidence supports the view that except for a short period after injury, rest has no effect on the natural history of back pain. A number of studies suggest that prolonged inactivity accentuates the problem and may increase the severity of the pain.[13,14] In spite of this evidence, bed rest, analgesics, the prescription of corsets, and the avoidance of physical activity are still the most commonly prescribed forms of medical treatment.[1,15]

There is no doubt that prolonged bed rest and inactivity brings about profound deleterious changes to the musculoskeletal system.[16,17] There is a decline in physical fitness, a marked reduction in muscle strength, a reduction in joint range and flexibility, and a decline in bone mass in those individuals whose activity levels are severely curtailed.[16,18,19] All parts of the musculoskeletal system demand constant use throughout life and even into extreme old age to maintain their strength and efficiency. In the spine, the health of joints is largely dependent on repeated low stress movements. The intervertebral discs and the articular cartilage of the facet joints are dependent on the "stirring effect" of movement for the maintenance of adequate fluid transfer and nutrition in their avascular cartilage.[17,20] A habitual reduction in activity levels is inevitably associated with a decline in a person's ability to react appropriately to changes in the environment. A return to physical work, after a period of bed rest for chronic back pain, exposes an individual to risk of further back injury, since the individual's state of musculoskeletal fitness is much lower than it was when the back pain initially caused the person to stop work. Such individuals are weaker, less mobile, and fatigue more rapidly than before they stopped work and it is little wonder they often suffer an early recurrence of their back pain problem on return to work.[3,13] Much of the lost productivity in industry, resulting from work absence due to back pain, relates to the physical changes directly resulting from bed rest and inactivity.[15,20]

## PHYSICAL REHABILITATION

In recent years, an improved understanding of the relationship between back pain and activity and of the deleterious effects of prolonged disuse, has resulted in a new approach to treatment in many centers.[1,3,13] This approach concentrates initially on the need to gain a comprehensive "baseline" measure of back function and fitness and pain levels. Patients are then fitted into a program of intensive physical therapy appropriate to their physical status. This will often include a behavior modification program, aimed at rapid functional restoration and a return to work as soon as possible. The success of such programs can be measured by marked improvements in physical capacity and function and particularly by the ability to return to the workplace. Improvement during the course of the program should not be judged solely by the patients' subjective self-reports on their pain levels, since this is often modified substantially by legal, psychological, financial, and social factors.[21] It is important to note that at the conclusion of such programs of intensive physical reconditioning a significant reduction in subjective pain measures are consistently reported.[1,21–23] As a general rule, people who are physically fit recover faster from any musculoskeletal ailment.[22,24,25] Thus McQuade et al[25] have shown that the stronger the individual with chronic back pain, the less that person appears to be limited by the condition, and also that the higher the aerobic work capacity, the more active and flexible is that individual. They showed that reports of back pain intensity were not increased by exercise; indeed many subjects reported feeling better following vigorous activity. The recent advances in the intensive physical rehabilitation of patients of all ages with chronic back pain have developed principally from the treatment of young athletes with sports injuries.[3,24] It has been known for some years that athletes with severe musculoskeletal damage (including back injury) respond very well to intensive programs of physical treatment.[24,26]

## MEASUREMENT OF FUNCTION

Measurements of spinal performance have proved difficult to devise and slow to gain acceptance because of the complexity of the vertebral column, which consists of a multitude of small joints, covered by large fleshy muscles with overlapping attachments, allowing complex multiplanar movements.[27] However, it is now possible to measure many aspects of the movement behavior and mechanical capacity of the vertebral column by noninvasive technologies that have been verified in laboratory and clinical trials.[3,5,28]

### Measures of Physical Function

The following techniques are used to measure and assess physical function.

1. Ranges of lumbar movements, using instruments such as the lumbar spondylometer and rotameter[29,30]
2. Isokinetic trunk strength, using isokinetic dynamometers such as Cybex, Kin Com, and Isostation B200[23,28]
3. Measures of muscle endurance for trunk extensor and flexor muscles[23,25,31]
4. Measures of cardiovascular fitness and efficiency using standardized fitness tests[32]
5. Static and dynamic lifting using fixed loads or dynamometry[3,12,23]
6. Measures of functional capacity: these are usually especially constructed for each subject and reflect the working conditions to which it is expected they will return[2,13]
7. Dynamic obstacle course: a timed test stimulating activities of daily living, and requiring the person to complete the series of tasks in many different positions[3]

### Measures of Behavioral Function

The behavioral self-report measures available are many and different clinics use many combinations of them. They include such tests as the Oswestry low-back pain/disability questionnaire; visual pain analog scale; quantitative pain drawing; Minnesota Multiphasic Personality Inventory; and Middlesex Hospital Questionnaire.

Patients are measured prior to and at the conclusion of the intensive physical treatment programs and at regular intervals during the program. In addition, every aspect of their physical work activity is carefully monitored to assess ongoing performance levels. Regular follow-up assessment is done at 6 weeks, and 3-, 9-, and 12-month intervals after the conclusion of the programs.

## PHYSICAL TRAINING AND WORK HARDENING

After the initial measurement of full medical diagnosis and assessment, patients begin a program of intensive physical therapy and work conditioning for 8 to 10 hours a day over 3 or 4 weeks.[3,13] Each program is carefully tailored to meet the particular requirements of the entering individuals, and is closely monitored by appropriately trained staff. The patient's working day consists of a well-constructed mix of weight training, aerobic and fitness work, functional activity, relaxation and stress training, work hardening, educational instruction, and where appropriate, behavior modification. All programs emphasize active participation, encourage the individuals to continue to persist at their tasks irrespective of their back pain levels, and demand a progressive increase in work output as the program proceeds. Cardiovascular fitness is always included as a central element, since it plays a most important role in back injury and in prevention.[32,33]

There is always an accompanying back education component that teaches the patients about the structure, function, and pathology of the vertebral column. This segment needs to allow considerable opportunity for dialogue between educator and patients and seeks to ensure that patients develop a proper understanding of their particular back problem and its management. Thus the educational component should include both group and individual counseling. This is usually done by a clinical psychologist who may be using behavior modification, relaxation, and pain management techniques.

The whole thrust of these programs is directed toward preparing each individual for return to work. Thus specific programs of work hardening need to be constructed and implemented. The aim is to return the individual to the previous occupation wherever possible. At times, either the workplace requires modification or the patient requires retraining for a modified or different occupation. In these circumstances, the physical and occupational therapists should work in close harmony with the rehabilitation counselor and representatives of the patient's workplace.

Patients from occupations requiring heavy and/or repetitive lifting procedures are not precluded from such programs. All programs include substantial lift-training components. Recent research clearly indicates that most individuals can be trained to manage heavy, repetitive lifting tasks, using well-proven and long-known weight training techniques.[34] Thus the initial assessment procedure determines the type and duration of lifting activity that any individual will need to perform at work and trains that person specifically for that task. If, for example, the job requires the lifting of 10-kg legs of ham from a freezer and placing them on a shelf, then the individual is trained to a level so that they may adequately perform that particular task. The physical therapist ensures that the training initially uses low loads and lower repetitions. Progressively, the size of the loads and the numbers of repetitions are increased until a satisfactory standard is reached. These methods will generally ensure that the patient's strength and endurance capacities are progressively and rapidly increased.

Other work activities can be measured and appropriate training is provided in the same way as for lifting. The whole process of fitness for a specific occupation forms a most important part of the total rehabilitation process and is the goal to which the physical program is directed. This requires a close investigation of the worksite by the rehabilitation team, a proper assessment of the physical/ mental requirements of the task, and the subsequent development of a training program aimed at developing those skills in the injured worker. It must involve dialogue with management, and often leads to changes in the workplace so as to provide an ergonomically safer and more efficient worksite. Thus the heights of benches, tables, and chairs may need modification and often the ergonomist/ therapist is able to provide information on alternative techniques or facilities that might be used to help the worker perform the tasks more appropriately and safely. Where repetition of physical activity is a central part of the occupation, the employees and employers are educated as to the length and nature of pauses that are necessary throughout the working day to avoid fatigue and prevent musculoskeletal problems. It is important that pause activities and exercises be taught to the employee as an essential part of a job. The close cooperation of the employer is central to the success of this approach. Just as much as the employees need to be fit for the tasks that the job requires, employers need to understand the physical difficulties of particular tasks and appreciate the need for some alternative activity at appropriate times throughout the working day.

Similarly, a strong association has been shown between poor physical work skills, low levels of strength and endurance, and the incidence of occupational back pain and dysfunction.[13,35] By increasing the participant's strength, endurance, and cardiovascular fitness, together with improving the specific handling skills necessary for a particular occupation, there is usually a concomitant reduction in the level of back pain reported.[13,32] This provides a cogent argument for ensuring that physical rehabilitation programs are especially tailored to suit the work skills and requirements of particular individuals. While there are many physical exercises and activities that can be done in common within a larger group, there is no doubt that specific work hardening is an essential part of any program.[13]

## RETURN TO WORK

In Mayer's classic study[3,36] of objective assessment and intensive physical treatment at the PRIDE establishment in Dallas, Texas, 84 percent of his study group ($n = 62$) returned to work and continued at work for 12 months after the conclusion of the program. This compared very favorably with a return to work of 55 percent for his control group, and only 20 percent for those who dropped out of his initial cohort. Mayer's control group consisted of 38 patients, each with a similar history of chronic back pain, who were eligible for entry into the program, but where there was prolonged delay or refusal by their insurance companies to authorize participation. Continuing data for the PRIDE clinic show that the initial population is continuing in employment for some years after the completion of their initial treatment/education program.

However, the figures indicating an 84 percent return to work are higher than those obtained at most other clinics. In West Australia, data from a clinic[23] with a similar philosophy demonstrate a 60 percent return to work, with that group still retained in employment at the end of 12 months.

A recent retrospective cohort study by Saal and Saal[33] considered the functional outcome of an aggressive physical rehabilitation program in 64 patients with herniated lumbar discs. The underlying premise of the treatment was that patients should be involved in active rather than passive therapy. The study showed that 90 percent of the patients had a good or an excellent outcome based on measurement criteria and there was 92 percent return to work. Four of the six patients who required surgery were found to have spinal stenosis. The study demonstrated that patients with herniated lumbar discs can be successfully treated by intensive physical therapy and that surgery should be reserved for those patients in whom function has not been improved by aggressive physical rehabilitation.[33]

## SUMMARY

A review of the recent current literature reveals that patients with chronic low back pain react better to active rather than to passive treatment regimens. Indeed, the existing information demonstrates that rest, which is currently the most popularly prescribed treatment, often exacerbates rather than improves the condition of those with low back pain. Deyo et al[15] have shown that 2 days of bed rest after an episode of acute back pain is sufficient, and that further bed rest causes a significant decline in a patient's functional capacity. They believe that if a policy of no more than 2 days of bed rest was universally applied that there would be significant benefits for a community. These would be realized in terms of a reduction in the indirect costs associated with low back pain for patients and employees and that absenteeism would be substantially reduced.

## REFERENCES

1. Waddell G: Clinical assessment of lumbar impairment. Clin Orthop Relat Res 221: 110, 1987
2. Nachemson A: Work for all: for those with low back pain as well. Clin Orthop Relat Res 179:77, 1983
3. Mayer TG, Gatchel RJ, Kishino N et al: Objective assessment of spine function following industrial injury. Spine 10:482, 1985

4. Nachemson AL, La Rocca H: Editorial: Spine. Spine 12:427, 1987
5. Twomey LT, Taylor JR: Physical Therapy of the Low Back. Churchill Livingstone, New York, 1987
6. Andersson GJ: The biomechanics of the posterior elements of the lumbar spine. Spine 8:326, 1983
7. Frymoyer JW, Cats-Baril WC: An overview of the incidences and cost of low back pain. Orthop Clin North Am 22:263, 1991
8. Waddell G, Main CJ, Morris EW et al: Chronic low back pain, psychological distress and illness behavior. Spine 9:209, 1984
9. Grieve G: Modern Manual Therapy. Churchill Livingstone, Edinburgh, 1986
10. Corrigan B, Maitland GD: Practical Orthopaedic Medicine. Butterworths, London, 1983
11. Smith S, Mayer TG, Gatchel RJ, Becker TJ: Quantification of lumbar function. Part 1: isometric and multispeed isokinetic trunk strength measures in sagittal and axial planes in normal subjects. Spine 10:757, 1985
12. Mayer TG, Barnes D, Kishino ND et al: Progressive isoinertial lifting evaluation 1. A standardised protocol and normative database. Spine 13:993, 1988
13. Ganora A: Rehabilitation of work related back injury. Aust Family Phys 15:430, 1986
14. Deyo RA, Tsui-Wu YR: Descriptive epidemiology of low back pain and its related medical care in the United States. Spine 12:264, 1987
15. Deyo RH, Diehl AK, Rosenthal M: How many days of bed rest for acute low back pain? New Engl J Med 315:1064, 1986
16. Twomey LT: Physical activity and ageing bones. Patient Management 27:34, 1989
17. Lowther D: The effect of compression and tension on the behavior of connective tissues. In Glasgow EF, Twomey LT, Scull ER et al (eds): Aspects of Manipulative Therapy. 2nd Ed. Churchill Livingstone, Melbourne, 1985
18. Pardini A: Exercise, vitality and ageing. Ageing 344:19, 1984
19. Shephard RJ: Management of exercise in the elderly. Appl Sports Sci 9:109, 1984
20. Frank C, Akeson WH, Woo SL-Y et al: Physiology and therapeutic value of passive joint motion. Clin Orthop Relat Res 185:113, 1984
21. Gatchel RJ, Mayer TJ, Capra P et al: Quantification of lumbar function, part 6: the use of psychological measures in guiding physical function restoration. Spine 11: 36, 1986
22. Deyo RA, Bass JE: Lifestyle and low back pain: the influence of smoking and obesity. Spine 14:501, 1989
23. Edwards BC, Zusman M, Hardcastle D et al: A physical approach to the rehabilitation of patients disabled by chronic low back pain. Med J Aust 156:167, 1992
24. Cinque C: Back pain prescription: out of bed and into the gym. Phys Sports Med 17:185, 1989
25. McQuade KJ, Turner JA, Buchner DM: Physical fitness and chronic low back pain. Clin Orthop Relat Res 233:198, 1988
26. Saal JA: Rehabilitation of football players with lumbar spine injury. Phys Sports Med 16:61, 16:117, 1988
27. Bogduk N, Twomey LT: Clinical Anatomy of the Lumbar Spine. Churchill Livingstone, Melbourne, 1987
28. Nordin M, Kahanovitz N, Verderane R et al: Normal muscle strength and endurance in women and the effect of exercises and electrical stimulation, Part 1: normal endurance and trunk muscle strength in 101 women. Spine 12:105, 1987
29. Taylor JR, Twomey LT: Age related change in the range of movement of the lumbar spine. J Anat 133:473, 1981

30. Lindgren S, Twomey LT: Spinal mobility and trunk muscle strength in elite hockey players. Aust J Phys 34:123, 1988
31. Cady LD, Thomas PC, Korwasky RJ et al: Programs for increasing health and physical fitness in firefighters. J Occup Med 2:111, 1985
32. Cairns D, Mooney V, Crane P et al: Spinal pain rehabilitation: inpatient and outpatient treatment results and development of predictors for outcome. Spine 9:91, 1984
33. Saal JA, Saal JS: Non operative treatment of herniated lumbar intervertebral disc with radiculopathy: an outcome study. Spine 14:431, 1989
34. Sullivan S: Back support mechanisms during manual lifting. Phys Ther 69:38, 1989
35. Videman T, Malmivaara A, Mooney V et al: The value of the axial view in assessing discograms: an experimental study with cadavers. Spine 12:299, 1987
36. Mayer TG, Gatchel RJ, Kishino N et al: A prospective short term study of chronic low back pain patients utilising novel objective functional measurement. Pain 25: 53, 1986

# 11 | Lumbar Spinal Stenosis

Nils Schönström

## DEFINITION

The concept of spinal stenosis was first introduced almost four decades ago by Verbiest,[1,2] who described a radiculopathy caused by a narrowing of the lumbar spinal canal. There had been sporadic reports earlier in the literature of a peculiar disease with radiculopathy that was cured by laminectomy and where no obvious pathology was found during surgery.[3–6] With Verbiest's reports, however, a possible explanation for these early results was given, an appreciation of the importance of the narrow lumbar spinal canal slowly developed, and the concept of developmental narrowing of the spinal canal was accepted. A true congenital form, with a stenosis present at birth, had been described earlier by Sarpyener in 1945.[7] The term developmental, chosen by Verbiest, was intended to indicate that symptoms did not develop until the patient reached maturity. This form of stenosis was characterized by a short anteroposterior diameter between the posterior part of the vertebral body and the vertebral arch.[1] Later Epstein and co-workers[8,9] described narrowing around the spinal nerve as it was leaving the dural sac and on its way down the root canal under the pedicle and out through the intervertebral foramen. This form was called *lateral stenosis* and the original form of stenosis around the dural sac and the cauda equina was called *central stenosis*.

The work of Kirkaldy-Willis and co-workers[10] has shown that another common type of stenosis occurs as a consequence of degenerative processes in the three-joint complex (Fig. 11-1), that is, in the disc and the two zygapophyseal joints holding two adjacent vertebrae together. This type of stenosis has a different etiology from the type initially described by Verbiest, and it is now common

285

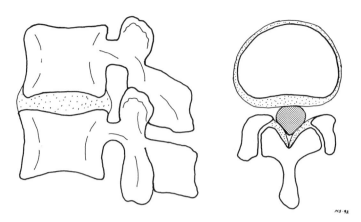

**Fig. 11-1.** The three-joint complex includes the disc, which is the joint between the vertebral bodies, and the two zygapophyseal joints between the posterior structures.

to distinguish between *developmental* and *degenerative* stenosis. Two reports described a prevalence ratio of about 10 to 1, comparing degenerative and developmental stenosis.[11,12] A broad definition of stenosis was given in 1976 by a group of authors where the stenosis was defined as "any type of narrowing of the spinal canal, nerve root canals or intervertebral foramina."[13]

From an etiologic point of view, in current practice we can generally distinguish at least seven different forms of lumbar spinal stenosis:

1. Congenital, which is present at birth[7]
2. Developmental, with a genetic disposition presenting itself with symptoms in adult life,[1,2,14] the most pronounced being a consequence of achondroplasia[15–17]
3. Degenerative, as a result of degenerative processes in the disc and facet joints[8–10,18]
4. Metabolic, as a consequence of pathologic changes in the bone substance (e.g., Paget's disease of the bone,[19] fluorosis, and diffuse idiopathic skeletal hyperostosis)[20]
5. Iatrogenic, usually postlaminectomy
6. Post-traumatic, with a distorted anatomy of the spinal canal as a consequence of trauma
7. Miscellaneous, such as epidural lipomatosis[21] and cysts of the ligamentum flavum[22]

From a morphologic point of view, lumbar spinal stenosis can be divided into central stenosis engaging the nerve roots of the cauda equina, and lateral stenosis disturbing the spinal nerve in the lateral recess, the nerve-root canal, or intervertebral foramina. Andersson and McNeill[23] clarified the "lateral anatomy," by dividing this region into three different zones related to the pedicle,

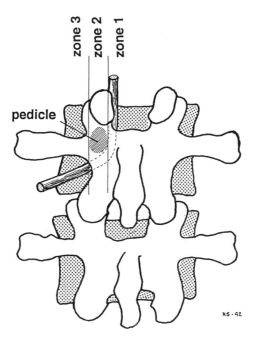

**Fig. 11-2.** The root canal containing the spinal nerve can be divided into three different zones in relation to the pedicle. (Adapted from Andersson and McNeill,[23] with permission.)

which is an important surgical landmark (Fig. 11-2). Zone 1 is the lateral recess; this is the area under the superior articular process medial to the pedicle. Zone 2 is below the pedicle and zone 3 is lateral to the pedicle. It is open to question if a mechanical disturbance of the spinal nerve in zone 3 should be categorized as stenosis.

## PATHOANATOMY

The developmental form of stenosis is characterized by a short pedicle and thick lamina, usually at multiple levels. Its most pronounced form is seen in achondroplastic dwarfs, where it is a common finding. The stenosis in achondroplasia is also different from other forms in that there is also a short interpedicular distance.[15] In the developmental form of stenosis, the emphasis is on an encroachment of the nervous structures by the skeletal structures. The stenosis is of a central type affecting the roots of the cauda equina and possibly the spinal nerve in the lateral recess (zone 1). According to Verbiest,[14] an anteroposterior diameter below 12 mm but over 10 mm is a relative stenosis where other problems, such as a herniated disc, will lead to symptoms. If the diameter is less than 10 mm there is an absolute stenosis capable of causing symptoms without the addition of any other factors. Measurement studies of skeletal collections show that these small dimensions are rare, indicating that developmental stenosis might be a rare disease.[24,25] A diameter of 13 mm or less was present in only 6.3 percent of Eisenstein's 433 skeletons.[24]

In the degenerative type of stenosis, the skeletal dimensions of each vertebra might well be within normal limits, but changes in the disc, ligamentum flavum, and zygapophyseal joints lead to narrowing of the spinal canal.[12] From a morphologic point of view, these changes can lead to both a central and a lateral stenosis as defined previously. These two types of stenosis will be discussed separately, but it is very common for central and lateral stenosis to occur together in the same individual.

The central stenosis in this group has three different components, often resulting in a typical trefoil shape of the spinal canal that can be present in the skeletal structure as well as being the result of a deformation of the dural sac by the surrounding soft tissues. A bulging disc, or sometimes a herniated disc, can cause an impression in the dural sac on its anterior aspect. From the posterolateral side, on both sides of the midline, enlarged zygapophyseal joints covered by a thick ligamentum flavum cause concave impressions (Fig. 11-3). Another common factor contributing to stenosis is an anterior or posterior slipping of one vertebra on the next. The pars interarticularis is often intact and the phenomenon is referred to as *pseudolisthesis* or *degenerative olisthesis/retrolisthesis*.[18] The slip can, in itself, be sufficient to cause stenosis, or it can significantly contribute to the deformation of the dural sac described previously as a result of soft-tissue encroachment.

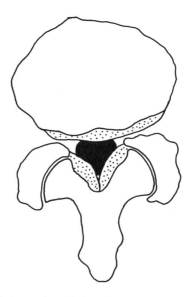

**Fig. 11-3.** The typical deformation of the dural sac at disc height is in the form of a trefoil.

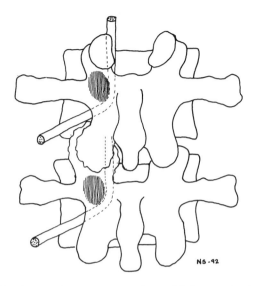

**Fig. 11-4.** Arthritic changes in one zygapophyseal joint can lead to impingement on two different spinal nerves: the upper nerve in zone 2 and the lower nerve in zone 1.

In the lateral type of stenosis, degenerative enlargement of a zygapophyseal joint can lead to encroachment on two consecutive spinal nerves.[26] It can either impinge on the nerve about it as it leaves the dural sac and passes out through the intervertebral foramen (in zone 2 in relation to the pedicle above), or on the next spinal nerve as it lies in the lateral recess (zone 1 of the next pedicle) (Fig. 11-4).

The metabolic type of stenosis is seen as a result of postmature growth of bone resulting in a central stenosis of much the same type as developmental stenosis.

The iatrogenic type of stenosis following surgery involves three different mechanisms: (1) new bone formation from raw bone surfaces after laminectomy or posterior fusion; (2) postlaminectomy membrane proliferation or cyst formation; and (3) instability caused by laminectomy with rapid degeneration and accentuated slipping between adjacent vertebrae (pseudolisthesis).

## PATHOPHYSIOLOGY

### Dynamic Concept in Degenerative Stenosis

The short description in the previous section gave a static picture of the basic changes leading to a degenerative stenosis. However, to understand the pathophysiologic description that follows, it is helpful to adopt a more dynamic concept of degenerative stenosis.

The three-joint complex formed by the disc and zygapophyseal joints is designed to permit movements between the vertebrae. Normally this is done in such a way that the space in the spinal canal and the nerve-root canals remains sufficiently large to accommodate the nervous structures inside it. We have shown in in vitro experiments that when a lumbar spine specimen was moved from full flexion to full extension, the transverse sectional area of the spinal canal was diminished by an average of 40 mm$^2$.[27] The same magnitude of change in the transverse area of the spinal canal was found after a shift in axial loading from 200 N of axial distraction to 200 N of axial compression. During the axial loading the spine was held in a neutral position. Since this is approximately equivalent to an increase in axial load of about 40 kg, the weight of a full-grown torso, it might represent the decrease in size of the spinal canal when a subject moves from lying down to standing up. These changes are well tolerated with a normal canal but it can have significant implications in a spine with a narrow canal.

It has been claimed that true hypertrophy of the ligamentum flavum is extremely rare.[28] This has led to the assumption that this ligament does not contribute to a central stenosis. However, several authors[29,30] have claimed that it has been their impression during surgery that it does play a role in the compression of the dural sac. In a measurement study, we have shown that the fully relaxed thickness of the ligamentum flavum is on average 2 mm greater than the ligament when distracted under 8 kg of load.[31] This is explained by the elastic behavior of the ligamentum flavum, which can contain as much as 80 percent of elastic fibers.[32] Thus, when the normal ligament is fully relaxed in extension, the resulting thickening can contribute significantly to a further constriction of an already narrow canal, even without hypertrophy of the ligament.

The spinal nerve in the lateral recess (zone 1) may or may not be affected by changes of posture and load. An increased backward bulging of the disc can increase pressure on the spinal nerve in the proximal part of zone 1, which is at disc height, but a few millimeters further distally, the vertebral body forms the anterior limit of this space and here the dimensions are constant during shifts in load or posture. Under the pedicle, in zone 2, however, great changes occur when the spine is moved from flexion to extension. In extension the superior articular facet moves upward, toward the pedicle where the spinal nerve is situated in the uppermost of the foramen. Normally, the foramen, which contains fat and vascular structures together with the nerve, is large enough to accommodate these changes. When there is degenerative enlargement of the superior articular process, the difference between extension and flexion might mean the difference between encroachment and no encroachment on that spinal nerve. In addition, when an axial load is applied to the spine over a period of time, creep in the disc results in a reduced disc height. As a consequence, there is a migration upward of the superior facet toward the pedicle above, with a risk of nerve impingement by an enlarged zygapophyseal joint.

This dynamic view of the size of the spinal canal and nerve-root canals is the key to understanding how changes in posture and load, which are problem free in a normal canal, can lead to symptoms when the canal is narrow. It also provides one explanation for the fluctuating nature of the symptoms that are so characteristic of lumbar spinal stenosis.

## Size of the Canal and Cauda Equina

Various measurements have been used to describe the available space in the lumbar spinal canal. The most frequently used measurement of the canal has been its anteroposterior diameter. The interpedicular distance has been proposed, but not generally accepted as useful, with the exception of stenosis in achondroplasia. The transverse area of the spinal canal, as outlined by the skeletal structures, has been used,[33] and this area will be reduced in cases with developmental stenosis. It is much less valuable in degenerative stenosis because the skeletal measurements could be normal despite severe stenosis, as described earlier. Based on a morphologic study in patients with central stenosis confirmed during surgery, we have found the transverse area of the dural sac to be the best measurement for confirming a central stenosis on transverse sections of the lumbar spine (Fig. 11-5).[12]

What about the size of the neural elements to be accommodated in the canal? In two in vitro experiments, we recorded this size expressed as the transverse area of the dural sac and its contents.[34,35] A carefully calibrated circular clamp was placed around the dural sac at the L3 level. A thin pressure-recording catheter was placed among the roots of the cauda equina inside the clamp. The clamp was tightened until the first sign of a pressure increase among the roots. The transverse area where this first pressure increase was noted was called *the critical size of the dural sac*. The critical size was surprisingly constant, among different individuals and using different measurement and experi-

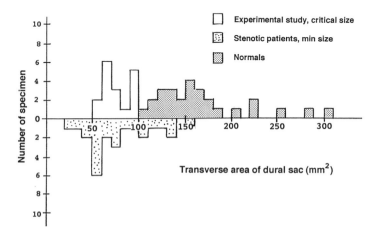

**Fig. 11-5.** The transverse area of the dural sac in one clinical and two experimental studies. (From Schönström,[41] with permission.)

mental procedures, at an average of 75 mm$^2$, with a standard deviation of 15 mm$^2$ (see Fig. 11-5). To reach a further pressure increase of about 50 mmHg among the roots, the clamp had to be tightened to reduce the area by another 19 percent below the critical size; to produce a pressure increase of 100 mmHg the area had to be reduced by an average of 26 percent below the critical size.

We concluded that the size of the spinal canal varies considerably between different individuals, but variation in the size of its neural content is small. We therefore defined central stenosis in terms of the size of the dural sac on computed tomography (CT) scans, based on our experimental data. No similar experiments have been done for lateral stenosis, and one has to rely on other methods, such as nerve-root blocks, to confirm the diagnosis.[36]

## Effect of Pressure on Nerve Roots

The pathophysiologic response to acute mechanical pressure on the nerve roots of the cauda equina has been investigated by Olmarker[37] in porcine experiments. A translucent pressure chamber was attached to the spine of the pig after laminectomy under general anesthesia. An acute pressure was applied to the nerve roots, using a balloon inside the chamber. The effects of a stepwise increase in pressure on the microcirculation of the roots was studied through the translucent chamber. The average occlusion pressure for the arterioles was slightly below the systolic blood pressure. It was also concluded that the flow in the capillary network was affected by venous stasis, which began to occur at low pressures of only 5 to 10 mmHg. A retrograde stasis could be responsible for disturbances of nerve function due to venous congestion. Observations of gradual decompression after initial acute compression revealed that the pressure levels had to go down to zero to obtain a full restitution of the blood flow. The possibility of edema and blocking of axonal transport are other mechanisms that may add to the disturbance of nerve function.

In an anatomic study on cadaver spines, Hoyland and co-workers[38] found a correlation between venous stasis in the intervertebral foramen and interstitial fibrosis in the corresponding spinal nerve. It seems possible that a chronic stasis can lead to edema as seen in the experimental study by Olmarker,[37] and over time this edema could be transformed into fibrosis. Thus the fibrosis seen by Hoyland et al[38] was interpreted as the end result of chronic nerve damage associated with venous congestion.

## Encroachment on Nerve Roots of the Cauda Equina

If we put the experimental information together, it is possible to create a hypothetical model for the pathogenesis of central stenosis of the degenerative type based on a dynamic concept.

The normal spinal canal has a reserve capacity over and above the space required for the contents of the canal, a concept introduced by Weisz and Lee.[39]

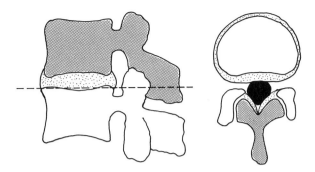

**Fig. 11-6.**   At disc height the spinal canal is made up of two adjacent vertebrae.

The smaller the canal the closer one approaches the critical size beyond which the nerve roots would be compressed. Canal narrowing occurs in most instances at the disc level, where the posterior boundary of the canal is formed on each side by a zygapophyseal joint (Fig. 11-6). The dural sac is usually deformed into a trefoil shape (see Fig. 11-3). Considering first the anterior aspect of the canal, a bulging disc can easily make an impression of 2 mm as a result of increased axial load (Reuber et al.[40]). The posterolateral impressions are made by enlarged zygapophyseal joints, with a possible further encroachment of 2 mm by the thickening of the ligamentum flavum that accompanies their relaxation in extension. Figure 11-7 shows how it can be calculated that an impression from the anterior aspect of 2 mm (disc) with a further 2 mm from the posterolateral aspects (ligamentum flavum) will reduce the area of the dural sac by about 40 percent, if the undeformed area is circular with 10-mm diameter.[41] Thus when the canal has reached the small dimensions of the "critical size," the normal changes in disc bulge and the thickness of the ligamentum flavum can reduce the remaining space considerably as a result of axial loading or extension of the spine. This was confirmed in our experiment with spine specimens in various postures and axial loads, described earlier.[27]

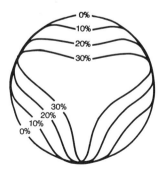

**Fig. 11-7.**   The trefoil deformation of the initially circular dural sac can be graded as a percentage of the initial diameter, whereby the magnitude of the deformation can be estimated. (From Schönström,[41] with permission.)

If the dural sac has already reached the critical size in flexion, when the canal size has its maximum, a further reduction of the available space by 40 percent as a result of extension could easily result in an acute pressure increase of over 100 mmHg among the nerve roots of the cauda equina.[35] The work of Olmarker et al[37] showed that this could lead to pronounced acute disturbances of nerve function. The chronic effects on the nerve roots are more unpredictable and a certain adaptation of the nervous structures to a narrow surrounding is possible. In our experiments with acute constriction of the nerve roots, we saw a creep downward with time of the initial pressure increase if the constriction was left constant.[35] One interpretation of this phenomenon could be that it was a result of a deformation over time of the nervous structures as a consequence of the sustained compression. However, with the dynamic concept described above, it is also justifiable to discuss acute changes in size superimposed on chronic deformation.

## THE CLINICAL PICTURE

### Clinical History

Spinal stenosis can be seen in all age groups, but its prevalence is greatest in patients over 60 years of age. Many of the patients with lumbar spinal stenosis have a long history of low back pain of a "mechanical" type, with sciatica and evidence of disc disease during their thirties and forties (Kirkaldy-Willis[26]). Symptoms are usually less pronounced in the fifties and they gradually become typical of established spinal stenosis in the sixties.

Although back pain is a common symptom, the clinical picture is dominated by various disturbances in the lower extremities. The principal complaint may be pain, but is more often described in terms of numbness, paresthesia, and weakness. Often the patient has difficulty in clearly expressing the quality of the symptoms. The sometimes bizarre nature of the symptoms can result in the patient being accused of malingering.

The well-known symptoms of neurogenic claudication are the unique feature of the disease and need special attention when taking the patient's history. These symptoms are usually brought on by walking and relieved by rest. The characteristic feature of neurogenic claudication is the influence of posture on physical activity. In this respect, neurogenic claudication differs from peripheral vascular claudication. Extension aggravates the symptoms whereas flexion facilitates the physical activity and diminishes the symptoms. Thus walking bent forward increases the maximum walking distance.[42] Riding a bike is often possible for considerable distances,[43] and leaning forward or squatting while resting relieves the discomfort. In one specific variant of this condition, the symptoms arise, not so much after walking or physical exercise, but simply by persistent extension of the back, even when standing still. This led Wilson[44] to define two types of clinical picture in stenosis, one postural type and one claudication type. He also stated that motor symptoms would often precede sensory changes, leading to "drop attacks," where during walking the patient gets a sudden weakness leading to a fall. A more infrequent symptom is a chronic cauda equina syndrome with genital pain and disturbances.

## Physical Examination

The physical examination follows the same principles as for all other problems of the lumbar spine with disturbances in the legs. Special emphasis is placed on a few points.

1. *The patient's ability to walk and perform other forms of physical activity and the influence of posture on these abilities:* The objective findings during a physical examination may be few at rest but could become more pronounced immediately after physical exercise or following a period of prolonged lumbar extension.

2. *The presence or absence of arterial disease:* Palpation of the abdominal aorta and auscultation for bruits in the iliac or femoral arteries are essential. Palpation of peripheral pulses and when necessary, recording of ankle blood pressure with the Doppler technique are also helpful.

3. Hip disease as degenerative arthritis is a common differential diagnosis in this age group and examination of these joints is recommended.[45]

Since the typical patient with lumbar spinal stenosis usually has few pathologic signs in the physical examination, the great importance of the examination is to exclude other serious diseases such as spinal tumors, neurologic problems with demyelinating or peripheral nervous disease, hip disease, and vascular problems. One should also bear in mind that in this age category it is quite possible to have various combinations of spinal stenosis with hip disease or vascular disease.

## Morphologic Examination of the Spinal Canal

A morphologic examination of the spinal canal is essential to confirm the diagnosis. On a plain x-ray of the lumbar spine the morphologic prerequisites for the disease can be identified. It is also important to exclude unpleasant surprises such as vertebral metastases. If any form of surgical intervention is contemplated, a more detailed analysis of the spinal canal and nerve-root canals is required.

### Myelography

Myelography has, ever since the syndrome was described by Verbiest, been the method of choice to analyze the dimensions of the canal and visualize any encroachment on the nerve roots. Despite the introduction of modern imaging techniques such as CT scanning and magnetic resonance tomography (MRT), myelography still has an advantage in certain respects. It gives a very good overview of the canal, which is essential to determine how many levels are affected and how surgery is to be planned. It also gives unique possibilities for dynamic investigations, with pictures in neutral, flexion, and extension as described by Sortland et al.[46] It is also possible to obtain pictures with various amounts of axial loading as proposed by Schumacher.[47] This not only helps us to understand the mechanics of the root compression, but can also assist in sharpening the diagnostic ability of the myelography by exaggerating the pathologic changes in borderline cases. The drawback of myelography is that it is an invasive procedure with attendant risks and discomfort for the patient, and it is also usually done as an inpatient procedure with the increased costs of hospitalization.

**Computed Tomography**

CT scans provide transverse cuts, perpendicular to the long axis of the spine, with excellent opportunities for a detailed analysis of the size and shape of the spinal canal and nerve-root canals. With an appropriate window setting of the machine, it is usually possible to visualize the encroachment on the nervous structures, also by the soft tissues such as the disc and ligamentum flavum. It is easy to appreciate the importance of the soft tissues in this respect by looking at Figure 11-8, which is a tracing from the CT scans of a patient

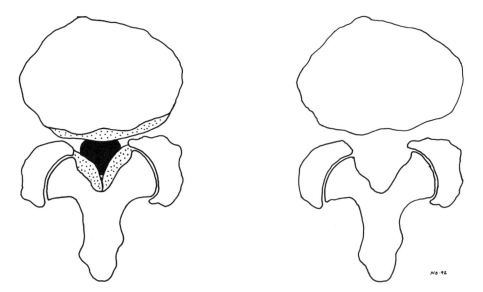

**Fig. 11-8.** Tracings from preoperative CT scans from a patient with central stenosis. The tracings are made with and without the soft tissues to emphasize the importance of the soft tissues in the deformation of the dural sac.

with a central stenosis of the degenerative type. Under certain circumstances an analysis of the influence of the soft tissues can be very difficult on CT scans (e.g., with very obese patients or after previous surgery in the area). Some of these difficulties can be overcome if the CT investigation is combined with myelography, so that a small amount of contrast remains in the thecal sac when the scans are done. Modern machines may also have the ability to provide sagittal views and three-dimensional reconstructions, which give significant contributions to the diagnostic information. In many centers today, it is customary to begin with the noninvasive CT scanning and proceed to myelography only if necessary. In terms of central stenosis, the measurement of the critical size of the dural sac, as outlined above, can be helpful in establishing the diagnosis. However, CT is still not suitable for dynamic investigations and one has to remember that with the patient lying down, the axial load is removed from the spine. Furthermore, to help the patients lie still and avoid distortion by movement, they are told to assume the most comfortable position. This means that they try not to provoke the nerve roots and in borderline cases the diagnosis can be missed. These deductions can be drawn from the concept of dynamic stenosis discussed above.

## Magnetic Resonance Tomography

MRT has the advantage of giving both an overview and a detailed analysis, both along the axis of the spine and perpendicular to it. It also gives unique information about the hydration of the discs and their state of degeneration. Furthermore it is noninvasive, cost effective, and without the dangers of ionizing radiation. The general impression is that MRT is better at depicting the soft tissues and CT scans are best for demonstrating skeletal structures. Surprisingly, one of the major contraindications for MRT is claustrophobia. Other contraindications are metal implants in the patient and especially cardiac pacemakers. MRT is not suitable for dynamic investigations in different postures or with axial loads.

It is a general belief that the morphologic analysis of lateral stenosis is more difficult than that of central stenosis, mainly because of the difficulty of clearly visualizing the interaction between the spinal nerve and the root canal. Van Akkerveken[36] has shown convincingly that nerve-root blocks can help in determining which spinal nerve is affected. This is of great importance in planning surgery so that the surgical trauma can be minimized.

## Diagnostic Synthesis

Diagnostic analysis is based primarily on the clinical history. The clinical examination reinforces the diagnosis, mainly by excluding other reasons for the symptoms, but also by helping to decide the level of lateral stenosis with rhizopathy. The morphologic evaluation of the spinal canal confirms the diagnosis and forms the basis for the planning of surgical intervention, if that is necessary. One cannot warn too much against overreliance on the morphologic analysis alone. A narrow lumbar canal without an appropriate clinical history does not justify the diagnosis of spinal stenosis! Even with an appropriate history and a narrow canal, it is absolutely essential to exclude other reasons for the symptoms, such as neurologic disturbances of other kinds, hip disease, and vascular problems. If surgery is contemplated, the risks of major lumbar surgery are only justified by a sound clinical diagnosis following a complete investigation and not simply by a morphologic confirmation of a narrow canal.

## TREATMENT

As with most forms of low back pain, with or without sciatica, good treatment is based on a correct clinical diagnosis and starts with conservative measures. A mild degree of numbness or weakness, combined with a gait where the patient prefers to walk somewhat bent forward, is by many people considered to be a natural consequence of old age. However, nowadays quality of life is an important issue and even a mild form of lumbar spinal stenosis is often a reason for a medical consultation. Usually, it is a natural anxiety about the possibility of serious disease, with a concern about a rapid decline in physical ability, that is the reason for the visit. Therefore it is important, even in the milder forms, to secure the diagnosis with a reasonable degree of care and to exclude a more serious disease. If this is done, sometimes the information about the spinal stenosis and some advice on how to live with it is all that is needed at this point. However, if the symptoms progress, a more active strategy is required. Considering that the symptoms by definition are brought on by encroachment on the cauda equina or the spinal nerves by the walls of the spinal canal or nerve-root canals, it could seem natural to contemplate surgical intervention as soon as possible when the symptoms have reached a certain level. However, surgery for this disease is not without risks, some patients do not obtain relief from an operation, and there is a risk of recurrence of symptoms. It is therefore worthwhile to discuss the conservative, nonoperative alternatives to surgery.

It has been shown by Johnsson et al[48] that even with clinical and radiologic signs of lumbar spinal stenosis, the prognosis was not bad even when surgery was not performed and the patients were followed up for at least 4 years.

The reasons for this are still obscure, because one has to assume that the degeneration responsible for the stenosis is likely to progress with time. However, emphasis should be placed on the importance of studying the natural history of any disease where major surgery is contemplated. I have no doubt that surgery has a well-defended position in the treatment of spinal stenosis and when symptoms are severe and progressive it is often the best solution. However, there is almost always time to undertake a period of conservative treatment and to evaluate its effectiveness. A conservative strategy could be based on the following modalities.

## Bed Rest and Reduced Physical Activity

Bed rest and reduced physical activity should be contemplated only in acute situations with severe back pain and sciatica. It is important to remember that in patients at a relatively advanced age, inactivity brings special risks. Bed rest for a maximum of 2 to 3 days can be an effective way of alleviating the pain of sciatica. This may be achieved by a reduced disc pressure, an increased size of the spinal canal due to reduced axial loading, or a reduction of an irritation of the nerve roots with increased blood flow after a reduction of pressure on the roots. However, with this kind of treatment, reduced physical strength comes rapidly and the accompanying mental inactivity does not help the patient's outlook. It is a potentially dangerous treatment in these respects, but can be justified and effective if the pain is severe.

## Corsets and Braces

The motive for the use of corsets and braces is to limit the motion of the different segments of the lumbar spine, thereby achieving a symptomatic relief. It may be argued whether a reduction in motion really is achieved by these devices, but in some instances they give relief. In a study from 1985, Willner et al[49] showed a positive effect of a rigid plastic brace on the symptoms of spinal stenosis and spondylolisthesis. A rationale could be that it helps to avoid extension, and may thereby avoid part of the insult on the nervous structures. It should be noted that they used a special jig to custom-fit the brace to the patient so that the best possible posture for symptomatic relief was obtained. They also excluded patients not suitable for treatment with a brace. This might be an alternative to the short bed rest described above, avoiding the hazards of bed rest.

## Physical Exercise

Different forms of physical exercise programs have for many years been part of the standard repertoire in the treatment of low back pain. They have been advocated for two main reasons: first, to strengthen the muscles controlling the movements of the lower back, achieving a better control of the motion segment, and second, to increase the sense of comfort and physical security that a general exercise program can give. This has been claimed to be the result of increased levels of endorphins reducing the pain level.

Since this is mainly a geriatric clientele, exercise programs should be individualized and monitored to avoid an increase in pain level as a result of the program. As has been mentioned several times the symptoms are usually aggravated by extension and, in my opinion, extension exercises should be avoided in spinal stenosis. Riding a properly adjusted bicycle is usually a good way of getting proper exercise and also gives a method of alternative transportation when walking is difficult. It is important to restore and strengthen the patient's physical function, and at the same time to educate patients on how to use their body so as to avoid irritation of the nerve roots.

## Drug Therapy

In an acute exacerbation of back pain with sciatica, drug therapy is often a good alternative if the nerve roots or spinal nerves have been irritated by prolonged intermittent compression producing "inflammation." According to Rydevik and co-workers,[50] edema in the nervous structures is part of the disturbance caused by acute compression. A period of 3 to 6 weeks of anti-inflammatory treatment, usually with a nonsteroidal anti-inflammatory drug (NSAID), may reduce the symptoms. If a reduction of edema is achieved, the space available for the nerve roots is greater. This is especially important in the case of a narrow canal where dynamic factors play an important role. One must make sure that there are no contraindications to that form of treatment, such as a tendency to gastric bleeding.

It is usually a good policy to use simple analgesics like paracetamol, instead of more potent drugs that carry a risk of making the patient dependent on the drug. Spinal stenosis is a more or less chronic condition and long-standing medication with analgesics is always a problem. It should only be instituted together with other conservative treatment modalities and should be carefully monitored with very precise instructions on dose and length of medication from the treating physician.

## Back Schools and Other Education

Knowledge about the disease and the mechanisms behind the symptoms helps the patient to deal with the problems of the disease. Whether this information is delivered by the treating physician, the physiotherapist, or in an organized form such as a back school, is not the main issue. In my experience, the physiotherapist is the best suited to give this kind of information, which can be organized in a very practical format, together with an individualized physical exercise program. Sometimes a geriatric clientele responds better to individual instruction. The goal is to make the patients aware of how to deal with existing symptoms and how to avoid acute exacerbations by adjusting their style of living, if possible, without reducing their activity level or quality of life.

The conservative treatment strategy is based on whether the patient presents during an acute exacerbation or in the chronic phase. If acute problems are present, a few days of bed rest combined with suitable drug treatment would be a good start. Alternatively, a period with a rigid brace, individually fitted according to the principles of Willner et al,[49] could be of help. If the patient presents without acute symptoms, or once these have settled, a change in lifestyle should be instituted, avoiding harmful postures and with an individualized and carefully monitored exercise program. A good conservative program together with some optimism often leads to a significant improvement.

## Surgical Alternatives

If conservative treatment fails to achieve a tolerable level of discomfort, or if progressive neurologic deficit threatens the patient's activities of daily life, surgical treatment should be considered.

The aim of surgery is to relieve the discrepancy in size between the spinal canal and its neural content. This is achieved by removing parts of the wall of the spinal canal or nerve-root canals. The main procedures in central stenosis are laminectomy or laminotomy, where the whole lamina or part of the lamina is removed. After that the ligamentum flavum is removed and in a few instances the anterior canal is decompressed by a discectomy. There are variants in these procedures, where the laminae are merely opened and hinged outward on a lateral attachment and left in that position. It has also been suggested that the lateral portion of the ligamentum flavum should be saved and a decompression be confined to removal of the skeletal structures posterior to it, with the aim of providing a soft-tissue barrier between the raw bone surfaces and the nerve roots. To achieve a good decompression it is often necessary to sacrifice the inner third of the zygapophyseal joint.

In lateral stenosis, a decompression by a foraminotomy has been the method of choice. Various forms of undercuts, taking only the most anterior part of the superior articular zygapophyseal joint, has been developed in order to save as much as possible of the zygapophyseal joint and avoid secondary instability.

It is common to perform a combination of both types of procedures. In both cases there is a delicate balance between achieving a good decompression and causing a significant instability. Secondary instability is a common postoperative finding, and therefore various types of fusion of the decompressed segment should be considered. The development of transpedicular screw fixation has provided the surgeon with methods of providing mechanical stability until a solid bony fusion of the stabilized segment is achieved.

Despite the combination of decompression and fusion, there is always a risk of a recurrence of the symptoms after surgery. Two common factors are new bone growth from the raw surfaces after partial resection and a progression of the degenerative changes responsible for the disease in the first place. A postsurgical instability can significantly add to these problems. However, with a successful outcome of the surgery there is a good relief of the symptoms with a dramatic improvement in the quality of life for the patient.

## REFERENCES

1. Verbiest H: A radicular syndrome from developmental narrowing of the lumbar vertebral canal. J Bone Joint Surg 36B:230, 1954
2. Verbiest H: Further experiences on the pathological influence of developmental narrowness of the bony lumbar vertebral canal. J Bone Joint Surg 37B:576, 1955

3. Bailey P, Casamajor L: Osteoarthritis of the spine as a cause of compression of the spinal cord and its roots; with report of 5 cases. J Nerv Ment Dis 38:588, 1911

4. Elsberg CA: Experiences in spinal surgery. Observations upon 60 laminectomies for spinal disease. Surg Gynecol Obstet 16:117, 1913

5. Kennedy F, Elsberg CA, Lambert CI: A peculiar and undescribed disease of the nerves of the cauda equina. Am J Med Sci 147:645, 1914

6. Sachs B, Fraenkel J: Progressive ankylotic rigidity of the spine. J Nerv Ment Dis 27:1, 1900

7. Sarpyener MA: Congenital stricture of the spinal canal. J Bone Joint Surg 27:70, 1945

8. Epstein JA, Epstein BS, Lavine LS et al: Sciatica caused by nerve root entrapment in the lateral recess: the superior facet syndrome. J Neurosrug 36:584, 1972

9. Epstein JA, Epstein BS, Lavine LS et al: Lumbar nerve root compression at the intervertebral foramina caused by arthritis of the posterior facets. J Neurosurg 39:362, 1973

10. Kirkaldy-Willis WH, Wedge JH, Yong-Hing K et al: pathology and pathogenesis of lumbar spondylosis and stenosis. Spine 3:319, 1978

11. Getty CJM: Lumbar spinal stenosis. The clinical spectrum and results of operation. J Bone Joint Surg 62B:481, 1980

12. Schönström NSR, Bolender NFr, Spengler DM: The pathomorphology of spinal stenosis as seen on CT-scans of the lumbar spine. Spine 10:806, 1985

13. Arnoldi CC, Brodsky AE, Cauchoix J et al: Lumbar spinal stenosis and nerve root entrapment syndromes, definition and classification. Clin Orthop Relat Res 115:4, 1976

14. Verbiest H: Neurogenic intermittent claudication in cases with absolute and relative stenosis of the lumbar vertebral canal (ASLC and RSLC), in cases with narrow lumbar intervertebral foramina, and in cases with both entities. Clin Neurosurg 20:204, 1973

15. Gelman MI: Cauda equina compression in acromegaly. Radiology 112:357, 1974

16. Lutter LD, Lonstein JE, Winter RB et al: Anatomy of the achondroplastic lumbar canal. Clin Orthop Relat Res 126:139, 1977

17. Lutter LD, Langer LO: Neurologic symptoms in achondroplastic dwarfs—surgical treatment. J Bone Joint Surg 59A:87, 1977

18. MacNab I: Spondylolisthesis with an intact neural arch: the so-called pseudospondylolisthesis. J Bone Joint Surg 32B:325, 1950

19. Weisz GM: Lumbar spinal canal stenosis in Paget's disease. Spine 8:192, 1983

20. Johnsson KE, Petersson H, Wollheim FA et al: Diffuse idiopathic skeletal hyperostosis (DISH) causing spinal stenosis and sudden paraplegia. J Rheumatol 10:784, 1983

21. Lipson SJ, Haheedy MH, Kaplan MM et al: Spinal stenosis caused by lipomatosis in Cushing's syndrome. New Engl J Med 302:36, 1980

22. Abdullah AF, Chambers RW, Daut DP: Lumbar nerve root compression by synovial cysts of the ligamentum flavum. Report of four cases. J Neurosurg 60:617, 1984

23. Andersson GBJ, McNeill TW: Lumbar Spine Syndromes. p. 11. Springer-Verlag, Vienna, 1989

24. Eisenstein S: The morphometry and pathological anatomy of the lumbar spine in South African Negroes and Caucasoids with specific reference to spinal stenosis. J Bone Joint Surg 59B:173, 1977

25. Postachini F, Ripani M, Carpano S: Morphometry of the lumbar vertebrae. Clin Orthop Relat Res 172:296, 1983

26. Kirkaldy-Willis WH: Managing Low Back Pain. Churchill Livingstone, New York, 1983
27. Schönström NSR, Lindahl S, Willén J et al: Dynamic changes in the dimensions of the lumbar spinal canal. J Orthop Res 7:155, 1989
28. Yong-Hing K, Reilly J, Kirkaldy-Willis WH: The ligamentum flavum. Spine 1:226, 1976
29. Towne EB, Reichert FL: Compression of the lumbosacral roots of the spinal cord by thickened ligamenta flava. Ann Surg 94:327, 1931
30. Yamada H, Ohya M, Okada T et al: Intermittent cauda equina compression due to narrow spinal canal. J Neurosurg 37:83, 1972
31. Schönström NSR, Hansson TH: Thickness of the human ligamentum flavum as a function of load. An in vitro experimental study. Clin Biomech 6:19, 1991
32. Nachemson AL, Evans JH: Some mechanical properties of the third human lumbar interlaminar ligament. J Biomech 1:211, 1968
33. Ullrich CG, Binet EF, Sanecki MG et al: Quantitative assessment of the lumbar spinal canal by computed tomography. Radiology 134:137, 1980
34. Schönström NSR, Bolender NFr, Spengler DM et al: Pressure changes within the cauda equina following constriction of the dural sac. An in vitro experimental study. Spine 9:604, 1984
35. Schönström NSR, Hansson TH: Pressure changes following constriction of the cauda equina. An experimental study in situ. Spine 13:385, 1988
36. Van Akkerveken PF: Lateral stenosis of the lumbar spine. A new diagnostic test and its influence on management of patients with pain only. Thesis, University of Utrecht, 1989
37. Olmarker K: Spinal nerve root compression. Nutrition and function of the porcine cauda equina compressed in vivo. Acta Orthop Scand, suppl. 242:1, 1991
38. Hoyland JA, Freemont AJ, Jayson MIV: Intervertebral foramen venous obstruction. A cause of periradicular fibrosis. Spine 14:558, 1989
39. Weisz GM, Lee P: Spinal canal stenosis. Concept of spinal reserve capacity: radiologic measurements and clinical applications. Clin Orthop Relat Res 179:134, 1983
40. Reuber M, Schultz A, Denis F et al: Bulging of lumbar intervertebral disks. J Biomech Eng 104:187, 1982
41. Schönström NSR: The narrow lumbar canal and the size of the cauda equina in man. Thesis, University of Göteborg, 1988
42. Dyck P: The stoop-test in lumbar entrapment radiculopathy. Spine 4:89, 1979
43. Dyck P, Doyle JB: "Bicycle test" of Van Gelderen in diagnosis of intermittent cauda equina compression syndrome. Case report. J Neurosurg 46:667, 1977
44. Wilson CB, Ehni G, Grollmus J: Neurogenic intermittent claudication. Clin Neurosurg 18:62, 1971
45. Bohl WR, Steffe AD: Lumbar spinal stenosis. A cause of continued pain and disability in patients after total hip arthroplasty. Spine 4:168, 1979
46. Sortland O, Magnaes B, Hauge T: Functional myelography with metrizamide in the diagnosis of lumbar spinal stenosis. Acta Radio, suppl. 355:42, 1977
47. Schumacher M: Die Belastungsmyelographie. Fortschr Röntgensrt 145:642, 1986
48. Johnsson KE, Rosén I, Udén A: The natural course of lumbar spinal stenosis. Clin Orthop Relat Res 279:82, 1992
49. Willner S: Effect of a rigid brace on back pain. Acta Orthop Scand 56:40, 1985
50. Rydevik BL, Pedowitz RA, Hargens AR et al: Effects of acute graded compression on spinal nerve root function and structure. An experimental study on the pig cauda equina. Spine 16:487, 1991

# 12 | Low Back Pain in the Workplace: An Ergonomic Approach to Control

*Margaret I. Bullock*
*Joanne E. Bullock–Saxton*

Low back pain (LBP) is one of the most common disorders seen today and many studies of its incidence have revealed that it may occur in as many as 80 percent of the population.[1,2] Biering-Sorensen[3] has also pointed out the high prevalence of LBP associated with work. Although the information on the importance of various workplace factors to the occurrence and etiology of LBP is incomplete, workers in many occupations complain of tension in the shoulders and in the upper and lower back, which interferes with their workplace performance.

According to Rowe,[4] 85 percent of LBP sufferers have intermittent attacks of disabling pain every 3 months to 3 years and, as work absence is often consequential on industrial injury, this high incidence is costly to industry. Yu et al[5] have drawn attention to the economic consequences of LBP and indeed, according to some estimates, in a plant with 1000 employees, an absenteeism rate of 5 percent would cost about $1 million per year.

Back pain can arise from many causes, including those related to pathologic problems elsewhere in the body, or to a traumatic incidence in which some component of the vertebral system is injured. However, in many instances, back pain develops unexpectedly without disruption of the normal daily pattern of activity. In such cases, it might be assumed that local degenerative changes or conditioning from previous postural or vibratory stress had increased the susceptibility to a sudden onset of symptoms.

Some authors believe the back to be particularly susceptible to early degenerative phenomena.[6–8] If degeneration is advanced, insignificant amounts of trauma may precipitate the onset of pain in a person with no previous history of back disorders. This is confirmed if the figures for industrial accident reports are considered. In a study of 148 workers from a British company presenting to the physiotherapy department with back pain, Strachan[9] found that 35 percent of cases could name no known reason for the onset of pain. In a further 14 percent of cases, an unexpected onset of pain occurred during the performance of an everyday task that had previously presented no problem.

It is difficult to diagnose and classify back pain and injury. Many variables may be involved in the cause of LBP, including physical characteristics; the experience of the worker; the demands of the task; organizational, social, and cultural influences; the characteristics of the work environment; and the outcomes of the injury. Furthermore, causes of LBP are not necessarily physical. Back pain experienced by the worker may be based on a mixture of organic and psychological causes, as well as social disturbances that may be influenced by the cultural background of the person.

Such a multifactorial problem demands resolution through a variety of measures and often by a group of people with differing but complementary skills. A physiotherapist is one of such a team. The physiotherapist's role includes both therapeutic activities and rehabilitation and prevention of injury, and concern with the latter process implies an understanding of the objectives and principles of ergonomics.

Ergonomics is concerned with ensuring that the work place is so designed that work-induced injuries, disease, or discomfort are prevented and safety is ensured, while efficiency and productivity are maintained or increased. Work stress problems at home, school, or at the place of employment need attention and often require the cooperative activity of representatives of a number of disciplines, such as engineering, psychology, medicine, and physiotherapy, to provide suitable solutions. Physiotherapists fit into this study of man–machine–task relationships because of their special ability to analyze body movements in detail and to evaluate postural abuse during dynamic situations.[10] The physiotherapist can help to eliminate misuse of the body and assist in the design of equipment and work areas so that the situations so arranged are better suited to the physical well-being of the person using them.

Bullock[10,11] has described the many facets of the preventive role of the physiotherapist, which include such responsibilities as job analysis; work posture monitoring; task design; personnel selection and placement; education; supervision of work methods; influencing of motivation and attitudes; and provision of appropriate activity breaks, exercise, and physical fitness programs. Although only physiotherapists with further education in the practice of ergonomics are likely to act as consultants to industry, all physiotherapists have a part to play not only in health prevention, but also in the prevention of injury or re-injury in clients under their care. The high incidence of LBP in the community and in clients presenting for physiotherapy suggests that methods of controlling it, whether associated with work, home, school, or leisure, should be addressed by the physiotherapist.

Prevention of LBP or injury relies on an understanding of the factors that may contribute to that pain, the implication of those factors for the production of LBP, and an appreciation for the rationale for use and the relative effectiveness of different approaches that may be taken to control the risk factors. These aspects are considered in this chapter.

## WORKPLACE FACTORS ASSOCIATED WITH LOW BACK PAIN

It appears that a number of vocational factors are associated with mechanical injuries, although individual factors and abnormalities also play a part. Andersson[12] has proposed that these factors include physically heavy work, static work postures, frequent bending and twisting, lifting and forceful movements, repetitive work, and vibrations.

Manning and Shannon[13] suggest three possibilities to explain how these factors could produce pain in the low back: abnormal strain on a normal back; normal stress on an abnormal back; and normal stress on an unprepared normal back.

Postures adopted during activity and developed over a period of time appear to have a major association with the presence of LBP. For example, Andersson[12] suggests that prolonged sitting, driving of vehicles, and bent-over work postures seem to carry an increased risk of LBP. It is generally accepted that certain occupational and postural stresses on an already inflicted back will produce further episodes of pain.[2,14]

The stresses of vertical compression, horizontal shear, rotary torque, or a combination of these are determined by the initial, final, and intermediate postures of the person, the velocity of movements, and the load carried by the subject during the task performed.[15] Nachemson et al[16] consider that mechanical stress has at least some role to play in the etiology of LBP syndrome.

### The Influence of Position

It is interesting to note that attempts have been made to calculate the load on the lumbar discs in different positions on the body. Nachemson[17] found an increase in load from lying, to standing to sitting. He also found that forward leaning increased the load. Nachemson[17] considered that these high stresses produced within the lumbar disc possibly play a role in the occurrence of posterior annulus ruptures and that dynamic forces would increase the magnitude of the stresses on the annulus. Such findings could be reflected in the results of Kelsey's experiments,[18] where it was demonstrated that sedentary occupations were conducive to the development of herniated lumbar discs, most especially among those aged 35 years and older, and more specifically among those who sat for half of the time or more at their jobs.

Physiotherapists need to be aware of the implications of postural load for LBP and the importance of providing relevant advice that could help to reduce postural stress. In their consideration of the features of work that influence postural load, special attention needs to be given to demands for sustained positions, bent-over work postures, and the influence on posture and activity of the seated position.

## Sustained Positions

Occupations involving light work with sustained postures have been reported to have a high incidence of back ache. Partridge et al[19] have claimed that sustained bent-over working postures are likely to precipitate back pain, whereas Magora's study[20] indicated that the incidence of back ailments was extremely high in occupations involving prolonged sitting of longer than 4 hours or sustained standing in one place.

Static work is characterized by slow contractions with heavy loads or by long-lasting holding postures. In a strong static contraction, the blood supply is impaired and waste products accumulate in the muscles. According to Grandjean and Hunting,[21] this is the reason for acute pain in the static preloaded muscle. If this is repeated frequently and for long periods of time, chronic pains may result. These are due to pathologic changes not only in the muscles, but also in the connective tissue of tendons, joint capsules, and joint ligaments. This may play a part in the postural backache suffered by workers who are not able to carry out normal movement during their working day. Corlett and Manencia[22] have argued that because many muscle groups are involved in holding a posture, it is possible that their relative contribution to the total supporting force required is changed during the period for which the posture is held. The importance of avoiding or reducing the duration of static muscle stress can therefore be appreciated.

## Bent-Over Work Postures

Investigations indicate that LBP is more frequent in people with predominantly bent-over work postures, where the load on the back is increased. It should be noted that when the lumbar spine is flattened as in the stooped position, the zygapophyseal joints are less able to resist compressive forces and the majority of the intervertebral compressive force must be resisted by the disc. Kisner and Colby[23] attribute postural pain to the mechanical stresses on various structures when a faulty posture is maintained for a lengthy period. Twomey et al[24] have explained how the process of creep in flexion occurs when the spine is loaded in full flexion for a sustained period. These authors have pointed out that if such loads are prolonged beyond 1 hour, with minimal activity into another position, as may occur in some occupations, there may be a considerable degree of extrusion of fluid from the intervertebral discs, the articular cartilage of the zygapophyseal joints, and the spinal ligaments. Twomey and Taylor[25] suggest that it may take many hours of rest for fluid to be reabsorbed into the soft tissues, and their shape re-established. These considerations reinforce the need to maintain the natural forward curve in the lumbar region during working activities and explains why it is inadvisable for those with LBP to sit leaning over a desk. Furthermore, opportunities for a change of position should be provided.

## Seated Postures and Activities

The cause of the high incidence of back pain in sedentary workers is not entirely clear since those with back pain may have elected employment in a sedentary occupation.[26] On the other hand, it may be the sedentary life-style itself that contributes to the onset of symptoms.

Grieco[27] has noted that because of the automation and integration of previously physical tasks, much heavy manual work has been replaced by fixed postures, particularly the sitting position. However, the attention given to controlling risks in heavy manual work has not been applied to other aspects of work postures. The prolonged sitting posture has brought with it a new problem, not only for the workplace, but also for life-style in general. Janda[28] has attributed this sedentary life-style and associated decrease in movement to the development of muscle imbalances, which he believes often predispose workers to LBP.

Physiologic and epidemiologic studies have demonstrated that prolonged sitting work can cause lower back pain.[29] In studying the alterations of the lumbar curve related to posture and seating in various positions, Keegan[30] noted that the reduction of the lumbar curve in some positions tends to force the central portion of the lower lumbar discs posteriorly by hydraulic pressure from anterior wedging. Such flattening of the lumbar curve could be caused by the tightening of the posterior thigh and gluteal muscles during hip flexion, due to their attachment to the ischium, the sacrum, and the ilium. Keegan's results[30] emphasize the fact that sitting with a 90° angle at the hip joints causes considerable strain at the lumbosacral junction, which would be increased by further hip flexion. Bodguk and Twomey[31] have explained how in sitting, due to the decrease in lumbar lordosis, the intervertebral discs are compressed.

Flattening of the lumbar spine also occurs in the sitting position when the legs are stretched out in front of the body. This can occur when a seat is too deep. If the person sits well back to make use of the leg rest, the knees do not reach the edge and the legs must be extended further than normal. This pulls on the muscles behind the thighs, tilting the pelvis backward and flattening the lumbar spine. Sitting with the legs stretched out because the seat is too low has a similar effect. Selecting a chair that is the correct height and depth and that has a low back support to encourage forward movement of the pelvis and maintain the lumbar curve is therefore critical in ensuring comfort and safety.

Driving a vehicle, an occupation involving prolonged sitting, also presents a risk of LBP. Kelsey[18] observed that driving for long periods of time often requires prolonged sitting in a seat with insufficient support for the low back and with legs extended, in a position subject to the vibration from the road and mechanical stress from starting and stopping. The absence of power steering in such circumstances can create a substantial risk to the operator, where the application of pushing and pulling forces on the steering wheel could induce major spinal stresses.

Andersson et al[32] consider that for the seated operator, maneuvers such as the gear shift and preparation for clutch depression can also increase load on the lumbar spine and can increase the myoelectric activity of the erector spinae muscles. These researchers found that lifting the lower limb to place the foot on the pedal placed stress on the lumbar spine due to the contraction of the psoas major muscle, whereas intradiscal pressure of the third lumbar disc was found to increase markedly during the depression of the clutch. Nachemson[33] had previously found that myoelectric activity in the psoas muscle corresponded with an increase in the intradiscal pressure in the lumbar spine. This suggests that a clutch pedal, which requires greater activity of the psoas muscle (due to a high location above the floor), may produce more stress in the lumbar spine than a lower-placed pedal.

Such findings are particularly relevant to drivers of heavy vehicles, such as trucks and tractors, in whom the incidence of LBP is high. They support the findings of Bullock,[34,35] who determined the optimal relationship of a pedal to the operator in terms of minimal spinal movements. Among her recommendations was the use of a pedal that required minimal hip flexion and abduction to reach it. Advice to drivers with LBP should include recommendations either for selection of trucks or tractors with suitably designed pedal locations or for incorporation of appropriate modifications to the seat/pedal relationship to avoid excessive lumbar movement during pedal use.

## Vibrational Conditions

Workers such as bus and truck drivers and heavy equipment operators are subjected to continuous vibration. The effect of vibration on height, implying spinal load, has been demonstrated by a number of researchers,[36,37] and the high frequency of low-back complaints among truck drivers and drivers of work machines has focused interest on a possible relationship between LBP and vibration. Troup[2] has advised that epidemiologic data suggest that the longer the time spent driving, the greater the risk of back trouble. Kakosky[38] has asserted that "vibration transferred from a machine to the human body may cause discomfort, a reduction in performance or even injury," whereas exposure to whole body vibration is listed as one of the factors causing LBP at work.[39] Control of vibrational conditions is therefore an important aspect of prevention in industry.

The greatest dynamic load on the trunk and probably on the spine occurs when it is vibrated at its natural frequency. Stress is therefore likely to be greatest when the seated body is vibrated vertically in the range of 4 to 8 Hz.[2] In a truck, vertical vibration is the dominant vibratory mode and occurs in the range of 2 to 15 Hz. To prevent vibration in the range of 4 to 8 Hz, firm cushions should be supplied and the seat should be suspended to give it a natural frequency of less than 1.5 Hz.[2]

## Effect of Other Musculoskeletal Injuries in the Workplace

The LBP syndrome may sometimes present a wide variety of neuro-orthopedic signs.[20] Some of these manifestations are the result of the underlying process causing LBP, while other clinically objective signs may be related either directly or indirectly to the actual cause of the LBP. For example, sacrolumbar postural disorders, affections of the hip and knee joints, foot deformity, unequal length of the lower limbs, muscle contractures, or poor muscle coordination and function have all been found to be accompanied by LBP.[40-42] The interrelationships between the lumbar vertebrae, sacrum, pelvis, and femur are prime factors in standing posture as well as during activity and it is not surprising that strains in one area can lead to stresses in another.[43]

Magora[20] found that 11.4 percent of LBP patients had at least a mild degree of limitation of movement in the hip, whereas only about 2 percent of the controls had mild unilateral or bilateral limitations. This discrepancy points to a possible connection between hip lesions and LBP. This could be explained by a secondary postural disorder and possibly by the compensatory degree of additional mobility and use demanded of the lumbosacral spine.

The influence of injuries in the lower limbs on the development of LBP must be considered by those concerned with prevention. Slipping and tripping are common industrial accidents and occur also in the domestic situation.[13] The incidence of ankle and knee sprain that is often associated with these accidents should alert the attending physiotherapist to the possibility of future LBP, so that appropriate preventive measures can be taken. Bullock–Saxton[44] has demonstrated that the function of muscles around the hip and low back changes significantly after ankle sprain and has recommended attention to normalizing muscle imbalances and then the application of sensory–motor programs, such as those advocated by Janda and Vavrova.[45] Such an approach would ensure maintenance of proprioception as well as muscle function. This recognizes that the maintenance of the correct upright posture depends on the coordinated activity and endurance of many muscles and that muscle control is largely automatic. But, as Roberts[46] pointed out, after injury or during disease, altered neural activity reaching the central nervous system is likely to influence the automatic mechanisms for muscle control. In time, the person may develop new patterns of muscle activity and this in turn may lead to muscle imbalance, unusual postures, or interference with the capacity to carry out certain movements. Much can often be learned about the nature and location of an injury from the changes in posture and movement patterns that follow it. Unfortunately, such new patterns may persist long after the original injuries have healed, leaving abnormalities of gait and posture attributable to habit.[46]

Active programs for prevention of LBP should include proper consideration of the long-term implications that could occur in areas remote from the site of injury, and should include comprehensive assessment and management of the musculoskeletal system following lower limb injuries.

Muscle weakness and muscle imbalance may also develop as a result of injury, through poor postural habits or through overactivity or underactivity of certain groups of muscles involved in work or play. Once an imbalance has occurred, Janda and Schmid[47] believe that changes in muscle function play an important role in the development of many subsequent painful conditions of the motor system, such as LBP syndromes. They are an integral part in the postural defects that can be associated with work. These authors argue that the activity of individual muscles is not of such great importance as their coordinated activity within different movement patterns. As a result of their clinical observations, they suggest that certain muscles appear to respond to pain by tightness and shortening, while others react by inhibition, atrophy, and weakness.

It has been observed that imbalance between muscles often starts to develop in the pelvic–hip complex.[47,48] Here, an imbalance develops between shortened and tight hip flexors and trunk erectors in the lumbar region on the one hand, and weakened gluteal and abdominal muscles on the other. Muscles that become tight or hypertonic are readily activated in most movement patterns and this is reflected by their earlier recruitment during movement. The changes in muscle length and recruitment patterns are considered to lead to anteversion of the pelvis, together with lumbar hyperlordosis and slight flexion in the hip. This in turn may cause unfavorable changes of pressure distribution on the discs, joints, and ligaments in the lumbar region and hip joints.

These views tend to confirm Micheli's impression[49] that many young athletes with LBP have relatively tight musculotendinous and ligamentous structures about the low back, hips, and knees. He has observed that many appear to have relative weakness of the anterior muscles including the abdominals, and a tightness of the hip flexors and anterior elements of the hip. It should be remembered, however, that on the other hand, many young gymnasts with back pain of either a spondylogenic or mechanical nature have a great flexibility although they can have relatively weak abdominal muscles. Micheli[49] suggests that this weakness may represent a relative musculotendinous imbalance. The influence of a muscle imbalance on the recruitment of muscles about the pelvis may be the most salient point, where a tendency to decreased pelvic stability and control is noted. The possibility of these muscle imbalances needs to be recognized by the physiotherapist involved in designing activity exercise programs for individual clients or for groups in industry or sport.

## Manual Handling and Lifting

Although mechanization has been introduced into many areas of work, prolonged heavy manual work is still necessary within some workplaces, particularly in relation to loading and unloading or to transferring goods. Further, lifting and carrying in the home or in leisure activities is not an infrequent activity. The relationship between heavy manual work and the frequency of LBP is a much discussed subject. For example, Troup[7] found a combination of flexion and rotation when lifting to be the most common cause of back pain at work. Stubbs[50] has also noted that LBP arising from manual handling is a constant hazard in the industrial environment. Workers with back pain lose more days from work when their jobs involve heavy loads[51] and, because pre-existing lumbar spine conditions can be aggravated by heavy loads, it follows that loads on the lumbar spine should be kept as light as possible.

Occupations involving only occasional lifting have also shown a high incidence of back pain.[14] Magora[20] claims that infrequent physical demands and sudden unexpected movements such as a rapid stretch, flexion, or rotational movement gives ". . . more low back pain often than continuous heavy work." That this may be related to poor execution of the task is supported by the evidence that a moderate amount of daily lifting was not found to influence the rate of back ache.[20]

The load on the spine during a lift is related to a number of factors, including the weight of the object to be lifted, the horizontal distance from the body from which or to which it is lifted, the height or vertical distance of the lift, the frequency of lifting, the duration or period of lifting, the speed of the lift, the body posture of the worker, and the bulk of the object lifted.

It has been argued that lumbosacral strain when lifting can occur through lifting a load too heavy for the person's physical strength or lifting a load within the person's strength capacity, but in an incorrect manner. Goldberg et al[52] have suggested that lumbosacral strain can also occur through improperly arching the spine into a lordotic position once the load is lifted. The proposal that the method of lifting may be an important factor in the production of LBP has come from a number of authors. For example, Chaffin and Park[53] have stated that the stresses induced at the lower back during weight lifting are due to a combination of the weight lifted and the person's method of lifting. The latter may be due to the person's approach or to work situations that impose restrictions on the way a lift may be performed.

Physiotherapists need to give some consideration to lifting methods in their prevention program, and they need to be aware of the potential hazards of the various approaches to lifting. Advice about manual handling depends on many factors, but in particular, must be approached in terms of the individual person's capacities and movement abilities.

Gravitational forces acting on the load held in the hand and the person's body mass create rotational moments or torques at the various articulations of the body. The skeletal muscles are positioned to exert forces in such a manner that they counteract these torques. The amount of torque at any joint is depen-

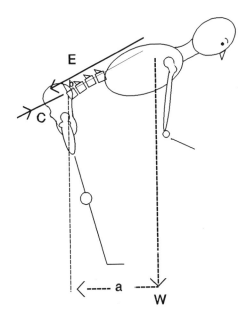

**Fig. 12-1.**   Extensor muscle force in a stooped position:

$$E(= -C) = \frac{W \times a}{b}$$

*E*, extensor muscle force; *W*, weight of upper body and load; a, moment arm of body weight; *b*, moment arm of the extensor muscle force; and *C*, compressive force acting longitudinally through the vertebral bodies and discs.

dent on the product of the force tending to rotate the segments and the moment arm of that force (i.e., the distance from the joint to the force vector measured normal to the force vector), as shown in Fig. 12-1. The magnitude of the moment arm varies with the person's posture. If the load lifted is held close to the body, the moment arms are small and the resulting torques at the joints are small. If the load is held away from the body, the large moment arms will cause large torques. This emphasizes the importance of positioning the body close to the load, which also has implications for both access and the bulk of the object.

Studies[54] have shown that during weight lifting, the bending moment at the lumbosacral junction can become quite large. To counteract this torque, the muscles of the low-back region, primarily the erector spinae group, must exert correspondingly high forces, since they operate on small moment arms. The high forces generated by the low-back muscles are the primary source of compression forces on the lumbosacral disc.

In lifting, the greatest stresses occur at the beginning when the inertia of the weight has to be overcome and the load accelerated. This is why it is important for the person to be in a position to move freely into the upright posture with the load. It is not wise to start a lift in an awkward position, which will prevent a smooth lift. Storage of items and arrangement of the workplace are important factors in this respect.

The trunk extensor muscles act strongly around the vertical but they do not work when the back is fully flexed and only commence their activity after 30° of extension. Electromyographic (EMG) studies[55-57] have demonstrated the electrical silence of the erector spinae in the fully flexed position, the activity of hip extensors as the trunk begins to rise, and the later vigorous activity of the erector spinae as the load nears the vertical. That is, return to the upright position from a flexed posture is begun by the hip extensor muscles rather than the lumbar spine extensors so that the posterior part of the disc, intervertebral disc, and the posterior vertebral ligament are not protected by actively contracting trunk muscles during the early stages of lifting from a flexed position. The likelihood of damage is therefore greater if load is placed on the back in this position. This emphasizes the value of initiating a lift through movement of the legs rather than the trunk. Further, where a stooping position is prolonged, muscles fatigue and their supporting function is decreased. Again, this places a greater demand on the posterior aspect of the intervertebral disc and the posterior ligaments. It has been argued that continued work from a flexed posture could ultimately produce strain and could predispose to LBP.

Disc damage has been linked with sudden high loading of the spine, especially in flexed postures (e.g., when a worker catches a heavy load). This can also occur when one of two partners loses grip on an object being lifted, so that the remaining partner unexpectedly receives an increased load. For this reason, group lifting needs careful coordination, in terms of number of personnel used, size of lifters, understanding of the proposed movements, appreciation of destination, preliminary position and grip to be used, and action commands for lifting, carrying, and lowering.

Speed of movement in lifting and handling may also be important, for if the movement is not adequately under muscular control, additional stress may be suddenly imposed on the spinal ligaments and a sprain may occur. Work demands that require rapid transfers of weights should be avoided.

For those who lift from a knee flexed position, the principal muscle work involved in raising the load relates to the extension of the knees and hips. Because the trunk is held more closely to the vertical, the vertebral column is not placed in a position of vulnerability. If some movement does occur in the spine, it is through a range where the distance of the combined load and weight of the trunk from the center of gravity is small and the effort required by the extensor muscles is less than that required if the trunk were horizontal.

Probably the major problem with the knee action lift is in whether the person has sufficient strength in the extensors of knees and hips to raise the load. These muscles work most efficiently and effectively when the joints are at 90°. If the person squats before lifting, the extensor muscles are placed in a position of mechanical disadvantage and it may be very difficult for the person to raise up to standing. This highlights the need to provide hip and knee extensor exercises in a prevention program.

Noting the challenges to the validity of the recommended lifting method with straight back and bent knees[53] and to the practical utility of such a method,[58] Parnianpour et al[59] applied a lifting stress calculator to individualize and optimize the lifting technique and to take into account clinical complaints. Parnianpour et al[59] reported that this model showed variability of knee joint and back joint angles for different loading conditions, but they emphasized that although the idea of distributing loads between the knee and the back according to a patient's symptoms may be appealing, there is a limited number of postures that can be assumed to carry out a lift in view of the physical characteristics of that load. These experimenters could find no single "safe" method of lifting, supporting previous assertions of the inadequacy of training in proper lifting techniques in reducing LBP and the possibility for greater success in injury prevention through the redesign of the task or workplace.

## ERGONOMIC APPROACHES TO PREVENTION OF LOW BACK PAIN

When the physiotherapist's approach to LBP is solely that of "treatment," the focus is on helping the individual to regain function or compensate for its loss. De Jong[60] has criticized this limited approach in which the physiotherapist aims to minimize the effect of sensory or physical impairment on movements, believing that while it may resolve immediate problems, it ignores the influences of attitudes and environments on the experience of disability. A broader approach, that of disability management,[61] is concerned not only with developing the abilities of those who are disabled, but also with changing attitudes of the professionals and employers to disability. Thus, in disability management, obstacles occurring in the environment are removed in order to restore the individual's working capacity. Such programs incorporate mechanisms commonly used in ergonomics to prevent the occurrence of disability. Because LBP is a multifactorial problem, a team approach is necessary to provide adequate management. Modes of treatment need to be varied according to the individual circumstances.

The emphasis on prevention in ergonomics is on risk control. This relies on the identification of risk factors associated with injury, evaluation of those risks, and implementation of controls that take those risks into account. Following a job analysis, corrective and preventive measures can include such features as advice, education, and training in ergonomic principles; a program of instruction for newcomers to the workplace; redesign of equipment and the work environment; changes in organization and work methods; relaxation and exercises; stress relief; and appropriate assessment and treatment should symptoms occur.

## Job Analysis

Through risk analysis, those aspects of the work situation that represent a risk to the worker can be identified and assessed, so that areas of risk can be placed in order of priority. Three basic approaches are usually adopted in risk identification: analyses of statistics, consultation with relevant personnel, and surveys and observations in the workplace. Statistics such as incidence of accidents and injuries can reveal where and in what jobs specific injuries have occurred. The frequency and severity of injuries relative to the number of employees, the hours worked, or the areas of work can be examined, and injury incidence relative to location, occupation, or task can reveal areas of greater priority for risk assessment and risk control.

Discussion with the personnel involved often helps to reveal problem areas. Because of their intimate knowledge of the work site and the particular task to be performed, the person at risk for musculoskeletal injury has information on potential hazards that may not be apparent to management until after an accident occurs.

Surveys and observations at the workplace can be carried out using simple checklist approaches or by implementing more complex procedures. Checklists provide a focus for examining specific problem areas and may deal with general issues, or more specifically with the type of handling task or the methods of carrying out a task by the operators. Checklists may provide a basis for appraising design of equipment, work space, or the environment, and they may also be used to review the approach to supervision and work organization.

Luopajarvi[62] has pointed out that when workers study their work and workplace actively through the use of worker checklists, they are able to learn the guidelines and, because of their personal involvement, become more motivated. They reflect the form of teaching that emphasizes active participation and learning by doing.

The approach to work analysis has been well described by Luopajarvi.[63] From the point of view of physical risk factors that may lead to LBP, analyses of work load that relate to observation of work postures and movements are most relevant. Direct visual observations, in which postures adopted by the worker are recorded, or more advanced methods of incorporating computerized data recording and possibly involving photography and videotaping may be used. Using work sampling methods, the postures may be observed at predetermined intervals, so that a profile of the work demands may be gained. Analyses can reveal the frequency of stressful postures or movements that could lead to LBP.

Special attention should be paid to the availability of adequate space for the worker's operation, the availability of access for the worker to equipment and storage areas, and the height relationships between the worker and the work surface that could influence the degree of static work posture.

Physiotherapists should apply their understanding of body mechanics to analyze the dynamic posture of the person during performance of their activity. The stability, symmetry, and quality of alignment of the posture assumed and the way in which movements undertaken follow the principles of good posture could be appraised. Details of whether the sequence of movements in various body parts was appropriate; whether satisfactory posture was maintained throughout the activity; and the duration, range, direction of, and resistance to individual specific movements could be determined. These appraisals, with or without the quantitative measures gained during work posture monitoring, would help to clarify the operational demands on the posture and on the musculoskeletal system, leading to the development of suitable modifications for the preservation of posturally safe working conditions.

## Education and Training

Perhaps more subtle than the effects of physical factors on the worker is the potential risk associated with lack of knowledge in relation to work demands. Here, the adequacy of communication, education, and teaching is important. Within the overall program of risk control, employee education has been shown to reduce lost work time.[64] Training workers to recognize and avoid hazards during manual work, to improve coordination and handling skill, and to develop an awareness of their capacity for handling or tolerance for postural stress without LBP is of considerable value.[65] However, poor techniques established after years of habit are very difficult to break.

Bullock[66] has outlined the objectives and possible content of educational programs that may be used for the various categories of worker in industry, and has highlighted the need to use different approaches in educating work supervisors and managers, so that all personnel understand their role in prevention. Supervisors have an added responsibility for risk control and need more guidance not only in methods of reducing work demands, but also in gaining the cooperation of workers.

Objectives for education depend on the program recipients and their type of work, but in most cases, educational programs will need to address the concept of ergonomics, the mechanism of injury relevant to the workplace, and approaches to injury prevention applicable to it. Participants would also be encouraged to question the suitability of their own environment.[66] For example, when guidance about lifting and handling was given, the person would be encouraged to ask whether the job itself needed to be done, whether it might be done more effectively by a machine, whether the frequency of handling material or the distance moved could be reduced, and whether the nature of the load needed to be considered. Participants would also be advised to query the number, capabilities, and lifting habits of people involved in handling the task. It is important that workers are encouraged to examine the situation itself before deciding on how to cope with a particular lift or method of handling.

It is recommended that workers be shown those positions and movements that could be potentially dangerous in their own working environment, and that they be given the opportunity of developing sensible and safe methods of handling and lifting under guidance. Most importantly, those who are involved in manual handling and lifting should be taught how to use their own body power in an appropriate way. This implies that there is sufficient space in which to move and room in which to place the feet and to coordinate the total movement of feet, body, arms, and load during a transfer. The need for suitable exercise and physical fitness must also be emphasized in education programs.

Special attention needs to be given to the education of new employees in an industry or of workers transferred to new manual tasks. Early training in appropriate approaches to movement and to safe working techniques could help to control back injury.

# Design

It has been claimed that the most important way in which ergonomic principles can be applied for prevention of injury is through design, in which all factors that affect the performance of a task are considered, to avoid its presenting a risk to the health and safety of the worker. An important aspect in this regard is the participation of workers in decision making about their own working place. The physiotherapist must be sure to involve the worker in discussions about design needs and improvements that would contribute to safety as well as effectiveness.

Developing a more effective design for a work operation or work method requires an appreciation for the purpose and requirements of the task, as well as the rules that govern design of working techniques matched to individual needs. In particular, these principles relate to the following points: (1) the avoidance of extreme positions of the trunk or shoulders; (2) the use of flowing dynamic movements rather than rigidly held static positions; (3) the importance of relaxing muscles not required for a particular task; and (4) the need to distribute heavy work loads over as many joints and muscles as possible.

The characteristics of the operators and the task are of prime consideration in planning a workplace. One of the most important aspects of the ergonomic design approach is the concern for careful specification of the worker–task relationship, and this demands an appreciation for the variations in body size. Basic requirements of size and shape should be established so that the appropriate height of equipment and workplace relative to the operator and the task demands can be determined, so that posture will be adequate and excessive static muscle work for the trunk muscles avoided. Reference should be made to anthropometric studies that define the range of dimensions relevant to the particular worker population and to the demands of the task. Where a workplace is to be used by many people, adjustability over a range of dimensions relevant to the users needs to be incorporated into the design.

The design of the work process is important also. It should ensure that prolonged fixed postures are avoided, that the worker is not required repeatedly to manipulate heavy objects, that movements demanded by the process do not require rapid acceleration or deceleration, and that there is varied activity by the one worker, combining gross and fine movements.

To avoid some of the musculoskeletal problems that may be associated with poor positioning in sitting, attention has been given to seat and table design. However, although many new ergonomically designed chairs and work tables have been provided for those involved in office work, many of which provide sufficient adjustability to accommodate the large variety of sizes found in workers, this adjustability is not always the case for many industrial activities.[67] In circumstances where the worker is involved in prolonged activity requiring some precision or dexterous work, a large amount of torso and upper extremity mobility is needed, while support for the lower torso and lower limbs is needed to avoid muscle fatigue and circulatory problems. This dual requirement for good postural support together with a capacity for adequate reach and vision, makes the chair and workplace design more complex.[67]

The seated posture should preferably be such that the person can work with the trunk erect; with the lower back supported by the back rest; with the elbows at the side of the body; where practicable, with forearms horizontal or inclined slightly downwards; without excessive bending of the neck; and without pressure being exerted on the underside of the thigh from the front of the seat, when the feet are flat on the floor and knees at right angles.

The seat design should allow for comfortable postural adjustment and should also allow adequate space for the buttocks below the back rest, for the legs if stretched out and for the knees and thighs under the bench or desk. The lumbar support should be firm and should not restrict movement of the vertebral column or the arms. Preferably, the back rest should be clear of the sacrum below and the shoulder blades above and should conform to the forward curvature of the lumbar region. Appropriate pelvic stabilization can also be provided by slightly inclining the seat surface and ensuring adequate support for both feet on the floor. Williams et al's study[68] has shown that with a lumbar support to increase lordosis in sitting, back pain can be significantly reduced.

The relationship of the seat to the work bench or the desk is also important in terms of preventing back injuries, as a too high bench requires the work to be done with arms raised, which is likely to lead to increased lumbar lordosis, while a too low bench encourages stooped working positions. In terms of function, the recommended table height is related to the position of the elbow, which in turn depends on the activity. Where forces need to be exerted through the arms, the person should be in a standing position. The greater the force to be applied, the more elbow extension is necessary. A working surface should be at the correct height for the task and, where the position is likely to be maintained for long periods, the work surface should be sloped toward the worker to reduce the need for stooping.

Care needs to be taken about the design of activities carried out in the sitting position. For example, pedal use in sitting, whether in industry, agriculture, or general transport, can be a risk factor for LBP. Where the line of action of the pedal is vertical, the hip extensor muscle activity needed for pedal depression may demand excessive stabilization forces in the trunk. As a result of extensive experimentation, Bullock[35] recommended that for the seated operator a pedal path should be at 45° to the horizontal, continuous with the "hip to foot on the pedal" line. Troup[2] also recommended that the line of action for pedal depression should pass from the foot through the hip joint and that the back rest should firmly resist the tendency of the pelvis to rotate.

Ergonomic guidelines have been provided for various aspects of work. For example, McCormick and Sanders[69] and Chaffin and Andersson[70] have provided guidelines for the maximum holding time of a static forceful exertion, while Eastman Kodak Company,[71] McCormick and Sanders,[69] and Grandjean[72] have provided ergonomic guidelines for lifting. The maximum allowable lifting for particular situations has also been recommended in a number of ergonomic texts.[69,72] Appreciation for the relationship between heavy manual work and

LBP led to guidelines being developed by the National Institute for Occupational Safety and Health (NIOSH).[73]

Dul and Hildebrandt[74] have reviewed the guidelines outlined by a number of authors concerned with ergonomics and the protection of the low back. Their conclusions suggest that limitations exist in the currently available guidelines and recommend the need for their validation. These authors highlight the need to advance knowledge about the relationship between back load variables such as EMG signals of back muscle activity, biomechanical torques or forces, intra-abdominal pressure, intradiscal pressure, and the long-term incidence of LBP. Dul and Hildebrandt[74] emphasize the need for the development of guidelines that will focus specifically on the prevention of LBP.

Work should be designed to be safe and also to suit the population involved in it. Through introduction of ergonomic principles, adverse handling stresses should be able to be minimized, the cause of postural backache should be removed, and vibratory stresses reduced.[65] The implications of certain design features for LBP and a knowledge of factors that can relieve back pain are necessary in approaching the design of techniques for specified physical activities.

## Work Organization

Although these areas are vitally important to the physical well-being of the worker, other risks associated with the work activity must be appraised. These include the effects of work organization, such as the way work is scheduled, the particular demands on the worker of peaks of activity, and the time allowed for carrying out an activity. Similarly, attitudes to occupational health and safety held throughout the organization, which may have an influence on the provision of assistance for heavy work tasks (in terms of additional personnel or appropriate equipment) and the arrangements made when workers are feeling fatigued as a result of the heavy work demands, need to be appraised.

To be effective, a prevention strategy should focus on the necessary organizational change that will ensure problem identification, documentation, and solution. A work environment must be created that will ensure the participation of the workers, ensure the proper coordination of all preventive measures, encourage both the development of skills and the observance of principles relating to safe manual handling, and that will integrate injury prevention with work procedures and work organization. Indeed, some prevention programs have failed in the past because they have had too exclusive an emphasis on specific lifting technique instructions, too little coordination between functions affecting occupational health and safety, and too little involvement by administrators and management in the prevention process.

## Exercise

It has been acknowledged that there are minimal as well as maximum acceptable work loads in keeping with safety of worker performance. Although emphasis is placed on loads that are beyond the capacity of the worker, it must also be appreciated that too little activity may be an eventual cause of LBP or injury. Magora[20] found the smallest incidence of back pain in a group of policemen who underwent intensive physical training before acceptance into the police force and had to maintain this fitness throughout their career.

Prevention programs should incorporate instruction and guidance in exercises for a number of purposes. For example, in addition to providing education in movement, programs can include advice on methods of general and specific relaxation, exercises to provide active work for muscles maintained in a state of static contraction during the work period, specific exercises to strengthen muscles concerned with lifting and handling, as well as exercises for general physical fitness. Particular attention should be paid to the correction of muscle imbalances and to the strengthening of postural muscles.

Although appropriate design of a job minimizes many of the factors leading to LBP, much of the responsibility for protection of the back must rest with the person. Back pain and back injuries do not only occur in the working environment, but may also occur out of working hours. It is therefore important that all people receive some education not only in ergonomic design, but also in correct approaches to movement, so that they can apply them to their leisure activities, whether it be sport, gardening, or sitting as a spectator.

Activity programs should also emphasize the importance of changing both position and work activity during the working hours. Opportunities for job rotation that allow a change in muscle activity should be provided by management.

## Prevention of Reinjury

The effectiveness of a man–machine system depends on the way in which the mechanical design of the equipment and workplace matches the capacities of the operator. Physiotherapists concerned with the care of the LBP patient should gain an appreciation of the various demands placed on the body by work, home, or leisure activities. Through assessment of relevant attributes such as joint flexibility, muscle strength and endurance, and functional capacity, they should provide advice about modifications of the work environment or the work method that would acknowledge any limitations of the operator.

### Work Site Visits

In considering how, when, and where the worker with LBP may resume work activities, details of the work environment and work activities, as provided by the job analysis, give an understanding of the demands placed on the worker.

This understanding of work demands provides the basis for development of safe and effective methods for the operator's performance of work, which should control risk factors arising from inadequate design of the work process.

Where visits can be made by the physiotherapist to the work site for supervision of work methods, the opportunity for correction of operating difficulties or potentially damaging postures provides reinforcement of good work methods and encourages consultation by the worker who may be uncertain of the correct approaches to prevention. Consultations with a person's foreman may result in the adaptation of the job for the period of rehabilitation.

### Assessment of Functional Capacity

To protect the person against exacerbation of injury, knowledge of their functional capacity—possibly changed by the incidence of the LBP—needs to be gained. Isernhagen[75] has emphasized that for the physiotherapist to provide correct and comprehensive information about a person's functional capacity, the appropriate design of functional capacity assessments is essential. She points out that the best functional capacity evaluators test the total person so that all aspects of movement and movement patterns can be observed. As proposed by Janda[76] in his rule of horizontal and vertical generalization, Isernhagen[77] outlines how a dysfunction in one area (e.g., the knee) may affect normal body mechanics and lead to injuries in another area (e.g., LBP).

The importance of evaluating body movements in the context of work and life situations is also highlighted by Isernhagen.[77] Thus tests of strength, endurance, range of movement, balance, and coordination should be related to relevant work activity. This positive approach, in which the person's level of capacity is assessed, leads to specifications of activities that may still be achieved by the worker.

Functional capacity assessment can provide information that would be helpful in relation to advising the LBP patient when return to work activity is safe and how much can be done. Isernhagen asserts that such an assessment can act as a guide to patients to reach their full maximum potential. She explains that later assessments provide the background to graduated return to work that is at a higher but safe functional level.

Watson et al[78] suggest that the ergonomist's approach to assessing human ability in relation to work demands is appealing in that it seeks to measure interactions between the employee and the work place through the structured, systematic examination of functional items relating to both. These authors developed the Activity Matching Ability System (AMAS), whereby criteria are identified against which measures could be set. They highlight the need for instruments or assessment techniques that measure differences in functional ability. Watson et al[78] believe that the ability assessment offers clinicians a potential instrument for identifying functional deficits and for monitoring functional outcome and change, because it implies that treatments may be focused on restoring or compensating for functions vital to work performance.

**The Back School**

The "back school" was established at Danderyd Hospital, Stockholm, in 1970 as an efficient organization for LBP treatment.[79] The approach of the back school was based on the knowledge that LBP is often exacerbated by increased mechanical strain and on scientific research concerned with etiology of LBP, intradiscal pressure measurements, and epidemiology. Zachrisson–Forssell[79] used ergonomics and education as the main elements of this Swedish program. The back school aims to enable patients to play an active part in improving their working environment in order to reduce their back problem, to provide increased knowledge, so giving better understanding and reducing the risk of inappropriate therapy and reducing the demand for social, medical, and economic resources resulting from avoidable back pain. Through their controlled study, Berqguist–Ullman and Larsson[14] demonstrated a reduction in days lost from work through use of the Swedish Back School, which emphasized the application of ergonomic principles.

Back schools have also been developed in other countries, including Canada[80] and the United States.[81] Hall[80] placed a greater emphasis on encouraging a change of attitude in the person. His study revealed significant subjective improvement in 69 percent of those involved in the Canadian Back School.

The variability in success of back school programs may reflect the great diversity in physical, psychological, and social factors influencing people with LBP as well as the nature, intensity, and duration of pain, and the level of education of the participants. Responsiveness of clients to particular approaches may depend on whether the components of the program match individual needs, can elicit a reaction, or can motivate the client. Most back schools include discussions of anatomy and biomechanics, pain and its control, relaxation and stress management, and the importance of the person's own attitude and motivation to taking positive steps for risk avoidance. Many programs also rely on operant conditioning and major contributions from a psychologist. Back schools usually offer a program of 4 to 10 classes, at weekly intervals. Reinforcement after a period of applying principles learned in daily life is essential.

It must be acknowledged that the back school has not been seen as an effective approach to the management of LBP by all who have used it. For example, Lankhorst et al's study[82] of the effect of the Swedish Back School in chronic idiopathic LBP subjects and Donchin et al's comparison[83] of the effectiveness of the back school with a second intervention program produced results that question the value of the program in reducing LBP episodes.

Ergonomists, recognizing the limitations of educational programs such as these, have emphasized the importance of design changes in the workplace and of modifications to work organization.

## CONCLUSIONS

The application of the principles of ergonomics to the prevention of LBP has considerable value to the person at risk for injury. Because of the cost benefits of controlling back pain and days lost from work, it also has great value to productivity in the industrial situation.

The physiotherapist can contribute to this important area in a significant way. Encouragement of the worker to be aware of hazards in the workplace or in leisure activities and involvement in identification of risks can help to produce the motivation for the clients' participation in control of their own environment. Education in aspects of prevention, in methods of moving the body effectively and safely, and in minimizing or eliminating postural stress through careful design, are essential components of a program. Also important is the need to modify attitudes to occupational health and safety, so that an environment is created in which protection of the person's well-being is seen as vital by all. It is hoped that this positive attitude to prevention will be taken increasingly by those who are consulted by sufferers of LBP.

## REFERENCES

1. Pedersen OF, Petersen R, Statfeldt ES: Back pain and isometric back muscle strength of workers in a Danish factory. Scand J Rehabil Med 7:125, 1975
2. Troup JDG: Driver's back pain and its prevention: a review of the postural, vibratory and muscular factors, together with the problem of transmitted road-shock. Appl Ergon 9:207, 1978
3. Biering-Sorensen F: A prospective study of low back pain in a general population. 1. Occurrence, recurrence and aetiology. Scand J Rehabil Med 15:71, 1983
4. Rowe ML: Low back pain in industry. A position paper. J Occup Med 11:161, 1969
5. Yu T, Roht LH, Wise RA et al: Low back pain in industry an old problem revisited. J Occup Med 26:517, 1984
6. Hershenson A: Cumulative injury: a national problem. J Occup Med 21:674, 1979
7. Troup JDG: Relation of lumbar spine disorders to heavy manual work and lifting. Lancet 1:857, 1965
8. Wickstrom G: Effect of work on degenerative back disease. Scand J Work Environ Health, Suppl. 1:1, 1978
9. Strachan A: Back care in industry. Physiotherapy 65:249, 1979
10. Bullock MI: Ergonomics—a broad challenge for the physiotherapist. p. 3. In Bullock MI (ed): Ergonomics: The Physiotherapist in the Workplace. Churchill Livingstone, Edinburgh, 1990
11. Bullock MI: The physiotherapist's role in the control of industrial injuries. Control 1:69, 1974
12. Andersson GBJ: Epidemiologic aspects on low back pain in industry. Spine 6:53, 1981
13. Manning DP, Shannon HS: Slipping accidents causing low back pain in a gearbox factory. Spine 6:70, 1981
14. Berqguist–Ullman M, Larsson V: Acute low back pain in industry. Acta Orthop Scand, suppl. 170:1, 1977
15. Kumar S: Lifting and ergonomics. p. 183. In Bullock MI (ed): Ergonomics: The Physiotherapist in the Workplace. Churchill Livingstone, Edinburgh, 1990
16. Nachemson AL, Schultz AB, Berkson MH: Mechanical properties of human lumbar spine motion segments. Influences of age, sex, disc level and degeneration. Spine 4:2, 1979
17. Nachemson A: The effect of forward learning on lumbar intra-discal pressure. Acta Orthop Scand 35:314, 1965

18. Kelsey JL: An epidemiological study of the relationship between occupations and acute herniated lumbar intervertebral discs. Int J Epidemiol 4:197, 1975
19. Partridge RE, Anderson JAD, McCarthy JA et al: Rheumatic complaints among workers in Iran foundries. Ann Rheumatol Dis 27:441, 1968
20. Magora A: Investigation of the relation between low back pain and occupation. Scand J Rehabil Med 7:146, 1975
21. Grandjean E, Hunting W: Ergonomics of posture-review of various problems of standing and sitting posture. Appl Ergon 8:135, 1977
22. Corlett EN, Manencia I: The effect and measurement of working postures. Appl Ergon 11:7, 1980
23. Kisner C, Colby LA: Therapeutic Exercises: Foundations and Techniques. 2nd Ed. FA Davis, Philadelphia, 1990
24. Twomey LT, Taylor JR, Oliver MJ: Sustained flexion loading, rapid extension loading of the lumbar spine, and the physical therapy of related injuries. Physiother Pract 4:129, 1988
25. Twomey LT, Taylor JR: Flexion creep deformation and hysteresis in the lumbar vertebral column. Spine 7:116, 1982
26. Jayson NEV: The lumbar spine and back pain. Pitman Medical Company, Edinburgh, 1980
27. Grieco A: Sitting posture: an old problem and a new one. Ergonomics 29:345, 1986
28. Janda V: Movement patterns in the pelvic and the hip region with special reference to pathogenesis of vertebrogenic disturbances. Habilitation Thesis, Charles University, Pragve, Czechoslovakia, 1964
29. Pope MH, Frymoyer JW, Andersson GBJ: Occupational Low Back Pain. Praeger, New York, 1984
30. Keegan JJ: Alterations to the lumbar curve related to posture and seating. J Bone Joint Surg 35A:589, 1953
31. Bogduk N, Twomey LT: Clinical Anatomy of the Lumbar Spine. 2nd Ed. Longman, Singapore, 1991
32. Andersson BJG, Ortengrem R, Nachemson A et al: The sitting posture—an electromyographic and discometric study. Orthop Clin North Am 6:105, 1975
33. Nachemson A: Electromyographic studies on the vertebral portion of the psoas muscle. Acta Orthop Scand 37:177, 1966
34. Bullock MI: The determination of an optimal pedal-operator relationship by the use of stereo photo-gammetry. Biostereometrics: 290. Proceedings of the Symposium of Commission V International Society for Photogrammetry. Washington, 1974
35. Bullock MI: Musculoskeletal disorders in the workplace. p. 93 In Kumashiro M and Megaw ED (eds): Towards Human Work. Taylor and Francis, London, 1991
36. Sullivan A, McGill SM: Changes in spine length during and after seated whole body vibration. Spine 15:1257, 1990
37. Magnussen M, Almqvist M, Broman H et al: Measurement of height loss during whole body vibrations. J Spinal Disorders 5:198, 1992
38. Kakosky T: Vibration disease. Baillière's Clin Rheumat 3:25, 1989
39. Troup JDG: Causes, prediction and prevention of back pain at work. Scand J Work Environ Health 10:419, 1984
40. Stevens J: Low back pain. Med Clin North Am 52:55, 1968
41. Sypher F: Pain in the back. A general theory. J Int Coll Surg 33:718, 1960
42. Janda V: Muscles, central nervous regulation and back problems. p. 27. In Kerr IM (ed): The Neurobiologic Mechanisms in Manipulative Therapy. 1st Ed. Plenum Press, New York and London, 1978

43. Clayson SJ, Newman IM, Debevec DF et al: Evaluation of mobility of hip and lumbar vertebrae in normal young women. Arch Phys Med Rehabil 43:1, 1962

44. Bullock-Saxton JE: Changes in muscle function at hip and low back following chronic ankle sprain. p. 57. Proceedings of the 11th International Congress World Confederation for Physical Therapy. Vol. 1. Chartered Society of Physiotherapy, London, 1991

45. Janda V, Vavrova M: Sensory Motor Stimulation: A video, presented by JE Bullock-Saxton. Body Control Systems, Brisbane, 1990

46. Roberts TDM: The mechanics of the upright posture. Physiotherapy 398:404, 1969

47. Janda V, Schmid HJA: Muscles as a pathogenic factor in back pain. p. 1. Proceedings of the IFOMT Conference, Auckland, New Zealand, 1980

48. Jull GA, Janda V: Muscles and motor control in low back pain: assessment and management. p. 197. In Twomey LJ and Taylor JR (eds): Physical Therapy of the Low Back. Churchill Livingstone, New York, 1987

49. Micheli LJ: Low back pain in the adolescent: differential diagnosis. Am J Sports Med 7:362, 1979

50. Stubbs DA: Trunk stressors in construction and other industrial workers. Spine 6: 83, 1981

51. Schultz AB, Andersson GBJ: Analysis of loads on the lumbar spine. Spine 6:76, 1981

52. Goldberg HM, Kohn HS, Dehn T et al: Diagnosis and management of low back pain. Occup Health Safety, June 14, 1980

53. Chaffin DB, Park KS: A longitudinal study of low back pain associated with occupational weight lifting factors. Am Ind Hyg Assoc J 34:513, 1973

54. Tichauer ER: The biomechanics of the arm-back aggregate under industrial working conditions. ASME 6:28, 1966

55. Schultz AB, Haderspeck-Grip K, Sinkora G et al: Quantitative studies of the flexion-relaxation phenomenon in the back muscles. J Orthop Res 3:189, 1985

56. Kumar S: The study of spinal motion during weight lifting. Ir J Med Sci 143:86, 1974

57. Kumar S, Davis PR: Spinal loading in static and dynamic postures: EMG an intraabdominal pressure study. Ergonomics 26:913, 1983

58. Graveling RA, Simpson GC, Sims MT: Lift with your legs, not with your back: A realistic directive? In Brown ID, Goldsmith R, Coombes K et al (eds): Ergonomics International 85, Proceedings of the 9th Congress of the International Ergonomics Association, Bournemouth, England, Taylor and Francis, London, 1985

59. Parnianpour M, Bejjani FJ, Pavlidis L: Worker training: the fallacy of a single, correct lifting technique. Ergonomics 30:331, 1987

60. De Jong G: Independent living as an analytic paradigm. Aust Rehabil Rev 6:45, 1982

61. Galvin DE: Employer-based disability management and rehabilitation programs. Ann Rev Rehabil 5:23, 1985

62. Luopajarvi T: Workers' education. Ergonomics 30:305, 1987

63. Luopajarvi T: Ergonomic analysis of workplace and postural load. p. 51. In Bullock MI (Ed): Ergonomics: The Physiotherapist in the Workplace. Churchill Livingstone, Edinburgh, 1990

64. Tabor M: Reconstructing the scene: back injury. Occup Health Safety, February 16, 1982

65. Troup JDG: Bone mechanics of the vertebral column, its application to prevention of back pain in the population and to assessment of working capacity in patients with lumbar spinal disability. Physiotherapy 65:238, 1979

66. Bullock MI: Health education in the workplace. p. 9. In Isernhagen S (ed): Work Injury, Management and Prevention. Aspen Publishers, Rockville, MD, 1988

67. Chaffin D: Occupational biomechanics—a basis for workplace design to prevent musculoskeletal injuries. Ergonomics 30:321, 1987

68. Williams MM, Hawley JA, McKenzie RA et al: A comparison of the effects of two sitting postures on back and referred pain. Spine 16:1185, 1991

69. McCormick EJ, Sanders MS: Human Factors in Engineering and Design. McGraw-Hill International, Auckland, 1984

70. Chaffin DB, Andersson GBJ: Occupational Biomechanics. Wiley, New York, 1984

71. Eastman Kodak Company: Ergonomics Design for People at Work. Vol. 1. Lifetime Learning Publications, Belmont, 1983

72. Grandjean E: Fitting the Task to the Man. Taylor and Francis, London, 1980

73. National Institute of Occupational Safety and Health: Work Practices Guide for Manual Lifting. Publication 81-122, Government Printing Office, Washington, D.C., 1981

74. Dul J, Hildebrandt VH: Ergonomic guidelines for the prevention of low back pain at the work place. Ergonomics 30:419, 1987

75. Isernhagen J: Work injury, management and prevention. Aspen Publishers, Rockville, MD, 1988

76. Janda V: Introduction to functional pathology of the motor system. p. 39. In Bullock MI (ed): Proceedings of the VII Commonwealth Games International Conference. Vol. 3. University of Queensland Press, Brisbane, 1982

77. Isernhagen J: The role of functional capacities assessment after rehabilitation. p. 259. In Bullock MI (ed): Ergonomics: The Physiotherapist in the Workplace. Churchill Livingstone, Edinburgh, 1990

78. Watson H, Whalley S, McClelland I: Matching work demands to functional ability. p. 231. In Bullock MI (ed): Ergonomics: The Physiotherapist in the Workplace. Churchill Livingstone, Edinburgh, 1990

79. Zachrisson-Forssell M: The Swedish back school. Physiotherapy 66:112, 1980

80. Hall H: The Canadian back education units. Physiotherapy 66:115, 1980

81. Mattmiller AW: The California back school. Physiotherapy 66:118, 1980

82. Lankhorst GJ, Van de Statd RJ, Vogelaar TW et al: The effect of the Swedish Back School in chronic idiopathic low back pain. Scand J Rehabil Med 15:141, 1983

83. Donchin M, Woolf O, Kaplan L et al: Secondary prevention of low back pain, a clinical trial. Spine 15:1317, 1990

# 13 | Lifting and Back Pain

*M. Scott Sullivan*

Epidemiologic studies have identified heavy manual labor as a major risk factor for the development of low back pain.[1] According to Kelsey,[1] one major risk factor for developing acute intervertebral disc prolapse is frequent lifting of objects weighing 25 lb or more. The risk is greater when objects are held away from the body while lifting, and when twisting of the trunk occurs during lifting.[2] Further evidence supporting lifting as a cause of low back pain stems from reports that sudden onset of low back pain is frequently preceded by an event involving manual lifting.[3,4]

Physical therapists frequently administer treatment to individuals with back injuries who return to jobs involving manual lifting. In addition to performing physical therapy assessments, physical therapists frequently evaluate patients' abilities to return to work through the use of functional capacities evaluations. These evaluations usually involve assessments of patients' abilities to lift manually. Physical therapy treatments are frequently complimented by patient education[5] and work-conditioning programs,[6] which have been developed to prepare the patient to safely tolerate the physical demands of the job. These programs frequently spend a great deal of time teaching proper lifting technique.

In recent years physical therapists have also become more involved in back-pain prevention programs involving pre-employment screening and back schools for workers.[7] The pre-employment screening programs often involve analysis of the critical demands of the jobs and measurement of the worker's physical capabilities to perform these tasks. Pre-employment screening is frequently used in industries with jobs involving manual lifting. Back school education programs instruct participants in basic spinal structure and function, basic mechanical principles, and proper body mechanics during lifting in an effort to prevent back injuries. Because physical therapists evaluate lifting ability and instruct patients and workers in lifting techniques, it is imperative for the physical therapist to have a working knowledge of the relationship between (1) lifting

329

and low back pain, (2) biomechanics of lifting, and (3) current theories of back support mechanisms employed during lifting.

Physical therapists also need to analyze critically the reliability and validity of lifting assessments performed in clinical and industrial settings, but exploration of the topic is beyond the scope of this chapter.

The purposes of this chapter are to consider the current literature on the biomechanics of lifting and the back support mechanisms, to discuss mechanisms of back injuries while lifting, and to offer rationale for instructing patients and industrial workers in lifting technique.

## BIOMECHANICS OF LIFTING

The forces acting on the spine during lifting may be estimated by the use of free body diagrams and static equilibrium equations. The free body diagram uses known quantities of certain variables to predict unknown quantities of other variables. For example, the biomechanist can predict joint reaction forces and muscle force requirements needed for a person to lift a given weight, by using some of the following information: the body positions during the lift, weight of the person and of the load lifted, acceleration of the body and the weight, ground reaction forces, and a variety of anatomic measurements. Some of the earlier biomechanical studies of lifting were limited by the available technology, and need to be considered within this perspective. State-of-the-art equipment is available to measure positions and acceleration at very short intervals of time. This increased accuracy of measurement of known variables increases the accuracy of predicting the unknown variables.

Joint reaction forces can be broken down into components of compression and shear. For the purposes of this chapter, the compression component of the spinal joint reaction forces is discussed, because the magnitude of the compressive forces are much greater than the shear forces. Because of the large magnitude of the compression component of the joint reaction forces during lifting, and the potential of these forces to injure the spine, these forces have been widely examined in the literature.

When the spine is modeled as a cantilever, contraction of the erector spinae and other back muscles produces an extension moment at the lumbar spine to balance a flexion moment produced by the forwardly inclined upper body and a weight held in the hands. Since loads are usually lifted a considerable distance in front of the lumbosacral joint, the flexion moment produced by even modest weights can be very large. For example, in Figure 13-1 a person with an upper body weight of 450 N holds a 200 N object 40 cm anterior to the L5–S1 joint. The center of mass of the upper body is 25 cm anterior to the L5–S1 joint, and the erector spinae and multifidus muscles are, on average, 5 cm posterior to the joint axis. The flexion moment about the L5–S1 joint is 192.5 Nm.

When static equilibrium is assumed, the sum of all forces must be equal to zero. To balance the moments, 3850 N of force must be produced by the musculature in the opposite direction (see Fig. 13-1).

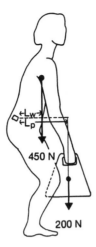

**Fig. 13-1.** Static equilibrium equations use known variables to predict an unknown variable, which in this case is the muscle force required to balance the moments generated by the upper body and the weight. This is expressed in the following equation:

$$\sum \text{moments} = 0$$
$$(W \times L_w) + (P \times L_p) - (M \times L_M) = 0$$
$$(450 \text{ N} \times 0.25 \text{ m}) + (200 \text{ N} \times 0.4 \text{ m}) - (M \times 0.05) = 0$$
$$112.5 \text{ Nm} + 80 \text{ Nm} = M \times 0.05 \text{ m}$$
$$192.5 \text{ Nm}/0.05 \text{ m} = M$$
$$M = 3850 \text{ N}$$

(Adapted from Nordin and Frankel,[64] with permission.)

This back muscle force is the major contributor to the compressive component of the joint reaction forces at the spinal joints; the weight of the upper body and the weight lifted add to the joint compression to a lesser extent.

The previous example estimated joint compression forces for a person standing still. When the body is accelerating, as it does during lifting, the moment produced by the weight and upper body is greater, and thus greater back muscle forces and joint compression forces result.[8,9]

In 1957 Perey[10] demonstrated that postmortem lumbar vertebrae and/or their cartilaginous end-plates will be crushed by compressive loads of 5000 to 11,000 N. Using the static equilibrium analysis from above, the compressive strength of these postmortem vertebrae would be exceeded if weights greater than 110 kg were lifted. This is precisely what was believed in 1957: a man lifting more than 250 lb should crush his lumbar vertebrae. However, competitive weight lifters were known to lift more than 250 lb without incurring back injuries. This apparent paradox sparked a series of studies to search for support mechanisms that would protect the spine from high compressive forces.

More recent studies of vertebral compression strength, however, have shown that the vertebrae in some cases are able to withstand compression forces of 14,000 N.[11] It is possible that vertebrae can be strengthened to even greater levels. For example, in a sample of eight elite weight lifters, Granhed et al[12] found bone mineral content of lumbar vertebrae to have a strong, positive correlation to the amount of heavy lifting performed over a 1-year period. Considering that bone mineral content has a positive correlation ($r = .86$) with ultimate compression strength in cadaveric vertebrae,[13] it is highly probable that the compressive strength of the vertebrae in these weight lifters is proportional to the amount of lifting performed over time. The results of the study by Granhed et al should be interpreted with caution because of the small sample size, and may only apply to extremely high levels of physical activity.

There is a high degree of variability in vertebral compressive strength,[10,11,13,14] which may be largely dependent on the intensity and type of physical activity in which individuals participate. Theoretical arguments for the need of spinal compression-sparing mechanisms during heavy lifting often neglect the ability of the vertebra to increase in strength in response to gradual increases in loading.

Intervertebral discs, contrary to popular belief, are very resistant to large compressive loads. In vitro experiments have demonstrated that the cartilaginous end-plates and the vertebral bodies fail under high compression loads prior to the intervertebral discs.[10,13,14] However, with frequent repeated loading over a period of 5 to 7 hours, cadaveric intervertebral discs will fail,[14,15] even when loaded under simulated physiologic range of motion (ROM), with forces as low as 1300 N.[15] It can be concluded that the intervertebral discs are resistant to high compressive forces but will eventually fatigue under repeated loading. The extent to which the results of these laboratory studies reflect the response of discs to physiologic loading in the living is unknown.

As stated earlier, joint compression forces are largely attributable to the force generated from the back muscles. It is logical that, in young healthy people, the compression strength of the vertebra must bear some proportionality to the tensile-producing capabilities of the muscles. If this were not the case, the vertebrae would be damaged by routine physical activity.

During most routine activities, a healthy person's vertebrae are strong enough to withstand the reaction forces produced by the body's own musculature. An exception may be made for generally healthy older women who have greater incidence of osteoporosis than the general population. Individuals who participate in strenuous activities build stronger tissue in response to loading; this is true of both the vertebrae[12] and the back muscles.[16] Animal studies have demonstrated that the ultimate tensile strength of ligamentous tissue also increases with increased activity.[17] Because of this tissue mutability in response to overload, arguments have been presented by some researchers that there is no need for theoretical explanations of compression-sparing mechanisms.[18,19]

Although mechanisms to reduce compression on the joints may not be necessary to explain human lifting ability, theoretical arguments for their existence have led to numerous studies of lifting, including studies measuring intraabdominal pressure (IAP). It is worth exploring these studies for several reasons:

1. Increased IAP has been observed in individuals performing heavy lifts when they were given no instruction to increase IAP by breath holding, presumably because it has some beneficial effect.[20]
2. The use of inflatable abdominal corsets and weight lifting belts have been demonstrated to increase IAP during lifting.[20,21]
3. Competitive weight lifters report that the belts increase their sense of security and comfort during training and competition.[21]

These factors suggest that IAP may play an important role in lifting. Furthermore, other theoretical support mechanisms are worthy of discussion because they may add insight to how the spine functions during lifting whether or not they reduce compressive loads.

## THEORIES OF BACK SUPPORT MECHANISMS

### The Role of Intraabdominal Pressure

Bartelink[22] first proposed the theory of weight transfer to the pelvis through the thorax and abdomen as a means of sparing the spine excessive compression. He measured IAP on one individual during lifting, and found increases in IAP with increasing loads. He theorized that if the abdomen were pressurized by the contracting abdominal muscles while the glottis and anus were held tightly closed, weight could be transferred through the abdomen as if the latter were a fluid ball. Bartelink theorized that the load imparted through the trunk would be dispersed across the pelvic floor rather than through the vertebral column alone (Fig. 13-2).

Morris et al[20] proposed to test the hypothesis that the thoracic cavity and the abdomen, when pressurized, were capable of resisting part of the force generated in loading the trunk during lifting. The investigators measured intrathoracic and intraabdominal pressure and raw electromyographic (EMG) activity of the "deep back muscles," rectus abdominus, oblique abdominal muscles, and intercostal muscles while 10 subjects lifted weights ranging from 0 to 200 lb. The IAP was measured with open-tipped catheters placed in the stomach and the esophagus. The authors described the EMG only by stating that fine-wire electrodes were used. No information was reported on their recording equipment.

Morris et al[20] concluded that intraabdominal pressure increased with increasing loads. They speculated that the increase in IAP was reflexive; they reached this conclusion because they observed IAP increases, but had not offered the subjects any instructions to increase the IAP during lifting. By the use of static equilibrium analysis, Morris et al predicted that the IAP mechanism

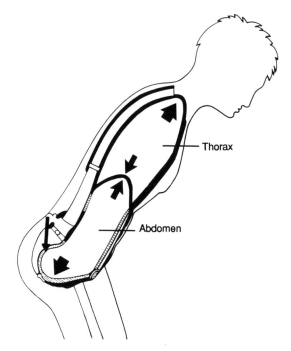

**Fig. 13-2.**    Raised intraabdominal pressure is depicted in the diagram. Load is theoretically transferred from the thoracic spine and the diaphragm, through the pressurized abdominal contents, to the pelvic floor. (Adapted from Kapandji,[65] with permission.)

reduced the compressive joint reaction forces at the lumbosacral junction by 30 percent.

Morris et al[20] also observed that the oblique abdominal muscles activity increased along with increases in IAP. When a corset was placed on the subjects to support the abdominal cavity, IAP increased, but there was little increase in the oblique abdominal muscle activity. This was an indication that the increase in IAP requires a firm abdominal wall, which was created by oblique abdominal muscle contraction in the absence of a corset.

There are several limitations of the study by Morris et al.[20] In their free body diagram and static equilibrium equation, the authors estimated muscle cross-sectional area indirectly through the use of tables in an anatomic text dating back to the year 1844. They did not account for changes in human nutrition, size, activities, and general health over the intervening century. They used the tensile capability of ankle muscles to estimate the tensile capabilities of the trunk muscles. Finally, they did not describe their recording equipment, nor report the reliability of their measurements. Given these limitations, it is difficult to accept their quantitative conclusions. Nevertheless, it appears from their data that IAP increased with increasing loads in all 10 subjects. The activity of the back muscles also appeared to increase with increasing loads. This may indicate that the IAP and the erector spinae activity work simultaneously to resist trunk flexion during lifting, although the degree to which these reported increases were attributable to measurement error is unknown.

McGill et al[21] studied the effects of breath holding and exhalation during lifting on the EMG activity of the erector spinae, abdominal, and intercostal muscles in six subjects. The EMG activity was normalized as a percentage of maximum voluntary contraction (MVC) for each muscle group studied. The raw EMG signals were obtained with surface electrodes and were processed to yield a linear envelope for each EMG signal. The IAP was measured by an intragastric catheter attached to a control unit, and vertical hand forces were measured by strain gauges in the handlebars of the lifting apparatus.

The authors demonstrated only a slight reduction in EMG activity of the erector spinae muscles when the abdomen was pressurized by the lifters holding their breath. This reduced EMG activity was not statistically significant. Using a complex computer algorithm, McGill and Norman[18] estimated that, on average, compression on the L4–L5 joint was reduced by 7 percent during lifting with the breath held.[21]

In the trial in which subjects lifted with belts, IAP was significantly greater than without the belt, but erector spinae EMG activity was not reduced, and compressive forces were not diminished at the L4 to L5 joint.

The authors did not describe whether the MVCs of the erector spinae and abdominal muscles was measured with the belt on. If MVC was measured with the belt off, it is conceivable that the pressure of the belt against the skin may have created an artificial increase in the EMG readout, thereby erroneously negating any compression-reducing effects of the belt. The results are inconclusive regarding EMG results in the trials with the belts worn. The IAP increased when subjects held the breath and increased further when belts were worn. The increase in IAP during lifting without a belt slightly reduced joint compression forces.

Andersson et al[23] studied in vivo intradiscal pressures and EMG activity and IAP on five men while they lifted 100 N. The purpose of the study was to examine the forces on the spine when lifting with the back flexed at the lumbar spine and with the back held in the upright position while the knees were flexed. In part of the study, one subject lifted the weight while performing a Valsalva maneuver. The authors found that the intradiscal pressure was not reduced, although there was an increase in the IAP. The intradiscal pressures were measured by use of a well-established procedure involving a pressure transducer inserted into the disc percutaneously; myoelectric activity was measured using integrated EMG, but measurement error was not reported for EMG.

In a later study, the same group investigated the effect of a Valsalva maneuver on intradiscal pressure and EMG activity of the rectus abdominus, oblique abdominal, and erector spinae muscles in four individuals.[24] The authors found that IAP increased with a voluntary Valsalva maneuver during all activities. In four of five activities, intradiscal pressure of the L3 to L4 intervertebral disc was also increased. The only activity in which intradiscal pressure was reduced involved subjects leaning forward 30° while holding 8 kg in the hands. This activity produced a mean intradiscal pressure of 1600 kPa. This was more than twice the intradiscal pressure produced by any other activity studied.

The reduction in intradiscal pressure with the Valsalva maneuver was only 150 kPa (0.9 percent). This reduction was less than 1 percent of total pressure, which likely represents little or no change in intradiscal pressure since the error in this measurement, under the best laboratory conditions, was ±0.5 percent.[25] The authors do not attempt to explain why intradiscal pressures were not increased in the one task. The results of this study suggest that increases in IAP, while subjects are in upright position, produce increases in intradiscal pressures.

The research on the IAP mechanism stems from an initial belief that the spine must be spared compression in order to remain uninjured during lifting activities. This belief is refuted by some of the recent literature. There is a strong argument raised that there is no need for a compression-sparing mechanism. If there is a need for a compression-sparing mechanism, the IAP mechanism is not likely to fill the role, since it has been demonstrated to increase intradiscal pressure, which is an indirect measure of spinal joint compression. Yet the consistent increases in IAP during lifting, and the popularity of weight lifting belts among competitive weight lifters, suggest that IAP plays some role during heavy manual lifting.

Weight lifters have been known to black out during extremely heavy lifting.[21] This phenomenon has been attributed to increases in IAP, which cause an impedance of blood flow in the major vessels. If the impedance of venous return increases the volume of blood contained within the vertebra, this increased blood volume in the vertebra might increase the compressive strength of the vertebral body. No research was found that investigated this theoretical construct.

## The Spine as an Arch

Aspden[26,27] has recently proposed a mathematic model that may explain the role of intraabdominal pressure during lifting. He proposes that the spine functions like a masonry arch. Aspden maintains that the predicted joint compression forces are greatly reduced when the spine is modeled as an arch rather than a cantilever. He proposes that, if stability is to be maintained, loads must be imparted through the cross section of the arch at all cross sections.[16] Aspden states that position of the spine is adjusted at each spinal segment under various loading situations, so that the thrust line is kept close to the center of the spine's cross section at all levels. This, he argues, is accomplished only if some degree of lumbar lordosis is maintained (Fig. 13-3).

Certain assumptions in Aspden's model have been refuted, such as the model's neglect for the joint reaction forces due to the contraction of the back muscles.[19] Aspden neglects these forces because he views the muscles as "intrinsic to the spine," whereas cantilever models view the muscle forces as "external" to the spine. Contrary to his argument that the muscles do not

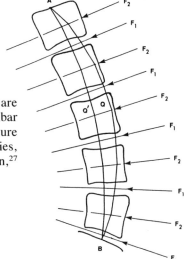

**Fig. 13-3.** The spine as an arch. AQB and AQ'B are thrust lines representing the load through the lumbar spine. $F_1$ and $F_2$ represent the intraabdominal pressure forces applied to the discs and the vertebral bodies, adding stability to the arch. (Adapted from Aspden,[27] with permission.)

produce tension in proportion to the loads carried, empirical evidence shows that the magnitude of myoelectric activity of the back muscles is proportional to the load held in the hands.[28]

The arch theory would not explain away high compressive forces if forces due to back muscle tension were included in the model. Additionally, isolated segmental activation of the back muscles has not been empirically demonstrated. Aside from the assumptions and limitations of Aspden's model, the arch theory helps to explain some previously unexplained phenomena.

For example, in the arch model increased IAP adds to stability of the spine by loading the convex side of the arch. Aspden mathematically demonstrated how increases in IAP also increase intradiscal pressures when the lordosis is maintained. This matches well with empirically demonstrated increases in intradiscal pressure when subjects performed Valsalva maneuvers while the trunk was in the upright position.[23] Aspden also explains why there is no increase in intradiscal pressure when subjects lean forward 30°[23]; in this position the anterior aspect of the lumbar spine is no longer convex, and the increase in IAP actually *reduces* intradiscal pressure, but also reduces the stability of the arch. Because there is reduced stability in the flexed posture, Aspden states that there is no improvement in mechanical advantage with increased IAP in a flexed position. If this is the case, Aspden[26,27] fails to explain why reflexive increases in IAP have been observed when subjects performed an isometric contraction of the back muscles while the trunk was flexed to 90° at the waist.[20]

If the spine does function as an arch, increases in IAP might add stability to the spine when the lumbar lordosis is maintained. The mathematic model of the spine as an arch does not explain the role of increased IAP in the flexed posture, nor does it adequately explain reduced compressive joint reaction forces when appropriate muscle tension forces are considered. Further research into this theoretical model is needed to draw any definite conclusions.

## Posterior Ligamentous
## and Thoracolumbar Fascia Models

Aside from concerns that dangerously large compressive loads on the spine occur during lifting, Gracovetsky et al[29] proposed that the back muscles lack the force-producing capabilities to balance the flexion moments produced during heavy lifting. This hypothesis has led them to introduce several new theories of back support mechanisms.

Gracovetsky et al[29] suggested that people who lift heavy weights reflexively flex the lumbar spine in order to impart tension of the "posterior ligamentous system" (PLS), thus allowing the system to create an extension moment. They argue that this is necessary because the muscles are not strong enough and the PLS has a better mechanical advantage than the muscle, which spares the spine undue compression. Their PLS consists of the supraspinous, interspinous ligaments, ligamentum flavum, the zygapophyseal joint capsules, and the thoracolumbar fascia.[29]

The model proposes that during trunk extension the erector spinae are not active until after the ligamentous system is engaged through active hip extension. As the erector spinae muscles contract and broaden within the envelope of the thoracolumbar fascia (TLF), they add tension through the TLF and increase its stiffness. The authors termed this phenomenon the *hydraulic amplifier mechanism*.[29]

Gracovetsky et al[29] believed that rises in IAP during lifting were produced by the contraction of the transversus abdominus and internal oblique muscles, whose major functions in lifting are to increase tension through the TLF.[30] The crisscross orientation of the fibers of the posterior layer of the TLF were believed to be capable of producing an "antiflexion moment" when tightened by the abdominal muscle contraction.[31] Figure 13-4 depicts the interaction of the mechanisms proposed by Gracovetsky et al.[29]

There are several limitations of the models presented by Gracovetsky et al. The first is their assumption that back muscles are not large enough to lift heavy weights. Their models determined muscle force capabilities by extrapolating muscle force-per-unit-area data from studies that did not specifically measure force production of back muscles. Nor did the authors state any limitations of the studies that determined these force capabilities. Gracovetsky et al[29,30] claim that these measures were substantiated empirically by isometric back extension force measurements. Unfortunately the study they cited measured isometric back extension force in the neutral, or lordotic, position of the lumbar spine.[32,33] Recent evidence demonstrates that back extension forces, produced isometrically, are much greater when the lumbar spine is flexed than when it is in a neutral position.[34] This fits well with lifting since the largest flexion

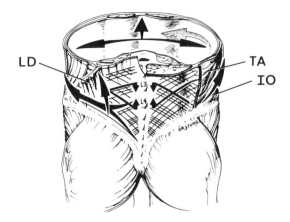

**Fig. 13-4.** Intraabdominal pressure, represented by the tri-radiate arrows within the abdominal cavity, increases tension along the transversus abdominus *(TA)* and internal oblique muscles *(IO)*. TA and IO insert onto the TLF, and along with latissimus dorsi *(LD)*, produce tension within the TLF. Due to the crisscrossing pattern of its fibers, the posterior layer of TLF produces an antiflexion moment on the lumbar spine. See text for further discussion. (Adapted from Sullivan and Jantzen,[67] with permission.)

moments occur at the early part of the lift, when the spine tends to be flexed and inertial forces must be overcome.[8–10]

Back muscle force production was probably greatly underestimated by Gracovetsky et al. Computed tomography (CT) measurements of cross-sectional areas of the back muscles and lengths of their lever arms have been reported for a sample of 13 young, healthy males.[35] Force production capabilities were predicted by use of estimates of force-per-unit-area of human muscle. Even though the limitations of these extrapolations are the same as expressed for Gracovetsky et al's work, the back muscles in this small sample were predicted to be capable of producing twice the moment predicted by Gracovetsky et al. It is interesting to note that McGill et al[35] predicted extensor moments of the back muscle to be as high as 490 Nm, and recent empirical data of isometric force production reveal a mean value of 465 ± 151 Nm, in a similar population.[34]

The hypothesis that ligaments counter the flexion moments about the spine during lifting has been refuted on the grounds that the combined tensile strength of the ligaments, coupled with very short lever arms, yields an extension moment of only 50 Nm.[36] This conclusion is based on average tensile strengths of tissue from cadaveric material.[37] With consideration of the large variability in tensile strength and lever arm distances, the magnitude of the forces produced during heavy lifting should still well exceed ultimate tensile strength of the strongest ligaments.

The abdominal mechanism theory in which the transversus abdominus muscle produces an extension moment through the TLF has been rescinded by those who originally proposed it.[38] The estimated ability of the transversus abdominus muscle to produce an extension moment through the TLF is only

7 Nm.[38] However, this does not imply that the TLF has no role in resisting lumbar spine flexion. It is important to realize that the TLF has the greatest mechanical advantage of any soft tissue posterior to the axes of sagittal plane rotation of lumbar spine, as it surrounds the muscles and ligaments. The TLF may be tensed, not only by the transversus abdominus and the back muscles contracting within its confines, but also by the latissimus dorsi, to which it is broadly attached.[31]

With regard to heavy lifting, there is little support for the back support models proposed by Gracovetsky et al,[29,30] and a fair body of evidence refuting their feasibility. No objective evidence was found to support the notion that the back muscles are incapable of lifting heavy loads. Also, there is no evidence to support the anecdotal accounts that, given the choice of lifting postures, people choose a flexed spine for lifting heavy loads. Contrary to these accounts, a study presented in the next section found that, when lifting extremely heavy weights, weight lifters avoided the full range of flexion, even when lifting with a "rounded back."[39]

## ELECTROMYOGRAPHIC ACTIVITY DURING LIFTING

### Flexion Relaxation Response

Studies of EMG activity of the erector spinae muscle group during spine flexion and extension from a standing position have found them to be active during the movement of flexion and electrically silent just prior to the end range of flexion.[40,41] This phenomenon is frequently referred to as the *flexion relaxation response*. This response has been reported in the transversospinalis group of lumbar spine muscles as well as the erector spinae.[42]

Kippers and Parker[41] reported that, during extension from the fully flexed position, electrical activity of the erector spinae muscles occurred *after* the lumbar spine began to extend. They explain that lumbar spine extension was facilitated by contraction of the hamstring and gluteal muscles, which rotated the pelvis backward on the hips. They hypothesize that extension of the lumbar spine is initiated via a rebound of the posterior ligaments.

The actual amount of extension of the lumbar spine at the initiation of the back-bent lift is debatable. Kippers and Parker report an average of 6° of lumbar extension prior to the return of erector spinae activity when subjects extended from full flexion.[41] When their measurement error is carefully considered, the average extension could have ranged from 2° to 10°.

Holmes et al[8] observed no lumbar extension until the erector spinae muscles were reactivated when subjects squat-lifted with fully flexed lumbar spines. They measured lumbar angular excursion by recording angular relationships between markers over the L3 vertebra and the hip. Therefore, they did not measure lumbar spine motion directly, and it is possible that the rebound phenomenon initiated extension to some degree.

Both of these studies also evaluated EMG response during extension movements when loads of 10 to 15 kg were lifted. As in unloaded conditions, movement was initiated via the rotation of the pelvis and the amount of lumbar extension produced prior to electrical activity of the muscles when rising from a flexed posture was nominal.

McGill and Norman[18] studied the EMG activity of the latissimus dorsi muscles during heavy lifting while subjects were positioned with the knees bent and back straight. They reported that the peak activity of these muscles was at the initiation of the lift. No studies were found that looked at EMG activity of the latissimus dorsi during lifts with the back fully flexed. It is possible that in this position the latissimus dorsi muscles initiate extension through their attachment to the TLF.

Cholewicki and McGill[39] measured vertebral motions via digitization of fluoroscopic images of the lumbar spines of four male weight lifters. Erector spinae muscle activity was monitored on an oscilloscope with surface EMG. The subjects flexed forward to the point at which myoelectric silence of the erector spinae muscles was achieved, the assumption being that in this position the ligaments bore the entire load of the trunk. Continuous fluoroscopic imaging was employed throughout the movement and recorded on videotape. Subjects then performed two dead-lifts (fully flexing at the trunk and extending to the upright position), under fluoroscopic imaging, with barbells of masses between 157 and 211 kg. Videotape of the fluoroscopic images were later digitized and angular and linear relationships between vertebrae were calculated for the unloaded and lifting conditions. Test–retest measurement errors of the angular and linear measurements were very small.

In all but one lift for one individual, the subjects flexed their lumbar spines to a position somewhat short of loading the ligaments. In the one lift during which the lifter flexed beyond the point of myoelectric silence, he adjusted his position at the request of the radiographer; the lifter also experienced pain during that lift. It can be concluded that in extremely heavy lifts performed by experienced weight lifters, the ligaments do not bear substantial loads. This holds true even when the spine appears to be fully flexed.

## Lumbar Posture and Electromyographic Activity

Several studies have compared EMG activity of the erector spinae and oblique abdominal muscles in kyphotic and lordotic postures during squat lifting.[43,44] Squat lifting is defined as lifting with the knees flexed and the back in a relatively upright position. Weight of the loads lifted ranged from 10 to 157 N. Each of these studies found the EMG activity of the erector spinae muscles to be greater in the lordotic posture, particularly at the early phase of the lift.[8,43] This peak activity of the muscles at the early part of the lift is attributed to the muscle forces needed to overcome inertia.[8,9,45] Delitto et al[43] found the oblique abdominal muscles to be active during the early phase of lifting regardless of the lumbar posture. They believed this abdominal muscle activity to be responsible for increased IAP and "enhancement of the thoracolumbar fascia" at the initiation of the lift.

Maintaining the lumbar lordosis during squat lifting has been advocated primarily because the muscles are well suited to produce high tensile forces and are able to adapt to sudden changes in loading conditions, whereas the ligaments are essentially passive structures and are limited in their ability to adapt to sudden changes.[43,44]

No studies of EMG activity of the psoas major during lifting were found in the literature, but two studies of the EMG activity of the vertebral portion of the psoas major under unloaded conditions have been documented. Nachemson[46] Studied EMG activity of the psoas major when a needle electrode was inserted into the muscle percutaneously with the aid of fluoroscopic visualization. Keagy et al[47] used implanted copper fine-wire electrodes applied to the muscle during abdominal-approach sympathectomies for treatment of intermittent claudication. Both studies used visual observation of raw EMG data on strip chart recorders to determine degree of muscle activity. Neither study reported the reliability of their classifications to determine difference in degree of muscle activity.

Whereas Nachemson[46] found the psoas major to be active in the upright position and while subjects bent forward 20°, Keagy et al[47] reported no activity of the muscle in these positions. Keagy et al[47] did find, however, that the muscle was most active when subjects laterally flexed to the side opposite the muscle, and when the subjects leaned backward. Since the insertion of the electrodes was visually observed by Keagy et al,[47] and since Nachemson's description of the action of the psoas major is paradoxical, I will accept the findings of Keagy et al[47] and attribute Nachemson's findings[46] to error associated with needle placement and/or electrical signals originating in other muscles.

It is possible, however, to speculate on the role of the psoas in heavy lifting. It is conceivable that the psoas major is actively stabilizing the lumbar spine when the spine is heavily loaded in the upright position. Individuals lean slightly backward while holding a heavy load. This "locking out" of the spine was observed by Cholewicki and McGill[39] when subjects reached the upright position at the completion of extremely heavy dead-lifts. Cholewicki and McGill[39] reported slight vertebral flexion at the upper lumbar levels at this final phase of dead-lifting. This upper lumbar spine flexion may be attributable to the contraction of the psoas major.

The stabilizing effect of the psoas major also seems to fit the arch model proposed by Aspden.[26] When the psoas major muscles contract simultaneously, they are ideally suited to load the arch through its cross section, thus adding stability. Measurements from CT scan images reveal that the psoas major has the largest cross-sectional area of any muscle surrounding the lumbar spine.[35] If form follows function, the vertebral portion of psoas major is likely to have a major role in stabilizing the spine. Further study is needed in order to draw any definitive conclusions of the role of this muscle during lifting.

## Stoop Lifting Versus Squat Lifting

Many studies have examined stoop lifting (back bent) in comparison to squat lifting (knees bent.[45,48–50] The squat lift is generally believed to be preferable to a stoop lift because it allows the subject to lift an object from between the legs, which has been demonstrated to shorten the horizontal distance of the load from the body and reduce the flexion moment at the lumbosacral spine.[9,45,50] The squat lift requires greater energy expenditure than the stoop lift because a larger portion of body weight is lowered and lifted than during stoop lifting.[45]

The evidence presented in this section suggests that none of the so-called back support mechanism theories can adequately account for significant reduction of joint compression forces during lifting. The current understanding of biologic response of spinal structures to loading suggests that, under routine loading conditions in healthy people, the vertebrae and discs should be able to withstand considerable compressive loads. These loads are largely attributable to the muscle forces that occur in response to flexion moments imposed on the spine.

Back muscle force production capability is highly variable.[51] These muscles are capable of producing the substantial extension moments needed to balance the flexion moments imposed on the spine by lifting heavy weights.[34] The back muscles, however, are not active when the lumbar spine is fully flexed,[41] and the ligaments have limited tensile strengths.[37] Therefore, heavy lifts are initiated with the spine in some degree of extension from the position where the flexion relaxation response occurs. Once the fully upright position is reached following heavy lifting, the back is "locked out" into extension.[39] This posture may be supported by contraction of the psoas major although direct evidence for this is lacking. Back muscles are most active during squat lifts in which the lumbar spine is held in a position of lordosis.[43]

Initiation of lumbar spine extension from a fully flexed position must be achieved through backward rotation of the pelvis initiated by the hip extensor musculature. Tension through the ligaments and back muscles pulls the spine toward the upright position until the muscles begin to contract; a rebound of the ligaments may initiate a few degrees of lumbar extension.

The ability of the posterior ligaments of the lumbar spine to withstand loads imposed on them during heavy lifting has been debated. The estimated average tensile strength of these ligaments combined suggests that their ability to resist flexion moments is extremely limited.[37] Empirical evidence shows that they do not play a role in resisting spinal flexion when experienced weight lifters perform extremely heavy lifts.[39]

Currently no theory adequately explains the role of increased IAP during lifting. The observed increases in IAP during lifting and the preference of competitive weight lifters to wear abdominal belts (which increase IAP during lifting), suggest that IAP has a role in supporting the spine. Explanations for this phenomenon can only be made by conjecture based on interpretation of the literature.

Cholewicki and McGill[39] demonstrated that the lumbar spine is kept in some degree of lordosis during extremely heavy lifts. It is possible that when the lumbar spine assumes a lordotic posture during lifting, increased IAP may play a role in adding stability to the spine by stressing the convex side of the lordotic arch. There is currently not enough evidence to conclude that the spine must function as an arch during lifting, nor that IAP serves the purposes described.

Average peak IAP was estimated to generate an extension moment of 16 Nm in six healthy weight lifters.[21] The posterior ligamentous system has been estimated to generate an extension moment averaging 50 Nm.[36] Therefore, based on averages, the total extension moment producible by IAP and ligamentous tension is estimated to be approximately 66 Nm. Average flexion torques produced by the unloaded trunk have been estimated at 40 Nm during kyphotic squat lifting[8] and 60 Nm when subjects stood with the trunk flexed to 30°.[28] Although the IAP and PLS mechanisms acting alone cannot produce enough extension torque to accomplish heavy lifts, acting together, they are able to resist full flexion of the trunk when handling light loads.

During stoop lifting the back muscles may limit the range of flexion at the lumbar spine. These muscles are probably active when heavy weights are lifted from a stooped position. The stoop lift requires less energy to perform, but does not allow the load to be held as close to the body as a squat lift with a staggered stance, and therefore increases the flexion moment.

Some of the in vivo experiments described in this section have the common limitation of a small number of subjects in the samples studied. The nature of these studies is such that finding a large number of volunteers may have been difficult to achieve. The reader should be aware of the potential for errors in determining the significance of results when small numbers of subjects are used. Furthermore it must be realized that the results of these studies are not generalizable to the general population, but may be valid for individuals matching the general description of the sample.

## BACK INJURIES AND LIFTING

An argument has been made to suggest that without any load-sparing mechanisms, individuals are capable of lifting heavy loads without sustaining back injuries. Why then, are people who lift on the job susceptible to back injuries? This question is not easily answered, and currently there are no studies that can directly identify a cause for back injuries that occur during lifting. Epidemiologic studies can measure the association of lifting to back injuries but do not claim to determine causation. By reviewing the epidemiologic data and laboratory studies of the response of the spine to loading, an attempt will be made to construct hypotheses for mechanisms of back injuries associated with manual lifting. These mechanisms fall into three basic categories: (1) lack of worker physical fitness relative to the job requirements, (2) twisting while lifting, and (3) unexpected loading.

## WORKER FITNESS RELATIVE TO THE JOB

Studies demonstrate that people with jobs involving heavy manual labor first experience low back pain within a few years of starting the job.[1] Additionally, Bigos et al[3,52] reported a trend of decreasing incidence of back injuries with increasing duration of employment. These studies may be confounded by factors such as workers with seniority have more to lose (i.e., retirement benefits) if they cannot work, and therefore may be less likely to report minor back injuries. Also, Bigos et al[52] found that workers who injured their backs had poor job appraisal ratings within the 6 months prior to injury than those who were not injured. They did not report on the interaction of the appraisal ratings with length of time on the job. Therefore, it is not known whether newer employees had poorer appraisal ratings than more senior employees, and if this had any effect on the report of low back pain. The potential for these variables to be confounded notwithstanding, it is possible that workers were injured because their bodies were inadequately trained for the physical stress of the job.

Chaffin et al[53] studied the ability to predict back injuries by using isometric strength testing in 551 industrial workers who performed manual lifting tasks. The investigators tested isometric force-producing capabilities of workers performing a simulated lift in the position in which the greatest amount of weight had to be lifted on the job. The incidence and severity of back pain occurring in these workers were recorded over 18 months following initial testing.

Those who could not produce isometric forces at least equal to the weight lifted on the job had three times the risk for developing back injuries than those who could produce force more than twice the weight lifted on the job. Those who could produce forces that were marginally greater than the weight lifted on the job were also at greater risk of injury than those who could produce isometric force more than twice the weight lifted. The study concluded that workers whose strength was not well matched to the amount of weight lifted were at greater risk of developing low back pain than those whose strength matched the job demands.

In a longitudinal study over a 3-year period, Cady et al[54] found that of 1652 firefighters, those who had higher indices of physical fitness had a significantly reduced incidence of back injuries than those with the lowest fitness indices. A major component of the index of fitness focused on cardiovascular fitness; flexibility and isometric extension force production in squat lift position were also included.

In contrast to the findings of Cady et al[54] and Chaffin et al,[53] Battié et al[55,56] prospectively studied risk factors of 3020 aircraft manufacturing employees over a 3-year period and found that neither "isometric lifting strength" nor cardiovascular fitness were predictive of low back pain. Possible explanations for the contrasting findings of these studies are differences in methodology, and different definitions of strength and cardiovascular fitness. Another explanation may be related to the differences in the work demands and the subjects in each study.

Battié et al[55,56] did not study the risk factors for specific jobs in either of their studies; they chose to study all plant workers rather than just manual workers. Battié et al state that the differences in their findings with those of Chaffin et al[53] and Cady et al[54] may be due to the knowledge that the specific demands of a job require specific types of fitness and strength. For example, to avoid back injuries, firefighters probably need more cardiovascular fitness while fighting fires than loading-dock workers. On the other hand, loading-dock workers may require more maximum force production during lifting activities than firefighters.

When workers have inadequate physical fitness in relation to the job demands, injuries during lifting may occur due to fatigue of the tissue following repeated loading. Human intervertebral discs have demonstrated weakening with repeated loads over several hours leading to failure of the tissue.[15] This weakening under repeated loading may hold true for human tissue under physiologic conditions.

Soft tissue may become fatigued from repeated loading throughout the day and may not be able to withstand the tensile forces that they withstood earlier in the day. Ligaments and muscles demonstrate viscoelasticity.[57,58] There is increased stiffness of the tissue and greater loads are withstood when the tissue is loaded at higher strain rates. This viscoelasticity helps to protect the tissue when large loads are imparted to the spine during accelerations that occur while lifting. People learn through experience that lifting objects rapidly allows them to lift more weight than if they lift slowly.

An example of acceleration loading when fatigued may be given of a homeowner building a new deck. When fatigued toward the end of the day, the person may rapidly "jerk" a plank as he lifts it in place. The homeowner does not realize that the acceleration imparted to the board created a larger flexion moment, which now must be overcome by the back muscles and other soft tissue. When the flexion moment is greater than the extension moment produced, two reactions may occur. The lifter may drop the object being lifted, or the lifter may attempt to continue lifting, ultimately bringing the tissues under strain to their failure point. Injured tissue may include muscle, ligament, joint capsule, cartilaginous end-plate, intervertebral disc, vertebrae, or hyaline cartilage of the facet joints.

When soft tissue containing nociceptors is mechanically strained, mechanical stimulation of the nociceptor should create some perception of discomfort. Individuals who injure themselves during repeated lifting often admit that they experienced mild back discomfort prior to the injury, which then produced extreme pain. Ignoring the body's warning signs may lead to overstress of the tissue, resulting in injury. Workers may have reasons to continue working despite experiencing mild pain or discomfort. They may want to demonstrate a certain level of productivity, may be distracted by other job stressors, or may need to finish within a given timeframe. These mental distractions may make workers less aware of the warning signs or the workers may ignore these signs in order to complete the task, making them susceptible to injury.

By contrasting the activities of trained weight lifters to those who lift in industry, it is possible to speculate on some causative factors of back injuries associated with lifting. Weight lifters rarely complain of serious back injuries, whereas industrial workers are plagued by low back pain.

Experienced weight lifters, unlike many industrial workers, can control many factors in their training routines. Weight lifters gradually work up to intense levels of training. They may begin their weight lifting careers by lifting moderate loads for short periods of time and then gradually increasing the amount of weight lifted, the speed of lifting, and the duration of training sessions. Conversely, industrial workers may participate in frequent lifting for a full workday as soon as they are hired, without allowing their bodies time to build a tolerance for frequent or heavy lifting.

## Twisting and Combined Movements

Kelsey et al[2] performed an epidemiologic study of lifting and twisting and the risk of developing injuries to the lumbar intervertebral disc. They used case-control design matching 241 patients with controls of the same gender, age category, and attending the same medical clinic for non-back pain complaints.

Prolapsed intervertebral disc was defined as surgical if a herniation was identified at surgery, probable if a cluster of clinical signs was positive on examination, and possible if limited signs were positive on examination. A structured interview was conducted on both case and control subjects.

The findings of the study demonstrate that persons who lift more than 11.3 kg more than 25 times per day were 3.5 times more likely to develop an intervertebral disc injury than those who do not lift. Additionally, the study found that twisting alone was not a risk factor for developing disc injuries but frequently twisting while lifting 11.3 kg or more increased the risk of disc injury to 3.1 times that of persons who never perform this activity. When workers keep the knees straight while frequently twisting and lifting more than 11.3 kg, the risk of disc injury is six times greater than when not exposed to this activity.

The results of this study must be interpreted with some caution because the following limitations threaten their validity. The authors did not report on the intertester reliability of the judgments of probable and possible disc prolapse, nor did they fully describe their structured interview, its validity, or test–retest reliability.

Axial rotation is limited in the lumbar spine by apposition of zygapophyseal joint surfaces.[59] These joint surfaces are subject to injury when loaded at the extremes of axial rotation. Injury to the hyaline cartilage has been demonstrated in vitro with forceful axial rotation.[60]

The combined movement of flexion and rotation of vertebral motion segments has also been demonstrated to injure intervertebral discs in laboratory experiments.[61] Flexion of a motion segment strains the posterior fibers of the annulus fibrosus. If rotation also occurs at the joint, the annulus is subject to injury because rotation is not fully restricted by the facet joints when the joint is flexed and rotation adds the strain on the annulus.

## Unexpected Loading and Acceleration

Back injuries may occur when a load, suddenly applied, creates a flexion moment of greater magnitude than the extension moment an individual's back can produce. This may occur when two people are carrying a heavy object together and one person drops his or her end of the load. Suddenly the other person is carrying the entire load, which is compounded by the sudden acceleration of the object as it is dropped on one side.

Another example of sudden loading may occur when individuals know they can lift a particular object, but the object is at a further distance in front of the individual than it is ordinarily. The increase in the effective moment arm of the object creates a flexion moment that the individual cannot overcome. If the individuals do not realize that they will not be able to lift the object, injury may occur as a strong effort is exerted against the immovable object.

## THE PROPER LIFTING TECHNIQUE

Physical therapists frequently instruct healthy workers and patients recovering from back injuries in "proper" lifting technique. Describing a single correct way to lift is not practical, as there are very many lifting situations in which people find themselves. However, there are some general principles that should be universally applied, and rationale for additional instruction should be considered on an individual basis.

General instruction should be fairly consistent for both workers and patients, as the therapist hopes to prevent the onset of low back pain in the worker and to prevent recurrence of low back pain with the patient. The approach to patients is somewhat different in that the therapist needs to instruct the patient in precautions to avoid overstraining the healing tissue in the acute and subacute stages of the injury.

## Universal Principles

### Test the Load

Prior to actually lifting an object, individuals should be instructed to test the weight of the object before attempting to lift. This will help the person be attuned to how much force will be required to perform the lift; it will also give the person an opportunity to see if attempting to lift the load creates any discomfort or pain.

## Hold the Object Close

The best way to limit the stress to the spine when lifting a given object is to hold the object as close to the body as possible; this reduces the length of the effective moment arm of the object, and reduces the flexion moment. Forces needed to overcome the flexion moment will be reduced.

In situations where individuals must lift with their arms extended in front of the body (i.e., a stationary obstacle is in the way), the job site should be redesigned. If the lift must be performed, the individual should be instructed to lock the back into some degree of lordosis and to flex at the hip joints rather than at the lumbar spine. This allows the spine to function as an arch and will allow the muscles to be active during the lift. The person should be aware of the lumbar posture and try to sense when the load is too great for the back muscles to hold the position of lordosis. When the back muscles cannot hold the lordotic position, the load should not be lifted; if the lift is attempted, the load will be transferred to the ligaments, which are not as strong as the muscles, and may be subject to injury.

## Do Not Twist

Kelsey et al[1,2] have demonstrated a greater risk for intervertebral disc lesions when twisting while lifting. Axial rotation of the spine while lifting may cause injuries similar to those created in the laboratory, which were described earlier in this chapter. In most cases there is no reason to twist the trunk while lifting, but workers or patients must learn to pay attention to their body movements to avoid subtle twists. In situations where a person is working in a confined space that dictates that one must twist while lifting, the workplace should be redesigned. If the lift must be performed with twisting, flexion of the lumbar spine must be avoided. Lifting with simultaneous flexion and axial rotation of the lumbar spine must be avoided at all costs.

## Other Principles to Consider

### Squat Lift Versus Stoop Lift

The choice of squat-lifting or stoop-lifting is rarely offered to clients by most physical therapists. Most back schools around the world train people to bend at the knees and keep the back straight. The problem is that once patients recover from a back-pain episode they probably do not follow these instructions. Kishino et al[62] recognized this and trained patients to lift however the patient preferred, and as the patients became stronger, gradually increased the magnitude of the load, the frequency of the lift, and the duration of the activity.

There is a more sound approach to the issue than either of the approaches described above. If squat lifting were always less stressful to the body than stooping, people would prefer to squat. But most people have to be instructed in squatting for light lifting. Squatting is much less energy efficient than stooping, as a greater portion of the body weight must be lifted along with the load during squat lifting. Perhaps workers are being efficient when they refuse to squat during every lift they perform. Careful observation of experienced industrial workers will reveal that they bend at the waist, or stoop most of the day when performing lighter lifts. There may be some degree of knee flexion depending on the person's hamstring length. Experienced workers will squat when they need to perform a heavy lift.

Stooping to lift only light loads is probably not dangerous under most conditions. In the section on Biomechanics of Lifting it was demonstrated that the ligaments, with the aid of IAP, should be able to withstand the moment produced by the upper body. When repeated stooping is performed by someone who is not accustomed to repetitive movements, fatigue of the ligamentous tissue might result in injury.

Studies of EMG activity of the spinal musculature during lifting suggest that heavy lifts should be performed by squat-lifting. The question remains, what is a heavy lift? This must be decided by the individual at the moment of the lift. Being attuned to the nociceptive signals being generated from the soft tissue, slight discomfort should be a signal that the load is too heavy to lift with the lumbar spine flexed. This may change over the course of time. For example at 9:00 A.M. 50 N is the threshold at which a given individual begins to feel slight discomfort when lifting with the back bent; at 3:00 P.M., after repeated lifting, this threshold may be 10 N. The individual should be trained to test the load first, and to be attuned to sensations emanating from the low-back area. When the slightest discomfort is felt, the individual should switch to a squat-lift.

During squat-lifting, ideally the feet should be staggered with one foot near a side of the object and one near an adjacent side. This allows the individual to bring the load between the legs, and reduces the effective moment arm of the object. Scientific investigations estimating loads on the spine with different postures found squat lifting, especially with a staggered stance, to be the most energy efficient, placing the lowest loads on the spine of all postures studied.[8,9,13,45,48,50]

## Lordosis Versus Kyphosis

The evidence presented in this chapter suggests that squat-lifting while maintaining some degree of lordosis is preferable for heavy lifts. The muscles are able to produce greater extension moments than the ligamentous and other systems combined. The amount of lordosis maintained may depend on the abilities and sensations experienced by each individual. With certain pathologies, such as spondylolysis, lifting in a full lordosis is likely to be painful. Finding a posture that is not flexed so far as to induce the flexion relaxation response, yet not in full lordosis, is probably a good posture for these patients. The patient's awareness of abnormal and painful sensations can guide the therapist and the patient to find the best lumbar posture for lifting.

In conditions in which an individual must lift an object without handles from the floor, maintaining a lumbar lordosis may be impossible. Many people are unable to squat deeply and maintain a lumbar lordosis because the length of the hamstring muscles will not allow both postures simultaneously (Fig. 13-5). In this situation the same principles should apply for stoop lifting. Individuals should test the weight of the object prior to lifting; if, while holding the object close to the body, they feel any discomfort when initiating the lift, the lift should be aborted.

## When Is an Object Too Heavy to Lift?

This question can be answered with some degree of common sense by using either a person's own kinesthetic sensations, or the observation of another. Heavier loads should be lifted by squatting with some degree of lumbar lordosis. When the lumbar musculature is unable to maintain the lordosis, or when the lift is initiated by the hips rising before the upper body carrying the load, the lift is too heavy to be completed safely. This is perhaps the best kinesthetic signal of which workers and patients should be made aware. If the lift is completed in the manner described, the back will be brought into full flexion, the erector spinae and multifidus muscles will not be active, and the ligaments will bear the load. If the muscles are not capable of producing the torque required to lift, then the ligaments are at risk for injury.

## Lifting Instructions for Patients Recovering from Low Back Pain

As with any injury, back injuries need to be treated cautiously at first and gradually progressed. Injured ligaments are repaired through inflammation and fibroplasia. In a study of isolated grade II injuries to medial collateral ligaments of sheep, collagen proliferation peaked at 6 weeks, but significant strength was regained in the tissue as early as 3 weeks.[63] The animals were allowed free activity in a large pen during the study. Using the results of this study and similar animal studies to predict human tissue healing times may not be valid.

Healing times for all human soft-tissue injuries cannot be easily assessed. A variety of factors must be considered, including the general health of the individual, the anatomy of the tissue injured, blood supply to the tissue, and the severity of injury. The physical therapist must rely on clinical information such as the patient's report of pain at rest, pain with palpation of specific areas, pain with gentle stress to the issues during examination, and observation of swelling and discoloration of the area to determine how healing is progressing. Minor injuries may be ready for repeated stress in less than 3 weeks, while more serious injuries may be repeatedly exacerbated at any time and the injury

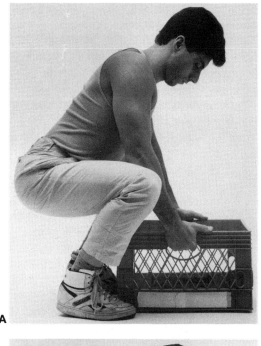

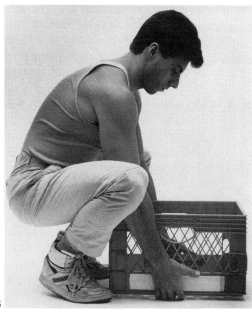

**Fig. 13-5.** **(A)** Lifting objects with handles or lifting objects raised off the floor may allow the lifter to maintain a lumbar lordosis. **(B)** When loads are lifted from the floor, short hamstring length may posteriorly rotate the pelvis, preventing the lifter from maintaining the lordosis during lifting. The lifter must carefully test the load before attempting to lift. See text for further discussion. (Adapted from Sullivan,[66] with permission.)

may start anew. My own clinical experience has been that therapists can begin to gradually stress tissue once the patient reports that constant pain at rest has been eliminated for at least 2 weeks, and when stress to the tissue during accessory motion testing to the area does not produce a lingering pain for more than a few minutes.

At this stage in the healing process the physical therapist should gradually progress the magnitude, duration, and frequency of repeated stress to the tissue. This can be accomplished by initially prescribing active range of movement exercises, progressing repetitions and duration, and later advancing to resistive exercises. Gradually stressing the ligamentous tissue in tension will induce increased tensile resisting capabilities.

As muscle performance capacity diminishes with rest, a program of resistive exercises for the trunk and lower extremity muscles should be implemented prior to starting light weight-lifting activities. A reconditioning program should be prescribed based on the requirements of the patient's job and the types of physiologic demands placed on the body when performing that job.

Instruction in proper lifting and precautions for determining safe limits of lifting should be presented to the patient with guidelines discussed earlier in this chapter. Exercises and activities that improve a patient's awareness of body postures, movement, and sensations should be implemented when instructing them in proper lifting. For example, when learning to squat-lift, a patient should learn to find the posture of the lumbar spine in which they experience the least discomfort during the activity. Patients are often comfortable lifting with lumbar spine in a lordotic posture. With some injuries, such as spondylolysis, patients may be uncomfortable in an extreme lordosis; the therapist should assist the patient in finding a position of comfort, while avoiding the extremes of flexion.

The biomechanics of lifting has been studied extensively and many theories of back support mechanisms during lifting have been proposed in the literature. Theoretical constructs based on the scientific literature suggest that the best ways to prevent back injuries while lifting are to match the worker and the job, such that demands of the job are within the capabilities of the person lifting; offer instruction in methods to reduce the moment created by the load; avoid twisting while lifting; and train workers to be more aware of their own kinesthetic sensations of posture, movement, and discomfort, while testing the load and lifting.

## REFERENCES

1. Kelsey JL, Golden AL, Mundt DJ: Low back pain/prolapsed lumbar intervertebral disc. Rheum Dis Clin North Am 16:699, 1990
2. Kelsey JL, Githens PB, White AA et al: An epidemiologic study of lifting and twisting on the job and risk for acute prolapsed lumbar intervertebral disc. J Orthop Res 2:61, 1984
3. Bigos SJ, Spengler DM, Martin NA et al: Back injuries in industry: a retrospective study II. Injury factors. Spine 11:246, 1986

4. Molumphy M, Unger B, Jensen GM, Lopopolo RB: Incidence of work-related low back pain in physical therapists. Phys Ther 65:482, 1985

5. Linton SJ, Kamwendo K: Low back schools: a critical review. Phys Ther 67:1375, 1987

6. Lett CF, McCabe NE, Tramposh A, Tate–Henderson S: Work hardening. p. 195. In Isernhagen SJ (ed): Work Injury: Management and Prevention. Aspen Publishers, Rockville, MD, 1988

7. Isernhagen SJ: Work Injury: Management and Prevention. Aspen Publishers, Rockville, MD, 1988

8. Holmes JA, Damaser MS, Lehman SL: Erector spinae activation and movement dynamics about the lumbar spine in lordotic and kyphotic squat-lifting. Spine 17: 327, 1992

9. Grieve DW: Dynamic characteristics of man during crouch- and stoop-lifting. p. 19. In Nelson RC (ed): Biomechanics IV. University Park Press, Baltimore, 1975

10. Perey O: Fracture of the vertebral end-plate in the lumbar spine. Acta Orthop Scand, suppl. 25:1, 1957

11. Porter RW, Adams MA, Hutton WC: Physical activity and the strength of the lumbar spine. Spine 14:201, 1989

12. Granhed H, Jonson R, Hansson T: The loads on the lumbar spine during extreme weight lifting. Spine 12:146, 1987

13. Hansson T, Roos B, Nachemson A: The bone mineral content and ultimate compressive strength of lumbar vertebrae. Spine 5:46, 1980

14. Adams MA, Hutton WC: Gradual disc prolapse: Spine 10:524, 1985

15. Gordon SJ, Yang KH, Mayer PJ: Mechanism of disc rupture: a preliminary report. Spine 16:450, 1991

16. Carpenter DM, Graves JE, Pollock ML et al: Effect of 12 and 20 weeks of resistive training on lumbar extension torque production. Phys Ther 71:580, 1991

17. Stone MH: Implications for connective tissue and bone alterations resulting from resistance exercise training. Med Sci Sports Exerc 20:S162, 1988

18. McGill SM, Norman RW: Positioning of the L4-L5 dynamic moment into disc, ligamentous, and muscular components during lifting. Spine 11:666, 1986

19. Adams M: Letter to the editor. Spine 14:1272, 1989

20. Morris JM, Lucas DB, Bressler MS: Role of the trunk in stability of the spine. J Bone Joint Surg 43A:327, 1961

21. McGill SM, Norman RW, Sharrat MT: The effect of an abdominal belt on trunk muscle activity and intra-abdominal pressure during squat lifts. Ergonomics 33:147, 1990

22. Bartelink DL: The role of abdominal pressure on the lumbar intervertebral discs. J Bone Joint Surg 39B:718, 1957

23. Andersson GBJ, Ortengren R, Nachemson A: Quantitative studies of back loads in lifting. Spine 1:178, 1976

24. Nachemson AL, Andersson GBJ, Schultz AB: Valsalva maneuver biomechanics: effects on lumbar trunk loads of elevated intrabdominal pressure. Spine 11:476, 1986

25. Nachemson A, Elfstrom G: Intravital dynamic pressure measurements in lumbar discs: a study of common movements, maneuvers, and exercises. Scand J Rehabil Med, suppl. 1:5, 1970

26. Aspden RM: Intra-abdominal pressure and its role in spinal mechanics. Clin Biomech 2:168, 1987

27. Aspden RM: The spine as an arch: a new mathematical model. Spine 14:266, 1989

28. Shultz A, Andersson GBJ, Ortengren R et al: Analysis and quantitative myoelectric

measurements of loads on the lumbar spine when holding weights in standing postures. Spine 7:390, 1982

29. Gracovetsky S, Farfan H, Lamy C: A mathematical model of the lumbar spine using an optimal system to control muscles and ligaments. Orthop Clin North Am 8:135, 1977

30. Gracovetsky S, Farfan H, Helleur C: The abdominal mechanism. Spine 10:317, 1985

31. Bogduk N, Macintosh JE: The applied anatomy of the thoracolumbar fascia. Spine 9:164, 1984

32. McNeill T, Addison R, Andersson G, Schultz A: Trunk strengths in attempted flexion, extension and lateral bending in healthy subjects and low back pain patients. Presented at the International Society of the Lumbar Spine, Goteborg, Sweden, May 1979

33. McNeil T, Addison R, Anderson G et al: Trunk strength in an attempted extension and lateral bending in healthy subjects and patients with low back pain. Spine 5: 529, 1980

34. Graves JE, Pollock ML, Carpenter D: Quantitative assessment of full range-of-motion isometric lumbar extension strength. Spine 15:289, 1990

35. McGill SM, Patt N, Norman RW: Measurement of the trunk musculature of active males using CT scan radiography: implications for force and moment generating capacity about the L4/L5 joint. J Biomech 21:329, 1988

36. Bogduk N, Twomey LT: The lumbar muscles and their fascia. p. 83. In Clinical Anatomy of the Lumbar Spine. Churchill Livingstone, Melbourne, 1991

37. Myklebust JB, Pintar FP, Ygandan N et al: Tensile strength of spinal ligaments. Spine 13:526, 1988

38. Macintosh JE, Bogduk N, Gracovetsky S: The biomechanics of the thoracolumbar fascia. Clin Biomech 2:78, 1987

39. Cholewicki J, McGill SM: Lumbar posterior ligament involvement during extremely heavy lifts estimated from fluoroscopic measurement. J Biomech 25:17, 1992

40. Floyd WF, Silver PHS: The function of the erectors spinae muscles in certain movements and postures in man. Physiology 129:184, 1955

41. Kippers V, Parker AW: Posture related to myoelectric silence of erectores spinae during trunk flexion. Spine 9:740, 1984

42. Donisch EW, Basmajian JV: Electromyography of deep back muscles in man. Am J Anat 133:25, 1972

43. Delitto RS, Rose SJ, Apts DW: Electromyographic analysis of two techniques for squat lifting. Phys Ther 67:1329, 1987

44. Hart DL, Stobbe TJ, Jaraiedi M: Effects of lumbar posture on lifting. Spine 12:138, 1987

45. Leskinen TPJ, Stalhammar HR, Kuorinka IAA: A dynamic analysis of spinal compression with different lifting techniques. Ergonomics 26:595, 1983

46. Nachemson A: Electromyographic studies of the vertebral position of the psoas muscle. Acta Orthop Scand 37:177, 1966

47. Keagy RD, Brumlik J, Bergan J: Direct electromyography of the psoas major muscle in man. J Bone Joint Surg 48A:1377, 1966

48. Andersson GBJ, Ortengren R, Nachemson A: Quantitative studies of back loads in lifting. Spine 1:178, 1976

49. Troup JDG: Dynamic factors in the analysis of stoop and crouch lifting methods: a methodological approach to the development of safe materials handling standards. Orthop Clin North Am 8:201, 1977

50. Anderson, CK, Chaffin DB: A biomechanical evaluation of five lifting techniques. Appl Ergonom 17.1:2, 1986

51. Delitto A, Crandell CE, Rose SJ: Peak torque-to-body weight ratios in the trunk: a critical analysis. Phys Ther 69:138, 1989
52. Bigos SJ, Spengler DM, Martin NA et al: Back injuries in industry: a retrospective study. III Employee-related factors. Spine 11:252, 1986
53. Chaffin DB, Herrin GD, Keyserling M: Pre-employment strength testing: an updated position. J Occup Med 20:403, 1978
54. Cady LD, Bischoff DP, O'Connell ER et al: Strength and fitness and subsequent injuries in firefighters J Occup Med 21:269, 1979
55. Battié MC, Bigos SJ, Fisher LD et al: Isometric strength as a predictor of industrial back pain reports. Spine 14:851, 1989
56. Battié MC, Bigos SJ, Fisher LD et al: A prospective study of the role of cardiovascular risk factors and fitness in industrial back pain complaints. Spine 14:141, 1989
57. Carlstedt CA, Nordin M: Biomechanics of tendons and ligaments. p. 59. In Nordin M, Frankel V (eds): Basic Biomechanics of the Skeletal System. 2nd Ed. Lea & Febiger, Philadelphia, 1989
58. Komi PV: Stretch-shortening cycle. p. 169. In Komi PV (ed): Strength and Power in Sport. Blackwell, London, 1992
59. White AA, Panjabi MM: Kinematics of the spine. p. 61. In: Clinical Biomechanics of the Spine. JB Lippincott, Philadelphia, 1978
60. Liu YK, Goel UK, Dejong A et al: Torsional fatigue of the lumbar intervertebral joint. Spine 10:894, 1985
61. Farfan HF: Mechanical Disorders of the Low Back. Lea & Febiger, Philadelphia, 1973
62. Kishino ND, Mayer TG, Gatchel RJ et al: Quantification of lumbar function part 4: isometric and isokinetic lifting simulation in normal subjects and low-back dysfunction patients. Spine 10:921, 1985
63. Laws G, Walton M: Fibroblastic healing of grade II ligament injuries. Histological and mechanical studies in the sheep. J Bone Joint Surg 70B:390, 1988
64. Nordin M, Frankel V: Basic Biomechanics of the Skeletal System. 2nd Ed. p. 197. Lea & Febiger, Philadelphia, 1989
65. Kapandji IA: The Physiology of the Joints. Vol. 3. p. 109. Churchill Livingstone, New York, 1974
66. Sullivan MS: Back support mechanisms during manual lifting. Phys Ther 69:38, 1989
67. Sullivan MS, Jantzen W: Enhancing of back support mechanisms through rehabilitation. Crit Rev Phys Rehabil Med 2:39, 1990

# 14 | Low Back Pain: Physical Treatment in Children and Adolescents

*Colleen B. Liston*

The implication that low back pain is prevalent in children is misleading. This chapter seeks to address issues in prevention of low back pain as well as providing guidelines for the management of those conditions that predispose to back pain. Initially, consideration of factors such as posture, flexibility, muscle strength, and motor development present background information required for assessment and intervention. Situations and disorders that present a risk to children in terms of low back pain are outlined. Finally, strategies in the prevention and physical treatment of low back pain in children will be indicated.

## POSTURE AND FUNCTION

Tachdjian,[1] Asher,[2] and Van Sant[3] report that alternate symmetry and asymmetry of posture can be expected in the first year of life. From about the age of 3 months (between 2 and 4 months), there is a change from a characteristic symmetrical posture throughout at rest, to asymmetry of the upper extremities. The asymmetrical tonic neck reflex predominates during this period, although there is frequent movement of the head and limbs out of this posture. By 6 months there is a return to symmetry when the infant is in supine and when seated using the forward supporting reaction.

In ventral suspension and in sitting, there is a gradual alteration in the posture of the spine from flexion to extension, which can be best observed in the sagittal plane. Support for the trunk is still required despite the increasing periods of activity of the upper extremities when the child is in the sitting position. At this state, the central nervous system has not matured sufficiently to allow for the balance of flexion and extension required to maintain vertical trunk posture.

Between 7 and 12 months, extension remains predominant, with the child now pulling to standing, standing, cruising along the furniture, then progressing to walk alone. The initially flexed lumbar spine posture now begins to develop the lordotic curve, as the child gains stability around the pelvis in order to ambulate.

In the toddler and preschool child, there is a period of exploring the environment, increasing gross motor abilities and the progressive development of fine motor skills. Although flexibility still predominates, strength increases with experiences in climbing, running, jumping, throwing, kicking, and the like. Symmetrical activity and exposure to a wealth of external stimuli result in the child moving, then progressively becoming increasingly adept and remaining far more active than the adult, even into their school years.

Few data have been recorded concerning range of movement and flexibility in children.[4] Adult norms are not relevant and demonstrate the urgent need for more normative studies to collect data for infants and children. It is important to be aware, for instance, that the normal cardinal planes of movement are rarely followed in infants. Prenatally and in early infancy, symmetrical diagonal movements are observed.

As with flexibility, muscle strength in children is rarely individually tested; rather, functional movements can be readily assessed and are a more appropriate indicator of strength and ability during this period of development. There is increasing capacity of the child to analyze input to be able to select, reject, and respond with attention to sensory feedback from the increasing range of activities. Isolated movements in the cardinal plane cannot be readily performed, nor can the child understand how to perform them until the teenage years are reached. This is especially the situation when assessing trunk muscle strength and in particular the abdominal muscles. Until excursion and fusion of the iliac apophyses there is poor fixation for these muscles. The young child naturally adopts a "swayback" posture of the trunk with overemphasis of the lordosis in the lumbar spine. In adolescence the forward tilt angle of the pelvis decreases from between 35° and 40° to approximately 20° in order to stabilize the pelvis. The earlier posture of increase in lordotic curve, protruding abdomen, and hyperextended knees may be perceived by parents as abnormal, although in the axial skeleton the most commonly detected asymmetry is that of scoliosis.

## SCOLIOSIS

Teachers (especially physical education staff and ballet instructors) as well as parents, may notice a "high shoulder," increased waist angle on one side, or pelvic obliquity revealed by the uneven level of the waist. This condition of

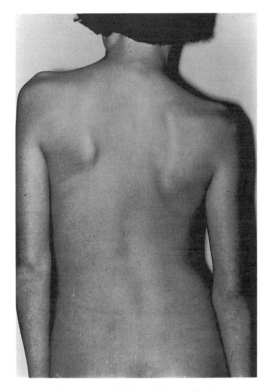

**Fig. 14-1.** Idiopathic scoliosis.

lateral curvature of the spine, with rotation in most cases, occurs in the thoracic and/or lumbar spine, either singly or in combination and may be convex to either right or left (Fig. 14-1). Often there is a double curve where the lesser curve compensates the greater. There is little evidence of low back pain reported by children with scoliosis.

If the scoliosis is postural and as the result of shortening of one leg, then a shoe raise may be prescribed to resolve the pelvic obliquity and straighten the spine. If the scoliosis is idiopathic then a review of appearance and x-ray is undertaken on a regular basis (three to six monthly). If there is an increase of the curve in an immature spine of about 30°, then a spinal brace may be advised, or, if within protocol, lateral electrical stimulation may be instituted. Exercises to maintain or improve flexibility and abdominal and back extensor strength are combined with the orthotic management. If there is a positive attitude to the whole regimen and there is compliance with brace wearing, stimulation, and regular effective exercises, then the scoliosis may be held at bay until skeletal growth is complete. If the scoliosis remains moderate at this time and there is reasonable symmetry in the trunk muscles, then the likelihood of reporting back pain at a level higher than that in the general population is unlikely.[5-7]

However, Afshani and Kuhn[8] report that persistent muscle spasm in congenital scoliosis caused by an osseous lesion on one side of a vertebra or the posterior end of a rib may result in pain. Where there is pain, radiography should be performed as well as other imaging modalities and systemic tests to determine the cause. The most common causes of painful scoliosis in children and adolescents are osteoid osteoma, benign osteoblastoma, pyogenic infection, eosinophilic granuloma, and aneurysmal bone cyst.[9-11]

## LOW BACK PAIN

### Epidemiology and Prevalence

Studies in low back pain are usually focused on adults and often within specific occupations.[12-17] The prevalence and epidemiology of low back pain in children and adolescents has had little attention. The limited data available are contradictory. Turner et al[18] found that less than 2 percent of children under 15 years of age presented to an orthopedic practice with low back pain. Similarly, King[19] also reported low clinical evidence of back pain in children, whereas Grantham[20] found in a 1977 study of male adolescent schoolchildren that 11.5 percent complained of backache. Fairbank et al[21] directly questioned 446 school students from 13 to 17 years of age and found that 115 (26 percent) reported a history of low back pain. Similarly, Balagué et al[22] found that of 1715 Swiss schoolchildren, 27 percent complained of low back pain. It is difficult to compare epidemiologic studies in children and adolescents because of methodologic dilemmas. Pain is a subjective phenomenon, and pain rating scales used for adults may not be appropriate. Simple occurrence or nonoccurrence may see minor pain, occurring infrequently, linked at times with severe, intractable pain. Parental reporting is unreliable.[23] The retrospective nature of most studies yields data with little meaning, and the age group studied may affect findings if the range is too small (for example Aro, et al's 1987 study[24] of psychosomatic symptoms in 14- to 16-year-olds).

A recent study by Olsen et al[25] reports data on low back pain prevalence in the United States. Of the 1246 adolescents aged 11 to 17 years (mean age, 13.6 years), 30.4 percent (95 percent confidence interval, 28.7, 32.2) reported experiencing low back pain at some time. The reporting rate was 30 percent in girls and 30.7 percent in boys (there were 601 girls and 641 boys). By 15 years of age, the prevalence was significantly greater ($p > 0.05$) in the black population who made up 24.4 percent of the group. A modified Fairbank et al[21] questionnaire was used. This retrospective study again begs the question about methodology and only 7 percent (8 percent of girls and 6.7 percent of boys) sought medical attention for their back pain.

Although the incidence of back pain in children and adolescents is generally thought to be low, if it is present it may indicate serious underlying pathology and is therefore of great significance.[18,26-29]

## Causes

Since degenerative changes are not common in the spinal structures in children,[27] the causes of low back pain vary from those usually seen in adults. Furthermore, assuming that psychogenic disorders may be responsible is also unwise, because emotional problems are rarely causative factors.[18,27,29]

Causes include infection, such as infective discitis and osteomyelitis; spondylolysis and spondylolisthesis; intervertebral disc herniation; Scheuermann's disease (in the lumbar spine this is often associated with pain[30]); and trauma (as in fractures, dislocations, soft-tissue injuries, overuse, and other athletic or recreational stresses or strains). Neoplasms in the lumbar spine are not common and include aneurysmal bone cysts, Ewing's sarcoma, osteoid osteoma, and lymphoma or more rarely a spinal cord tumor (ependymoma). Systemic disorders such as sickle cell anemia or acute lymphoblastic leukemia may also present with back pain as a major symptom.[8,31]

Discitis is seen most frequently in children less than 10 years of age (on average, 6 years).[19] The child may present unable or refusing to walk or sit and complaining of hip, leg, back, or abdominal pain. There is elevated erythrocyte sedimentation rate and white cell count and narrowing of the intervertebral space on x-ray. The adjacent vertebra has an eroded end-plate and magnetic resonance imaging (MRI) or computer tomography (CT) scan reveals the infection. Osteomyelitis may also be identified by MRI, so it is important for children to undergo relevant investigation procedures if they present as described above.

McKee et al[32] reporting on 63 cases of spondylolysis and spondylolisthesis found that these occur equally in males and females. If the defect in spondylolysis is bilateral (found in 75 to 85 percent of cases by Moreton[33]) then spondylolisthesis of varying degrees results. This condition presents in the athletically active adolescent, usually male.[34] Spondylolysis is commonly associated with gymnastics and diving, and in sports such as hockey, lacrosse, soccer, and football. As much as a 30 percent frequency has been reported in gymnasts[34] and in 30 to 70 percent it has been found to be a familial disorder.[35] Radiographic and CT scanning should be undertaken to clarify the diagnosis.

As previously indicated, degenerative changes are not commonly considered to contribute to findings of low back pain in children, although Tertti et al[36] report on a study of 39 14- to 15-year-old Finnish schoolchildren. They claim that disc degeneration was present in 38 percent (15) of their subjects who indicated low back pain on questionnaire. Disc protrusion was reported as being nearly always associated, and there was a positive correlation with Scheuermann's-type changes in 9 cases. These authors attribute their findings to constant load from continuous forward bending at a school desk, which may reduce nutrition to the growing disc. The changes interpreted from MRI may be attributed to fluid composition changes rather than true degeneration, although these may be a warning of degeneration to follow.[37–39]

Disc herniation is more common in adolescents than in younger (prepubescent) children.[40] It is most commonly found to occur suddenly in the athlete and after exertion, so in this sense is more often categorized as traumatic than degenerative. Bunnell[28] reports that two-thirds of adolescents experience local pain while the other third complained of sciatic pain. Delayed diagnosis is common because of the lack of neurologic evidence.[41] Afshani and Kuhn[8] recommend a comparative study of myelography, CT scan, and MRI in a large series of children with disc herniation to identify their relative usefulness.

Scheuermann's disease occurs in both the thoracic and lumbar spine. There is wedging of the vertebrae, irregularity of the end-plate, and narrowing of the disc space. This may be associated with herniation of the disc. Pain is associated more often if the condition presents in the lumbar spine, and is reported in 31 percent of male and 21 percent of female adolescents with back pain.[30] Schmorl's nodes (herniations) have been found in 30 percent of adolescents with Scheuermann's disease, and an important factor is that fusion of the ring apophysis to the vertebral body does not occur until around 16 to 18 years of age.[42]

Other congenital disorders of the spinal structures, such as stenosis and lumbar arachnoid diverticula, are rare and are not discussed here.

Mechanical causes of back pain in children and adolescents are the main group usually considered under the heading of trauma. Because of the range of recreational and competitive activities undertaken by an increasing number of young people, the risks are great. Common causes of pain are traumatic and stress fractures (of the posterior elements or body of the vertebra), discal injuries, interspinous process ligament strains, "kissing" spines, muscular strains, and iliac crest apophysitis.

A direct blow to the back in contact sports is the most common cause of fractures to the pedicles, pars interarticularis, and articular, transverse, or spinous processes. Excessive torsional loads to the lumbar spine may result in fracture of the inferior articular processes.[43]

Checking on spine instability, spasm of the paraspinal muscles, and aggravating factors (activity) will assist diagnosis. Chronic pain may result from persisting spinal instability and spinal fusion may be required later.[44] Leg length inequality causing back pain is corrected by shoe raise and strengthening muscles around the pelvis to ensure a level pelvis and equivalent trunk muscle strength.[45] Tenderness in the muscle rather than over the iliac crest differentiates muscles strain from iliac apophysitis. Kissing spines (lumbar interspinous process bursitis) has an insidious onset, is common in gymnasts, and caused by repetitive contact between the spinous process tips (commonly L4 and L5).[46] A differential diagnosis from acute ligament sprains may be made because the onset in this instance is likely to be acute and exacerbated by flexion. In bursitis, the pain decreases with flexion and increases with hyperextension.

Overuse injuries occur secondary to repetitive activities and unrepaired low levels of trauma resulting in soft tissue remaining shortened. These injuries may affect the immature disc, vertebral bodies, or muscles and ligaments around the spine.

Nocturnal pain and paresthesia may indicate a primary osseous neoplasm of the lumbar spine. Although these are rare (in a series of 1971 patients with musculoskeletal neoplasms, 29 [8 children] were spinal), back pain is the most common complaint.[47] Osteoid osteoma is the most prevalent,[48] with benign osteoblastoma, aneurysmal bone cyst, and Ewing's sarcoma occurring less frequently.[8] Scoliosis may be present and diagnosis may be made through radiography and CT scan for extent and differentiation. Ewing's sarcoma is prevalent in 5- to 15-year-olds; it is uncommon under 5 years of age. Since it is frequently associated with fever, leukocytosis, and localized pain, it may be misdiagnosed as osteomyelitis. Lymphoma accounts for 2 to 6 percent of primary malignant bone tumors in children.[48]

Progressive extremity weakness with back pain, or sensory or bladder disturbance in those with developmental problems (such as cerebral palsy) may indicate a spinal cord tumor. Spinal cord lesions include ependymomas, which are usually benign and often reached a large size before producing neurologic and back pain symptoms. Radiographic imaging and myelography precede CT scanning to provide full diagnosis. Encapsulated schwannomas, neurofibromas, and neurofibrosarcomas are malignant, metastasizing to the lungs and having a poor prognosis.[48]

Systemic disorders may present with back pain. Thus acute lymphoblastic leukemia may cause the young child to complain of severe low back pain that is intermittent and exacerbated by movement.[31] There may be inability to walk. Radiographic changes that may show demineralization, compression fractures, and thinning and breaking of cortical areas, associated with a low blood count, are diagnostic. However, these diagnostic elements occur *after* the symptom of back pain. Early in the progress of leukemia, the back pain often occurs in the absence of the other diagnostic elements. Thus there may be inaccurate diagnosis of tuberculosis or delayed diagnosis of the leukemia.

Tewari et al[49] report three cases of acute backache and rapidly progressive neurologic deterioration that had spontaneous spinal extradual hematoma. These are more common in the cervicodorsal region and are rare.

## Predisposing Factors in Sports and Recreational Activities

In the growing child and preadolescent there are five physical factors that predispose to injury in general. These are outlined and then information specific to low back pain will be provided.

1. *Muscle strength to bone length ratio:* Where bones are growing faster than muscles are increasing in strength, then attachment areas provide increased pressure to the bone. At growing points (apophyses), this can be a problem for those undertaking repetitive activities.

2. *Growth plate susceptibility:* Epiphyses (in the vertebrae) and apophyses on the vertebral ring and pelvis, for example, may be disrupted or distorted with stress from overloading or repetitive activity. Pain may result and there may be disruption to growth.

3. *Growth nonlinearity:* Greater load and stress in some activities may result from the disproportional size of the head to the rest of the body.

4. *Moments of inertia changes:* With the preadolescent growth spurt, the resistance to acceleration is affected and altered with the nonlinearity of growth. Hence some previously developed physical skills may decline temporarily, exposing the child (particularly the gymnast) to risk of injury.

5. *Delayed menarche:* Excessive training in young females leads to lack of estrogen production and delayed onset of menstruation. If this persists osteopenia may result as the bones are less able to absorb calcium.[50]

There is evidence that in the United States and Scandinavia half of the boys and around one-third of girls between 14 and 17 years of age are involved in organized, competitive sports.[51,52] The incidence of back pain is greater in those who are involved in athletics and gymnastics.[53,54] In Australia it has been reported that sports injuries double after the age of 12 years and increase by as much as six times after the age of 16 years. Rugby League, Rugby Union, Australian Rules football and soccer, netball, basketball, hockey, and cricket account for 75 percent of all sports injuries. Physical contact and human error account for 54 percent, the surface of terrain 31 percent, and equipment 15 percent. Forty percent are due to incorrect training or overtraining.[55]

Ballet dancers and gymnasts sustain back injuries from impact or floor contact, are hypermobile, exposed to hyperextension repetitive injuries, and have imbalance around the trunk and pelvis that further predisposes them to injury.[56–58] Hyperlordosis with tight lumbodorsal fascia and hamstrings and weak abdominal muscles are evident during the growth spurt and may persist to contribute to back injury and back pain in these young athletes.[59,60]

Keene et al[61] studied back injuries in 4790 college athletes competing in 17 sports over 10 years. Three hundred and thirty-three back injuries (a rate of 7 per 100) were sustained. Eighty percent occurred in practice, 6 percent in competition, and 14 percent in preseason training. Eighteen (5 percent) were in the area T11–L1, 286 (81 percent) L2 to L5, and the rest in the thoracic spine. Females had a higher rate of overuse injuries due to pre-existing conditions, and a greater number of injuries in the lumbar spine. Football and gymnastics produced significantly higher numbers of injuries (133 and 23, respectively). Track and basketball also produced significant numbers of acute and overuse injuries. Acute injuries were greater (59 percent) than overuse (12 percent). Twenty-nine percent of injuries were associated with pre-existing conditions. Muscle strains accounted for 60 percent of the injuries ($P < 0.001$) and these most frequently in football players (84, $P < 0.01$). Kissing spines and spondylolysis were significantly more common (8 out of 201 and 5 out of 201, respectively) in gymnasts ($P < 0.01$).

These figures are similar to those obtained by other researchers,[62–64] who found significantly greater numbers of muscle strain in wrestlers, football players, and gymnasts, with spondylolysis being diagnosed at an equivalent rate.

Thus it can be seen that predisposing factors for back pain in sports or recreational activities can range from the activities themselves, through physical factors related to the participants, to external factors such as the surface, or equipment or apparatus. The cause of pain may be an acute contact, impact, or stress injury. Shearing and friction forces may result in more chronic sprains, and strains and overuse or repetitive mechanical stress can be identified as predictors for pain.

## Predisposing Conditions and Postures

Some of the predictors in this category, such as leg length discrepancy and spinal deformity, have already been addressed. Specifically, scoliosis studies of the sequelae in adults with untreated scoliosis have been conducted by Nilsonne and Lundgren,[65] who reviewed 113 patients around 50 years after first being seen; Nachemson,[66] whose 130 patients were followed up on average after 35 years; and Collis and Ponseti,[67] who followed up 205 of 353 patients who had been reviewed by Ponseti and Friedman in 1950.[68] Nilsonne and Lundgren[65] found that 90 percent had back symptoms, Nachemson[66] reported backache was noted by 40 percent, and the third study stressed that although 54 percent of patients had backache complaints, this incidence was not considered to be higher than in the general population. Furthermore, only eight of the 205 had been hospitalized for their back pain.[67] Weinstein et al[69] confirmed these earlier findings of no higher incidence of back pain than in the whole population.

Pain is reported more commonly by those with scoliosis who have lumbar curves of over 50°, because such curves are progressive and so the likelihood of degenerative disc disease, and thereby pain, is greater.[26] Thus, a lumbar scoliosis of greater than 50° (Fig. 14-2) in an adolescent spine is an important predictor of back pain.

Dieck et al,[6] in conducting an epidemiologic study on any relationship between postural asymmetry and subsequent back pain, followed 903 young women who had been posturally assessed and charted according to deviations at the shoulder or waist, or from the midline. Reports of subsequent pain were not shown to be associated with the postural asymmetry. These authors sought to explain this finding in three ways. First, postural asymmetry may not exert a force of such a magnitude required to produce degeneration of facet joints or annular tears. Second, pre-existing pathology does not mean subsequent pain. Third, Wolff's law, which states that form follows function,[70] operates; that is, that any asymmetric loads on the spine are compensated for by adaptation of the rest of the body. Similarily, a study conducted by Hertzberg[71] of 302 persons who were examined at 16 years of age, when any postural deviations were noted, also revealed no consistent risk factor predictive of lumbar pain.

Cerebral palsy is a condition in which there is disorder of movement and posture because of injury to the developing brain.[72–76] There is little evidence documented about the incidence of back pain in cerebral palsy; however, scoliosis has been shown to be more prevalent in this population.[77–80] This may

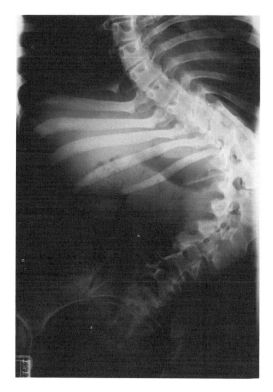

**Fig. 14-2.**   Untreated lumbar scoliosis.

be combined with kyphosis or lordosis or these latter two deformities may be present alone. When most children with cerebral palsy first sit, they exhibit a dorsal kyphosis that may become fixed. Significant hip flexion deformity is often present in those with lordosis. Furthermore, sitting ability may be affected by any of these deformities, and poor trunk control may be present as well. Inequivalence can give rise to "windswept" hips, pelvic obliquity, or rotation and interfere with the ability to sit (and stand).[81]

Moreau et al[82] reviewed adults with disabling spastic cerebral palsy and contractural hip deformity. Pelvic obliquity and scoliosis was present and led to loss of sitting balance in one-third of those with dislocation or subluxation (Fig. 14-3). Pain, chiefly in the hip, was present in 11 and for this reason and the importance of maintaining sitting function, surgical treatment in the more neurologically mature and athetoid subjects was recommended. Hoffer et al[83] reviewed 20 spastic cerebral palsied children who underwent osteotomy for pain and various degrees of hip dislocation. They remarked on the importance of a level pelvis for walking and especially for sitting as well as for reducing the amount of back pain experienced. It may be hypothesized that the resultant pelvic obliquity and scoliosis in the lumbar region of those with cerebral palsy may in time predispose these people to pain in that area, as well as in the hip.

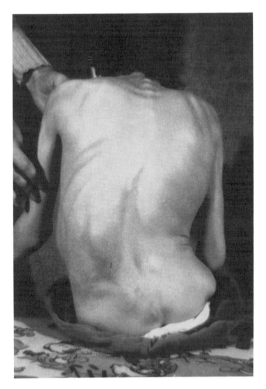

**Fig. 14-3.** Pelvic obliquity in cerebral palsy.

In fact, Hoffer et al[83] stress the importance of attending to the pelvic obliquity and scoliosis before any hip procedure is undertaken. Rosenthal et al[84] reported that of 50 ambulatory, adolescent subjects with cerebral palsy, 19 had scoliosis and of those only two complained of back pain. This contrasted with their study of idiopathic, scoliotic adolescents where 40 percent complained of back pain.

So despite a higher incidence rate of scoliosis in those with cerebral palsy, and despite the compounding factor of hip dislocation precluding sitting and leading to pelvic obliquity and scoliosis, the incidence of low back pain is not reported to be increased. The "windswept" hip syndrome is more likely to be associated with hip pain[85-88] (Fig. 14-4).

Stanitski et al[89] report that spinal deformity from neuromuscular imbalance, such as in cerebral palsy, may progress to cause pain. These authors present qualitative results of surgical management to correct spinal deformity, which led to elimination of back pain in all of those who complained of it preoperatively. Nevertheless, this was seen to be a "major therapeutic triumph," as many had difficulty indicating the exact area of pain because of inability to communicate effectively.

There is no other reported evidence of significant low back pain in other disorders in children and adolescents. These include those that predispose to

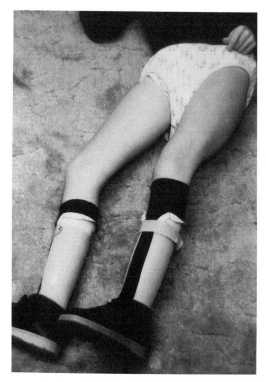

**Fig. 14-4.** Windswept hips in cerebral palsy.

spinal deformity such as spina bifida and muscular dystrophy. Nor has it been documented as prevalent in those children with systemic musculoskeletal disorders such as juvenile chronic arthritis.

As previously documented, pelvic obliquity and loss of sitting balance may result from unilateral hip dislocation or from scoliosis. Sitting posture is therefore of vital importance in any situations or conditions that predispose to the development of low back pain.

## Prevention

Prevention measures should always include primary prevention (attention to personal and environmental components of tasks), secondary prevention (early detection of predictors, such as those conditions and activities already outlined, in order to institute remedial action), and rehabilitation (to reduce chronicity and prevent recurrence). As for all injuries and predisposing factors for overuse and pain, common sense, knowledge, and understanding are the keys to success in prevention.

Good postural alignment is important in ensuring that optimum muscle length, flexibility of soft-tissue structures, and weight-bearing through joint surfaces are permitted. This should be especially observed during the growing years, since malalignment and inattention to the five factors predisposing to injury (and thence to low back pain if the injury is in the area of the lumbar spine), are ill-advised. Physical factors such as obesity, ectomorphism, leg-length discrepancy, hypermobility, and persistent or chronic sequelae from previous injuries, require special attention. A check to confirm that there is relaxed good posture, that muscles and ligaments around joints are equivalently flexible and strong, and that the child's physical characteristics are not likely to pose risks, should be undertaken.[50]

Understanding the risks from impact, friction, shearing, stretching, twisting, and loading forces will ensure that these factors are addressed. By avoiding repetitive, mechanical stresses and overuse, and by reducing the likelihood of injury from impact, twisting, and overstretching, fewer injuries and less low back pain will occur. Awareness of sound ergonomic practice during sport, recreational activities, when sitting at the school desk or in front of the computer, and when lifting, pulling, or pushing objects, is recommended.[90,91] Good preparation for sport and recreational activities is an important preventive strategy. Understanding and practicing the skills required should be accompanied by correct training techniques. Fitness should also be considered so that aerobic capacity is gradually improved by walking, cycling, swimming, and running. Under supervision, flexibility can be gradually increased so as to improve performance. Training for specific sports should ideally commence 4 to 6 weeks before the season starts.[92] The principles of warm-up and stretching, the use of suitable equipment, as well as respect for and adherence to any rules and safety precautions, are of vital importance in back-pain prevention.

Other factors to be considered include the mental attitude and psychological motivation of the individual. These vary between individual children and may be the cause of overexertion, roughness, disobeying rules, poor preparation, poor training, and overtraining. As well, the pressure of overenthusiastic coaches and parents may push the normal competitive urge in the 8- to 10-year-old to aggression. In the young elite dancer, the risk of back injury is increased by the demands of diverse choreography, long rehearsals, and the expected quality of the performance.

The inclusion of rehabilitation under the heading of prevention highlights the importance of the judicious management of acute conditions to prevent them from becoming chronic. Furthermore, education about avoiding postures and activities that are implicated as the cause of one's low back pain is important, as is the need for retraining to achieve these goals.[93]

Preventive measures should also be considered in those who have conditions that predispose to poor postural alignment, and perhaps subsequently to low back pain. For example, the child or adolescent wheelchair occupant must have comfortable, functional posture with optimal pelvic stability and postural support to facilitate the achievement of his or her full potential at school as well as in recreational activities and sport. Techniques to achieve this goal will be presented in the section on Management.

Strategies in prevention include screening; attention to environmental factors; education about postural, structural, and risk factors; preparedness; optimal management of acute injuries; and the possibility of retraining. Although prevention is preferable, knowledge about how to best manage back pain or predisposing factors is essential to avoid chronicity and long-term sequelae.

## Management

Management encompasses the physical treatment of low back pain in children and adolescents, as well as ideas and techniques that may be part of an overall management strategy.

In athletes it is necessary to understand the significance, location, and nature of mechanical low back pain. Furthermore, it is of assistance to know which injuries or conditions, likely to lead to low back pain, are associated with a particular age or a particular sport.[44] For example, sprains of interspinous ligaments and muscle strains occur at any age and in all sports. Differential diagnosis with the use of appropriate radiographic, imaging, and physical tests will ensure correct diagnosis to facilitate the choice of a management strategy and specific treatment.

Pain during standing while bent forward or in supine lying, especially in those with spondylolisthesis or spinal stenosis, has been found to be relieved by antilordotic rigid spinal braces in the older age group.[94] These would not allow movement required for full activity in children and adolescents, and unless the spondylolisthesis or spinal stenosis were severe or accompanied by marked pain, then such an immobilizer is unlikely to be recommended.

There is very little literature addressing physical treatment for low back pain in children and adolescents because the overall incidence of the condition is low. Those conditions that pre-eminently are the cause of back pain are generally tumors and fractures, where physical management is minimal.

In a paper concerning ballet dancers, Bryan and Smith[60] discuss the need for the dance instructor to understand proper body alignment and to be able to assess areas of weakness. The importance of close liaison with a therapist who understands the requirements of the instructor, and the physical, dietary, and psychological factors that impact on the dancer is stressed. It has already been reported that back injury is common in the ballet dancer. Treatment of acute injuries should follow traditional techniques of rest and ice, not heat and stretching, which may be recommended by some dance instructors. Rest may be seen to be impossible, so a reasonable timeframe to allow tissue healing and proper neuromuscular rehabilitation must be negotiated between the therapist, company director, instructor, and dancer.

Overall management may include assessment of aggravating and alleviating factors with an exercise program that is modified to take account of common aggravating factors. These include sensitivity of movement, static posture, and weightbearing. The dancer can be made aware of the range of motion that is pain free (for instance in the lumbopelvic region), in a variety of positions. Work within the pain-free range in standing, two-point and four-point kneeling, supine, and prone is undertaken to build up trunk control. Micheli,[95] Jull and Janda,[59] and Morgan[96] provide a range of techniques and examples for those specifically working with ballet dancers.

Similar strategies may be applied when working with gymnasts, wrestlers, and other team sports players who exhibit pain from overuse and repetitive injuries, or where predisposing hypermobility, kissing spines, and spondylolisthesis are factors.

In addressing the topic of the young patient, Farrell and Drye[54] drew attention to the knowledge that pain-sensitive structures in the intervertebral foramen and neural canal can be affected at any age.[97–99] Testing for adverse mechanical neural tension through passive neck flexion, straight leg raise, prone knee bend, and slump testing is advocated by these authors when young patients complain of low back pain. These tests are often not undertaken in adolescents, and "adverse neural tension" may be missed as a causative factor. Stretching techniques may be implemented and the patient taught to undertake slump sit stretches at home. If these are not included in a treatment regimen because of missed evaluation, it will not be surprising if other modes of treatment such as pelvic traction, knees to chest, hamstring stretches, and the like do not improve symptoms such as buttock cramping.

As in the management of all patients with low back pain, there are important guidelines to follow. Assessment is required to identify the pain category—for example, nonspinal, nonmechanical, acute mechanical, chronic anterior element, chronic posterior element, and so on. This will allow an algorithm to be followed where signposts can guide those involved in treatment to know where to go next. Sikorski[100] has suggested such an algorithm for use in decisions about physiotherapy intervention. The following is part of such an algorithm. (Adapted from Sikorski,[100] with permission.)

```
Low back pain? ──────→ No ──→   Exit
        ↓
      Yes
        ↓
Is it spinal? ────────→ No ──→   Referred pain?
        ↓
      Yes
        ↓
Is it mechanical?
        ↓
      Yes
        ↓
Is it acute? ─────────→ Yes ──→  Rest
        ↓
Is it postural? ──────→ Yes
        ↓               ↓
      No         Is it anterior element?  ──→ Yes → Extension program
        │               ↓
        │              No
        │               ↓
        │        Is it posterior element? ──→ Yes → Flexion program
        │               ↓
        │              No
        │               ↓
        │                        ┌─→ Yes → Isometric program
Is it movement induced? ←─┘      └─→ No → Mobilization program
```

As with any algorithm, this can become more complex and should provide alternate routes if the treatment is not helping or where other factors are involved. Awareness of the need to seek additional assistance through analgesics and/or immobilization should enhance the efficacy of treatment. Treatment choices should not only include specific exercise regimens, but also mobilization, manipulation, and education. Education is an essential element in any treatment, rehabilitative/preventive program for those with low back pain, after low back pain has abated, and for any adolescent or child who is involved in activities that predispose them to pain or if they have a predisposing condition.

Information about optimal postural alignment in the range of positions used in recreational and sporting activities, sitting, standing, lying, and so on, will assist the young person to be aware of and avoid situations that put them at risk of succumbing to low back pain. Specific education about maintenance of control around the pelvis and trunk, together with information about those types of chairs, beds, and so on that assist the maintenance of good postural alignment, should be given.

For those who require assistance because they spend much of their time in a wheelchair, and who have inadequate postural control for some reason, special advice should be given.

The basic principles of seating should be followed for a variety of reasons:

To provide a functional, comfortable position for hypotonia
To control spasm—as in adductor spasticity leading to hip dislocation
To provide some correction for spinal curvature
To assist a moderately handicapped child (e.g., with cerebral palsy) to develop postural control
To ease the task of handling/management

In all of these principles are the implicit goals of enhancing posture and function while providing pelvic stability to reduce the risk of low back pain from secondary lumbar scoliosis developing with pelvic obliquity.[101,102]

Description of specific techniques such as types of pelvic, groin, and thigh straps; lateral trunk and pelvic supports; harnesses and trunk straps; ramped, antithrust, and pressure cushions; and hillocks, pommels, and easements for ischeal tuberosities and the coccyx, are provided by Motloch,[103] Nelham,[104] Liston,[105] Liston,[102] and Fay et al.[106]

Awareness of the need to provide management programs for all members of the childhood and adolescent population who have, or are at risk of, developing low back pain, is the physical therapist's responsibility.

## CONCLUSIONS

Goodman and McGrath[23] provide profound insight into the failure of researchers to validate currently available low back pain survey instruments, such as questionnaires, used with children. For this reason the limited data in the area of low back pain prevalence in children and adolescents are inconsistent and confusing. Although scales have been developed for the clinical measurement of pain in children, these too remain to be validated on large numbers and across broad age ranges. Furthermore, studies to validate survey measures of disability in children and adolescents need to be undertaken.[107]

Few attempts have been made to quantify frequency and intensity of pain in this population, nor are there criteria available to indicate what is normal. Epidemiologic studies to provide normative data are required, as is an understanding of the role of family members' attitudes to pain and disability in themselves and others.[25]

To identify those children and adolescents who may be at risk of developing debilitating low back pain in adulthood, studies into the etiology of low back pain should be conducted. Knowledge of the associated risk factors, the severity of the pain, and the degree to which risk factors and severe pain are predictors for recurrence of low back pain and other sequelae, would assist in the provision of preventive measures.

Prevention is the most important strategy to adopt for all children and adults. Where there are obvious risk factors inherent within sports and recreational activities, or certain physical and psychological predisposing factors pre-exist, then education, training, and sensible practices are essential.

Attention to children and adolescents with the characteristics and conditions that put them at risk of developing low back pain includes screening, effective management, and retraining in many cases. No child or adolescent should go on to adulthood without a thorough understanding of those activities and practices that render them particularly vulnerable. Education in this area is required from an early age, to see awareness move to responsibility for the care of one's back being taken by the young. Poor role models, low priority in the education system, lack of awareness, and few incentives, mean that programs of back education in schools are rarely delivered. In many states and countries, government funding for this exercise is not seen as important. The absence of any data to support early intervention in terms of the education of children to prevent the high levels of low back pain and subsequent high costs for management in adults, especially in the workforce, is an issue that demands attention from researchers in the future.

# REFERENCES

1. Tachdjian M: Paediatric Orthopaedics. Vol. 2. WB Saunders, Philadelphia, 1972
2. Asher C: Postural Variations in Childhood. Butterworth, London, 1975
3. Van Sant AF: The child with orthopaedic problems. p. 495. In Payton OD, DiFabio RP, Paris SV et al (eds.): Manual of Physical Therapy. New York, Churchill Livingstone, 1989
4. Hensinger R: Standards in Paediatric Orthopaedics: Tables, Charts and Graphs Illustrating Growth. Raven Press, New York, 1986
5. Nachemson A: Adult scoliosis and back pain. Spine 4:513, 1979

6. Dieck GS, Kelsey JL, Goel VK et al: An epidemiologic study of the relationship between postural asymmetry in the teen years and subsequent back and neck pain. Spine 10:872, 1985

7. McCarthy R: Prevention of the complications of scoliosis by early detection. Clin Orthop Relat Res 222:73, 1987

8. Afshani E, Kuhn J: Causes of low back pain in children. Radiographics 11:269, 1991

9. Mehta M, Murray R: Scoliosis provoked by painful vertebral lesions. Skeletal Radiol 1:223, 1977

10. Amacher A, Eltomey A: Spinal osteoblastoma in children and adolescents. Child's Nerv Syst 1:29, 1985

11. Fakharini–Hein M, Griss P, Ludke A, Bittinger A: Rapidly developing scoliosis in an adolescent due to spinal osteoblastoma. Arch Orthop Traum Surg 107:259, 1988

12. Frymoyer JW, Pope MH, Clements JM, et al: Risk factors in low back pain. J Bone Joint Surg 65A:213, 1983

13. Biering-Sorensen F: A prospective study of low back pain in a general population. Scand J Rehabil Med 31:62, 1984

14. Lanier D, Stockton P: Clinical predictors of outcome of acute episodes of low back pain. J Family Pract 27:483, 1988

15. Nepomuceno C, Faught E, Langford K: Diagnosis and management of low back pain. Alabama J Med Sci 25:430, 1988

16. Kelsey JL, Golden AL, Mundt DJ: Low back pain/prolapsed lumbar intervertebral disc. Rheumatol Dis Clin North Am 16:699, 1990

17. Bengtsson B, Thorson J: Back pain: a study of twins. Acta Genet Med Gemellol 40:83, 1991

18. Turner PG, Green JH, Galasko CSB: Back pain in childhood. Spine 14:812, 1979

19. King H: Back pain in children. Pediatr Clin North Am 31:1083, 1984

20. Grantham VA: Backache in boys: a new problem. Practitioner 218:226, 1977

21. Fairbank J, Pynset PD, Van Poortyliet JA, Phillips H: Influence of anthropometric factors and joint laxity in the incidence of adolescent back pain. Spine 9:461, 1984

22. Balagué F, Dutoit G, Waldburger M: Low back pain in schoolchildren. Scand J Rehabil Med 20:175, 1988

23. Goodman J, McGrath P: The epidemiology of pain in children and adolescents: a review. Pain 46:247, 1991

24. Aro H, Paronen O, Aro S: Psychosomatic symptoms among fourteen to sixteen year old Finnish adolescents. Soc Psychiat 22:171, 1987

25. Olsen TL, Anderson RL, Dearwater SR et al: The epidemiology of low back pain in an adolescent population. Am J Public Health 82:606, 1992

26. Winter RB: The spine. p. 573. In Lovell WW and Winter RB (eds): Paediatric Orthopaedics. JB Lippincott, Philadelphia, 1978

27. Hoffman H: Childhood and adolescent lumbar pain: differential diagnosis and management. Clin Neurosurg 27:553, 1980

28. Bunnell W: Back pain in children. Orthop Clin North Am 13:587, 1982

29. Rosenblum B, Rothman A: Low back pain in children. Mt Sinai J Med 58:115, 1991

30. Alexander C: Sheuermann's disease: a traumatic spondylodystrophy? Skeletal Radiol 1:209, 1977

31. Samuda GM, Cheng MY, Yeung CY: Back pain and vertebral compression: an uncommon presentation of childhood acute lymphoblastic leukemia. J Pediatr Orthop 7:175, 1987

32. McKee BW, Alexander WJ, Dunbar JS: Spondylolysis and spondylolisthesis in children: a review. J Can Assoc Radiol 22:100, 1971
33. Moreton R: Spondylolysis. JAMA 195:671, 1966
34. Wiltse LL, Widell EH, Jackson DW: Fatigue fracture: the basic lesion in isthmic spondylolisthesis. J Bone Joint Surg 57:17, 1977
35. Libson E, Bloom RA, Dinari G: Symptomatic and asymptomatic spondylolysis and spondylolisthesis in young adults. Int Orthop 6:259, 1982
36. Tertti MO, Salminen JJ, Paajanen HEK et al: Low back pain and disk degeneration in children: a case-control MR imaging study. Radiology 180:503, 1991
37. Thompson JB, Pearce RH, Ho B: Correlation of gross morphology and chemical composition with magnetic resonance images of human lumbar intervertebral discs. Trans Orthop Res Soc 13:276, 1988
38. Erkintalo M, Laato M, Aho H et al: Correlation of MR imaging, radiographic, biochemical and histologic changes in healthy and degenerated human intervertebral lumbar disks. Radiology 173:314, 1989
39. Modic M, Herfkens R: Intervertebral disk: normal age-related changes in MR signal intensity. Radiology 177:332, 1990
40. Webb JH, Svien JH, Kennedy RL: Protruded lumbar intervertebral discs in children. JAMA 154:1153, 1954.
41. Zamani M, MacEwen G: Herniation of the lumbar disc in children and adolescents. J Pediatr Orthop 2:528, 1982
42. Banerian KG, Wang A, Samberg LE et al: Association of vertebral end plate fracture with paediatric lumbar intervertebral disk herniation: value of CT and MR imaging. Radiology 177:763, 1990
43. Farfan H: The torsional injury of the lumbar spine. Spine 9:53, 1984
44. Keene J, Drummond D: Mechanical back pain in the athlete. Comp Ther 11:7, 1985
45. Gofton P: Leg length disparity and back pain. J Rheumatol 12:747, 1985
46. Hazlett J: Kissing spines. J Bone Joint Surg 46:1368, 1964
47. Delmarter RB, Sachs BL, Thompson GH et al: Primary neoplasms of the thoracic lumbar spine: an analysis of 29 consecutive cases. Clin Orthop 256:87, 1990
48. Azouz EM, Kozlowski K, Martin D et al: Osteoid osteoma and osteoblastoma of the spine in children. Pediatr Radiol 16:25, 1986
49. Tewari MK, Tripathi LN, Mathuriya SN et al: Spontaneous spinal extradural hematoma in children. Child's Nerv Syst 8:53, 1992
50. Caine D, Lindner K: Preventing injury to young athletes. Part 1: predisposing factors. Aust Council Public Health, Educ Rec J March/April: 30, 1990
51. Paaganen H, Alanen A, Erkintalo M et al: Disc degeneration in Scheuermann's disease. Skeletal Radiol 18:523, 1989
52. Sward L, Hellstrom M, Jacobsson B, Peterson L: Back pain and radiologic changes in the thoraco-lumbar spine of athletes. Spine 15:124, 1990
53. Stanitski C: Low back pain in young athletes. Phys Sports Med 10:77, 1982
54. Farrell J, Drye C: The young patient. Occup Med 7:55, 1992
55. Department of Community Services and Health: Sports Injuries: Causes, Costs and Prevention. Better Health Program Report. Canberra, Australia, November, 1990
56. Grahame R, Jenkins JM: Joint hypermobility: asset or liability? A study of joint mobility in ballet dancers. Ann Rheum Dis 31:109, 1972
57. Bejjani F: Occupational biomechanics of athletes and dancers: a comparative approach. Clin Podiatr Med Surg 4:671, 1987

58. Russell B: A study of lumbopelvic dysfunction/psoas insufficiency and its role as a major cause of dance injury. Chiropract Sports Med 5:9, 1991
59. Jull G, Janda V: Muscles and motor control in low back pain. p. 253. In Twomey L and Taylor J (eds): Physical Therapy of the Low Back. Churchill Livingstone, New York, 1987
60. Bryan N, Smith B: The ballet dancer. Occupat Med 7:67, 1992
61. Keene JS, Albert MJ, Springer SL et al: Back injuries in college athletes. J Spinal Disorders 2:190, 1989
62. Snook G: Injuries in women's gymnastics: a five-year study. Am J Sports Med 7: 242, 1979
63. Semon R, Spengler D: Significance of spondylolysis in college football players. Spine 6:172, 1981
64. Snook GA: Injuries in intercollegiate wrestling: a five-year study. Am J Sports Med 10:142, 1982
65. Nilsonne U, Lundgren K: Long-term prognosis in idiopathic scoliosis. Acta Orthop Scand 39:456, 1968
66. Nachemson A: A long-term follow-up study of non treated scoliosis. Acta Orthop Scand 39:456, 1968
67. Collis O, Ponseti I: Long-term follow-up of patients with idiopathic scoliosis not treated surgically. J Bone Joint Surg 51A:425, 1969
68. Ponseti I, Friedman B: Prognosis in idiopathic scoliosis. J Bone Joint Surg 32A: 381, 1950
69. Weinstein SL, Zavala DC, Ponseti IV: Idiopathic scoliosis. Long-term follow-up and prognosis in untreated patients. J Bone Joint Surg 63A:702, 1981
70. White A, Panjabi M: Clinical Biomechanics of the Spine. JB Lippincott, Philadelphia, 1978
71. Hertzberg A: Prediction of cervical and low-back pain based on routine school health examination. Scand J Prim Health Care 3:247, 1985
72. Little W: On the influence of parturition, difficult labors, premature birth and asphyxia neonatorum on the mental and physical condition of the child, especially in relation to deformities. Trans Obstet Soc London 13:293, 1862
73. Solomons G, Holden RH, Denhoff E: The changing pattern of cerebral dysfunction in early childhood. Pediatrics 63:113, 1963
74. Schezer A: Current concepts and classification in cerebral palsy. Clin Proc Children's Hosp Nat Med Centre 29:143, 1973
75. Bobath K: The normal postural reflex mechanism and its deviation in children with cerebral palsy. Physiotherapy, November:1, 1974
76. Illingworth R: The Development of the Infant and Young Child. 8th Ed. Churchill Livingstone, London, 1983
77. Balmer G, MacEwen G: The incidence and treatment of scoliosis in cerebral palsy. J Bone Joint Surg 52B:134, 1970
78. Edmonson A: Postural Deformities. p. 1886. In Crenshaw A (Ed): Campbell's Operative Orthopaedics. CV Mosby, St. Louis, 1971
79. Samilson R, Bechard R: Scoliosis in cerebral palsy: incidence, distribution of curve patterns, natural history and thought on etiology. Curr Pract Orthop Surg 5:183, 1973
80. Bleck E: Deformities of the spine and pelvis in cerebral palsy. Clin Dev Med 52/ 53:124, 1975
81. Banks H: Cerebral palsy. In Lovell WW and Winter RB (eds): Paediatric Orthopaedics. JB Lippincott, Philadelphia, 1978

82. Moreau M, Drummond DS, Rogala E et al: Natural history of the dislocated hip in cerebral palsy. Dev Med Child Neurol 21:749, 1979
83. Hoffer MM, Stein GA, Koffman M, Prietto M: Femoral varus derotation osteotomy in spastic cerebral palsy. J Bone Joint Surg 67A:1229, 1985
84. Rosenthal RK, Levine DB, McCarrer CL: The occurrence of scoliosis in cerebral palsy. Dev Med Child Neurol 16:664, 1974
85. Bleck E: The hip in cerebral palsy. Orthop Clin North Am 11:79, 1980
86. Cooperman D: Hip dislocation in spastic cerebral palsy: long-term consequences. J Pediatr Orthop 7:268, 1987
87. McCarthy RE, Simon S, Douglas B et al: Proximal femoral resection to allow adults who have severe cerebral palsy to sit. J Bone Joint Surg 70A:1011, 1988
88. Clarke A, Redden J: Management of hip posture in cerebral palsy. J R Soc Med 85:150, 1992
89. Stanitski CL, Micheli L, Hall JE, Rosenthal RK: Surgical correction of spinal deformity in cerebral palsy. Spine 7:563, 1982
90. Liston C: Back schools and ergonomics. p. 279. In Twomey L and Taylor J (eds): Physical Therapy of the Low Back. Churchill Livingstone, New York, 1987
91. Liston C: Towards healthy Australians: schools and prevention of posture problems. Aust J Early Childhood 13:43, 1988
92. Lachmann S: Soft Tissue Injuries in Sport. Blackwell Scientific Publications, London, 1988
93. Anderson J: Low back pain—cause and prevention of long-term handicap (a critical review). Int Rehab Med 3:89, 1981
94. Willner S: Effect of a rigid brace on back pain. Acta Orthop Scand 56:40, 1985
95. Micheli L: Back injuries in dancers. Clin Sports Med 2:473, 1983
96. Morgan D: Concepts in functional training and postural stabilization for low-back patients. Topics Acute Care Trauma Rehabil 2:8, 1988
97. Maitland G: Negative disc exploration. Positive canal signs. Aust J Physiother 25:129, 1979
98. Butler D, Gifford L: The concept of adverse mechanical tension in the nervous system. Part 1: testing for dural tension. Physiotherapy 75:629, 1989
99. Garfin S, Rydevik B, Brown R: Compressive neuropathy of spinal nerve roots: a mechanical or biological problem. Spine 16:162, 1991
100. Sikorski JM: A rationalised approach to physiotherapy for low-back pain. Physiotherapy 10:571, 1985
101. Liston C, Freegard H: Principles, problems and practises of seating cerebral palsied clients. 13th Federal Conference of AAOT, Western Australia, Perth, August 15–18, 1984
102. Liston C: Seating cerebral palsied clients in Western Australia: a team approach to problem solving. Physiother Pract 2:11, 1986
103. Motloch W: Seating and positioning for the physically impaired. Orthot Prosthet 31:11, 1977
104. Nelham R: Seating for the chairbound disabled person: a survey of seating equipment in the United Kingdom. J Biomed Eng 3:267, 1981
105. Liston C: Seating for the disabled child in Western Australia. Proceedings of Seating and Posture Control Seminar T.A.D., New South Wales, Australia, 1983
106. Fay T, Lennox L, Dobie A, Williams S: Seating: you have to start somewhere. Cumberland College of Health Sciences, Sydney, 1990
107. Salminen J: The adolescent back. A field survey of 310 Finnish schoolchildren. Acta Paediatr Scand, suppl. 315:1, 1984

# 15 | Therapeutic Exercise for Back Pain

*Joe Farrell*
*Caroline Drye*
*Mike Koury*

The prevalence and financial impact of low back pain (LBP) in Western cultures is unquestioned among epidemiologists and practicing clinicians who regularly treat and study the disabling effects of spinal disease. Back injuries affect nearly 2 percent of all workers[1] and the costs exceed $16 billion per year in the United States.[2] Risk factors that predispose individuals to LBP are numerous. A study by the National Institute for Occupational Safety and Health (NIOSH)[3] reports that musculoskeletal injury rates increase significantly when heavy bulky objects are lifted, when the object is lifted from the floor, and when objects are lifted frequently. Other risk factors that may contribute to the growing epidemic of LBP include pushing,[4] pulling,[5] twisting,[6] slipping and tripping,[7] sitting,[8] loss of lumbar lordosis,[9,10] decreased strength of truncal musculature,[11] poor levels of physical conditioning,[12,13] and social variables such as drug and alcohol abuse.[14]

Since there are numerous risk factors and pathologic entities that contribute to LBP and associated symptoms, it is essential that the treatment of LBP should address the many causes of this disease process. For decades, considerable attention has been given to the role of exercise in the treatment of LBP. Recent studies support the premise that physical activity and exercise are beneficial for patients with back pain.[15–18] Active rehabilitation programs that emphasize exercise and patient participation appear not only to restore function, but in many cases may be associated with reduction in pain[19,20] and improved strength, endurance, and levels of fitness.[18] Lower extremity flexibility[21]; strength/endurance of muscle groups such as the abdominals,[11] spinal exten-

379

sors,[22] thoracolumbar fascia, latissimus dorsi, and abdominal obliques[23,24]; and lower extremities[25] all appear to be important in rehabilitation of the spine. Current research has shown that patients suffering from low back pain who underwent an aggressive exercise program were able to avoid surgical intervention, even in the presence of herniated nucleus pulposus (HNP) with radicular symptoms and neurologic signs.[26]

Physical therapists have traditionally played an important role as part of the rehabilitation team in prescribing exercise for patients presenting with both acute and chronic spinal pain. This chapter discusses the role of therapeutic exercise in the management of individuals with back pain. The following topics are emphasized:

1. The evaluation process that leads to successful exercise programs
2. Principles of therapeutic exercise training pertaining to spinal stability, strength, coordination, endurance, kinesthetic awareness, flexibility, and aerobic fitness
3. Progression of exercise
4. Functional training
5. The integration of exercise in overall patient management

## THE EVALUATION PROCESS

Numerous diagnostic labels may be given to patients with LBP.[27] However, clinical syndromes (e.g., sciatica or radiculitis) and diagnostic labels (e.g., HNP) do not consistently reflect functional disability. For example, patient A may present with sciatica extending to the lateral aspect for the foot in an S1 dermatomal distribution and be unable to sit for more than 5 minutes due to onset of lower extremity symptoms. Conversely, patient B with the same presenting clinical syndrome is able to sit through a 2-hour dinner prior to experiencing the same distribution of lower extremity symptoms as patient A. These patients have quite different functional limitations despite having the same clinical syndrome. In our clinical judgment it is likely that they will respond differently to exercise.

Successful treatment outcomes in response to exercise are dependent on methodical patient evaluation. Physical and functional limitations should be identified by carefully interviewing the patient and by performing appropriate physical and functional examinations. These provide the basis for realistic goal setting and the development of an individualized therapeutic exercise program.

### The Patient Interview

During the interview process, it is imperative that the clinician acquires an understanding of the patient's life-style and the specifics of his or her working environment. The patient should be questioned about the amount of time spent sitting or standing and the extent to which he or she must perform tasks such as lifting, pushing, pulling, carrying, reaching overhead, twisting, or working in awkward positions (often required of plumbers, aircraft maintenance workers, electricians, and so forth). Recreational activities should also be analyzed to determine which element of the activity is pain provoking (i.e., serving versus groundstrokes in tennis). It is also important to determine the extent to which the patient's normal activities are restricted by LBP, if the patient's goals include resumption of all of these activities, and how much time the patient can realistically devote to a home exercise program.

A detailed description of all of the patient's symptoms guides the examiner in determining which body regions should be emphasized during the physical and functional examination. These are easily recorded on a body chart.[28]

Determining the behavior of the symptoms during various activities will help to identify movements or postures that increase and/or decrease the patient's symptoms. This information also assists the therapist in understanding the types of exercises that may be indicated during subsequent treatment. For example, if sitting and/or driving most of the day aggravates the patient's symptoms, then instruction in proper sitting postures and spinal extension exercises may assist in controlling the symptoms. In addition, spinal extension performed many times per day would provide the patient with "pauses" from the flexion dominated lifestyle and assist in decompressing the posterior aspect of the motion segment.[29]

Patients may report problems with the position of their spine during activities (e.g., flexion versus extension), their tolerance to vertical loading (e.g., activities that increase vertical compression on the spine such as standing for long periods of time or carrying various objects such as groceries), sensitivity to pressure against the spine, and difficulty maintaining any position for extended periods.[30] If the patient's LBP is irritated by varying degrees of spinal flexion or extension, then careful attention will need to be paid to the amount of lordosis that is maintained during exercise and functional activities. Patients who are sensitive to tasks that increase the axial loading on their spine (lifting, carrying, prolonged standing or sitting) may need to avoid exercises that add to the compression on their spine. Strategies for "unloading" the spine will be discussed in the Treatment section.

Occasionally patients do not tolerate pressure directly against their spine because of acute tenderness. These patients will need to exercise in positions that decrease or avoid pressure on the spine (i.e., prone over a ball). Finally, if symptoms increase when any position is maintained for extended periods, then the exercise program will have to allow for frequent changes in posture.

Gathering sufficient information to understand how the problem affects the patient over the course of 24 hours is important for determining whether the patient will need instruction in sleeping positions, pacing of activity and exercise, and rest. Load-sensitive patients may need to plan to lie down at some point in the day to decrease the vertical loading forces on the vertebral column.

Asking questions regarding the patient's medical history, use of medications, or the results of special tests (i.e., x-ray, magnetic resonance imaging [MRI]) helps to identify specific contraindications to treatment and should ensure safety in the application of the treatment program. If a patient is hypertensive, grossly overweight, and has not exercised in 20 years, a vigorous exercise program would be difficult and dangerous, and lead to frustration and poor compliance on the part of the patient.

A thorough history of the current episode of spinal pain and any previous history of complaints related to the spine, guides the therapist in determining the nature (type of pathology), the extent of functional deterioration, and if the patient's symptoms are stable or deteriorating.[28] For example, if a patient reports that onset of lower extremity pain and paresthesias has occurred for the first time during the past year, or that each episode of LBP comes on with less provocation, then this may be indicative of a deterioration or worsening of the symptoms and the pathology. This information would alert the clinician that the intensity of the exercise and training program should be gentle until it is clear that exercise will not lead to further deterioration of the pathology or an increase in symptoms.

During the interview on previous medical history, the patient who has had previous episodes of spinal pain should be able to describe the type(s) of treatments that they have received (physical therapy, chiropractic, injections, medications, and so forth), the nature of previous exercise programs (e.g., flexion or extension, aerobic, various home programs), and whether or not these approaches have helped. The patient should demonstrate previous exercise programs because verbal description may not always be accurate. This will alert the clinician to exercises that were performed incorrectly or that have been detrimental to the patient's condition. Patients frequently have a limited understanding of the purpose of specific exercises and may not have complied with the instructions provided by the previous therapist.

Before progressing to the physical examination, the therapist should set priorities for the physical examination based on the patient's complaints of functional limitations, the severity (e.g., intensity of symptoms) and irritability of the symptoms (e.g., if the symptoms are easy or difficult to aggravate), the extent of the functional deterioration, and whether the patient's symptoms are stable or deteriorating.[28] Since the interview process is subjective, the astute clinician must take into consideration factors that may affect the information that the patient provides regarding his or her spinal problem. These factors include the patient's perception of pain, level of motivation, and potential avoidance behaviors associated with negative aspects of his or her life-style or work environment.[31,32] All of these factors can also impact on the patient's compliance with an exercise program.

## The Physical Examination

Data collected from the patient interview enable the clinician to plan and prioritize physical and functional examination procedures during the initial evaluation and during subsequent treatments. Typically all patients undergo active spinal range of motion (ROM) testing (flexion, extension, lateral flexions, and rotation). Motion testing helps to identify pain-provoking and pain-easing movement patterns and any restriction of movement. This also provides some baseline data from which to measure mobility and to assist in choosing the spinal position(s) that are safest and most comfortable for the initial exercise program. Improvement in spinal mobility has been shown to be a predictive variable in deciding a successful treatment outcome.[33]

The neurologic status and the presence of adverse neural tissue tension (ANTT)[34] should also be assessed. Passive neck flexion, straight leg raising, passive knee bend testing, and the slump test are performed depending on the nature of the patient's complaint.[28,34] These ANTT tests assist in confirming the contribution of "neural tension" to symptom provocation. In our experience many clinicians are unsuccessful treating spinal patients with exercise because signs of ANTT are not identified and treated.

Standardized muscle length tests[35] of the iliopsoas, rectus femoris, hamstrings, hip internal and external rotators, and adductor muscles should be performed because they indirectly affect the spine through their influence on pelvic and hip motion. Detailed biomechanical studies show that lower extremity flexibility is required for prevention of lumbar spine injuries.[36]

Muscles attaching more directly to the spine should also be tested for length restrictions. These include the latissimus dorsi, quadratus lumborum, and spinal extensors. The mobility of muscles that attach to the spine is important because shortened muscles lead to joint limitations (e.g., stiffness and loss of mobility) and may facilitate a pain cycle that is difficult to break.[37]

Many times muscle and joint restrictions in other regions of the body contribute to pain in the lumbar spine. For example, a golfer may be lacking mobility of the shoulder complex. This contributes to an alteration in the golf swing that may be contributing to lumbar pain. Clearly, the clinician should not limit mobility and muscle length testing to the muscles that most directly affect the lumbar spine. It is important to evaluate all possible contributing factors.

As an adjunct to specific manual muscle testing of the lower extremities and the trunk, it is helpful to test various functional activities that relate to the patient's functional limitations. Thus we routinely assess activities such as single-leg or double-leg lunge squats (Figs. 15-1 and 15-2) to test strength and endurance of the quadriceps and gluteals. The patient's control of the spinal column should be observed during these tests. A simple count of the number of repetitions performed prior to fatigue of the lower extremities or loss of control of the spine (Fig. 15-3) provides baseline data from which progress may be judged. Careful observation of these maneuvers may also confirm the suspicion of lower extremity joint or muscle tightness, which should be addressed in the ensuing exercise program.

If the patient must perform tasks at home or work that require repetitive pushing and/or pulling, then a loaded shopping cart or pulley system (Fig. 15-4) could be used to document the amount of weight the patient can safely move. Other functional activities should be assessed as indicated to determine the need for specific training in body mechanics. (e.g., rising from a chair, dressing,

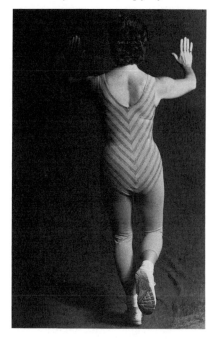

Fig. 15-1.    Single-leg squat.

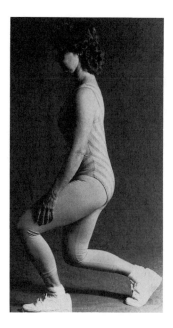

Fig. 15-2.    Double-leg lunge squat.

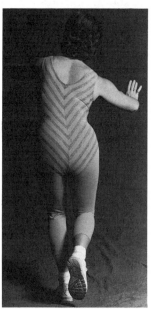

Fig. 15-3.    Single-leg squat with loss of spine control.

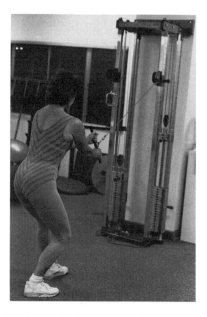

Fig. 15-4.    Pulley system for testing the amount of weight the patient is able to push/pull safely.

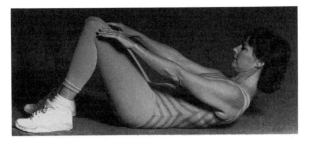

**Fig. 15-5.** Muscle test for rectus abdominus.

laundry-related tasks, carrying objects, getting in and out of a car, vacuuming, and reaching activities).

Lifting is a key functional activity for nearly any individual experiencing back pain. The clinician should be able to mimic most lifting situations with simple equipment (boxes, shelves, tables, weights). It is important to test the specific type of lift that the patient must perform at work or at home. Measurements should include the amount of weight lifted, the number of repetitions prior to experiencing symptoms, type of lift (e.g., floor to waist or waist to shoulder level), distance the load is carried, observation of spinal position (flexed or extended), and the ability to control the spinal position during the test (see Ch. 12).

Specific muscle strength and endurance testing of the truncal muscles may be measured by performing abdominal curls (Fig. 15-5) and diagonal curls (Fig. 15-6). The clinician can record the number of repetitions prior to fatigue or time an isometric hold in the test position to document the baseline measure. Back extensors may be tested through range (Fig. 15-7A & B) or isometrically (Fig. 15-8), prone extending over a pillow.

Figure 15-9 depicts a patient in a bridging position while the therapist applies alternating torsional forces to the pelvis. The assessment of torsional trun-

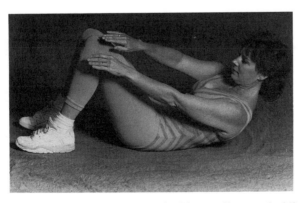

**Fig. 15-6.** Muscle test for abdominal internal/external obliques.

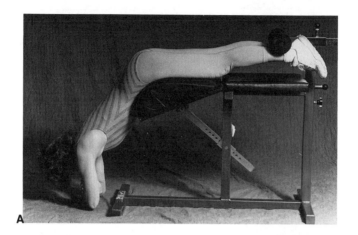

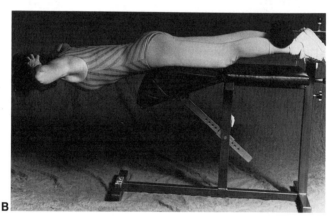

**Fig. 15-7.**  **(A)** Starting position to test back extensors through range. **(B)** End-range position to test back extensors.

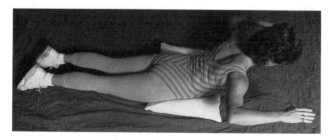

**Fig. 15-8.**  Isometric test for back extensors.

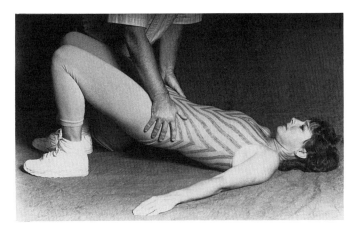

**Fig. 15-9.**  Bridge position with physical therapist applying torsional forces to pelvis.

cal resistance, which appears to activate a truncal cocontraction, is important because these muscles promote stability of the spinal column.[38]

Cardiovascular fitness may be measured by using a 6- or 12-minute walk test on a level surface or a standard protocol on a bicycle ergometer or treadmill.[39,40] The patient's heart rate and blood pressure should be monitored during the test to ensure that his or her response to exercise is appropriate for the particular age group. When using a walk test, distance covered and time prior to fatigue should be recorded. The time for the heart rate to recover provides another indicator of the patient's level of fitness.

The onset of back or leg pain may limit the patient's ability to perform aerobic testing to the point of fatigue. It is still helpful to document the time that elapsed during the test, the work load that was performed, and the heart rate and blood pressure responses during exercise in order to establish a baseline for future testing. The clinician should always screen patients for cardiovascular risk factors prior to performing even a submaximal stress test (heart rate kept under 75 percent of the predicted maximum heart rate). The American College of Sports Medicine[40] recommends that men over the age of 40 years and women over the age of 50 years should be evaluated by a physician prior to beginning any vigorous exercise program.

Palpation of the spine and associated soft tissues (e.g., posterior thigh/hamstrings) is another important aspect of the physical examination.[28] Palpation and passive movement testing yield information about joint and soft-tissue dysfunctions and the need to include manual therapy techniques within the treatment program. Manual therapy assessment and treatment may be helpful in restoring spinal mobility and decreasing pain as an adjunct to therapeutic exercise in patients suffering from back pain.[15]

The final component of the physical examination is the determination of the patient's spinal functional position (SFP). Morgan[41] describes the SFP as "the most stable and asymptomatic position of the spine for the task at hand."

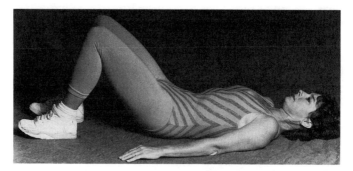

**Fig. 15-10.**    Hook-lying position with posterior pelvic tilt.

The patient is first assessed in a hook-lying position. Exploration of posterior (Fig. 15-10) and anterior pelvic tilting (Fig. 15-11) indicates whether the patient's symptoms are increased, decreased, or eliminated at any point in the range between spinal flexion and extension. The most comfortable position is by definition the SFP. This position is also referred to as "spinal neutral" by other practitioners.[26]

The SFP is not specifically related to the medical diagnosis; however, it is not unusual to see patients with stenosis or facet syndromes exhibit an SFP that is biased toward flexion of the lumbar spine. The critical factor is to find the lumbopelvic position that is most comfortable for the patient. This position may vary depending on the posture or activity performed by the patient (e.g., supine, sitting, or standing). The SFP may not be the same from day to day.[41] Identifying the SFP assists the clinician in determining the positions and the ROM in which the patient may safely begin to exercise. This will be discussed in detail in the subsequent sections.

## TREATMENT GOALS

At the conclusion of the physical and functional examination, the clinician should be able to analyze the presenting data and formulate realistic goals to

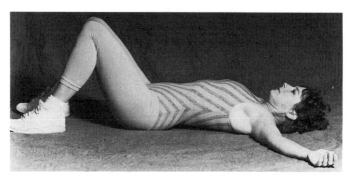

**Fig. 15-11.**    Hook-lying position with anterior pelvic tilt.

be addressed during the exercise/training program. Treatment goals should address specific improvements in strength, endurance, cardiovascular fitness, flexibility, and function. The goals are discussed with the patient in order to assist in understanding the relevance of the exercise program and to facilitate compliance with the treatment plan. An exercise program can only be successful if the patient is committed to participating.

Finally, a treatment plan is formulated that may include the use of other forms of treatment besides exercise (e.g., manual therapy, electrotherapy), instruction in back care, ergonomic principles applied to work-related tasks and activities of daily living, and supervised and independent exercise programs.

## PRINCIPLES OF EXERCISE RELATING TO BACK PAIN

### Self-Management

The major goal of any exercise program for the LBP patient is to teach the patient to control and prevent pain while normalizing spinal movement patterns during work, home, or recreational activities. Each patient should obtain the skills needed to apply the principles of back care to problem situations that confront them on a daily basis. Encouraging patient responsibility for long-term low-back management should assist in decreasing the economic cost of treating back pain.

### Stabilization

In recent years the term *spinal stabilization* has emerged in the literature. At times, this term has been described as rigid fixation to prevent movements of vertebral motion segments. However, we agree with Morgan[41] that it is impractical and rarely necessary to train patients to maintain their spine in one lumbar position during exercise and activities of daily living. As patients improve they are encouraged to exercise within the lumbopelvic ROM that is painless[40]; therefore, the patient is not maintaining a strict SFP throughout the treatment program.

Dynamic spinal stabilization in practice is a complex neuromuscular skill that necessitates continuous muscular adjustments to maintain a safe spinal position.[40] For example, as an individual lifts a box overhead the tendency is to extend the spine. The abdominals and gluteal muscles must work in concert to counteract this tendency to extend the spine.

Porterfield[42] defines dynamic stabilization as the ability of the patient to be active throughout the day without increasing symptoms. A cornerstone of our approach to exercise is to make every attempt to work the patient as vigorously as possible without increasing symptoms. As patients progress in their ability to control the SFP during various exercises, there should be a corresponding increase in the ability to perform activities of daily living without increasing symptoms.

## Kinesthetic Training

Kinesthetic awareness is often lost following injury to the spine and periods of relative immobilization, Therefore, the patient must be retaught to coordinate the spine during functionally related tasks. When patients are able to recognize small changes in the movement pattern and control the SFP, then they have begun to learn how to control their body in space. Repetition of these movements enhances the neurophysiologic process of learning.[43] The goal is to develop engrams for these activities and diminish repetitive trauma to the spine due to poor movement patterns.[44]

Substitution patterns[25] can arise due to muscle weakness and loss of spinal or lower extremity flexibility. They are accompanied by an inability to perform functional movements in a manner that is not pain provoking. Porterfield and DeRosa[45] define fatigue as substitution of muscle function and suggest that if a patient changes the spinal motion during performance of a task by altering body position, then the exercise should cease.

## Endurance and Strength

It is critical that an exercise program is progressed to the point where it adequately addresses the truncal and lower extremity strength and endurance that the patient needs to return to the rigors of specific life-style or work environments.[22,46] This is one of the basic principles of work-hardening programs. In addition, failure to adequately train the patient in functional activities is one reason for poor results of many exercise programs.[47]

## Exercise During the Pain Phase

During the acute phase of spinal rehabilitation, modalities such as ice, electrical stimulation, transcutaneous electrical nerve stimulation (TENS), traction and anti-inflammatory medications are often used to control pain. The patient is also given specific instruction in activities such as dressing, getting in and out of bed, sitting, and rising from sitting. This assists patients in learning how to protect their backs and prevent unnecessary microtrauma to the injured spine.

Manual therapy can be an important part of treatment during the acute phase of rehabilitation. It has been shown to be effective in treating acute back pain[48,49] and may assist in improving the spinal ROM necessary to begin therapeutic exercise. However, it has been our experience that it is important to implement active exercise as soon as possible in order to avoid deconditioning and loss of spinal and extremity ROM, and to prevent the development of abnormal movement patterns. Indeed, our experience has shown that many patients who cannot tolerate direct manual therapy techniques will improve rapidly with gentle strength training and ergonomic instruction.

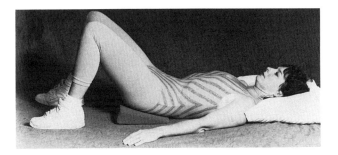

**Fig. 15-12.**    Passive prepositioning of the lumbar spine in flexion to maintain a safe SFP.

To begin the exercise portion of the rehabilitation program, patients must first learn the limits of their SFP so that they may gain an appreciation of the lumbopelvic positions that must be avoided. Initially the patient may not have the strength or kinesthetic awareness to prevent painful movements. Prepositioning the spine to prevent movement out of the SFP or range is often necessary. Morgan[41] describes two methods of prepositioning the spine. Passive prepositioning uses body and/or limb placement to avoid movement of the lumbopelvic region into painful positions. Minimal muscular effort is required and assistive devices (Fig. 15-12) help the patient to maintain a safe, painless SFP. Even during the pain control phase of rehabilitation the patient is then able to exercise the abdominals and upper extremities fairly vigorously (Fig. 15-13) with minimal risk of aggravating LBP.

As the patient learns to control the SFP, active prepositioning is used.[41] If the SFP is biased toward flexion, the patient will be instructed to actively maintain a posterior pelvic tilt by contracting the gluteals and abdominals instead of relying on passive prepositioning of the spine.

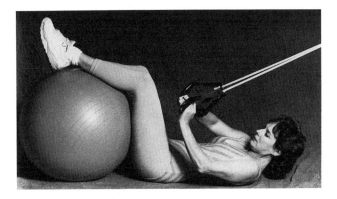

**Fig. 15-13.**    Diagonal pulls to exercise the abdominals and upper extremities while passively prepositioned.

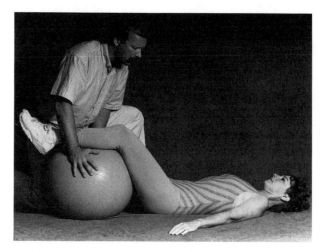

**Fig. 15-14.**   Rhythmic stabilization technique, prepositioning using gym ball. Resistance to trunk is provided indirectly through gym ball.


As kinesthetic awareness and pain control improves, other techniques are used to challenge the patient while maintaining a safe SFP. Alternating isometric and rhythmic stabilization techniques[50] are employed to facilitate truncal muscles in an isometric manner because movement through range is often pain provoking during the pain control phase of rehabilitation (Fig. 15-14). As spinal range of movement improves and the excursion of painless lumbopelvic motion increases, the vigor of the exercise program is increased.


## Treatment Progression

The exercise regimen should relate to the patient's specific functional goals. We explain to patients that to attain their goals certain skills must be mastered. For example, as an infant matures it must endure the exploration of the developmental sequence prior to learning to walk. Similarly, if the patient's long-term goal is to repetitively lift 40-lb boxes 4 hours per day, certain skills must be mastered prior to actually training the patient in the skill of lifting.

After patients learn the limits of their SFP in hook-lying, prone, side-lying, quadriped, and standing positions, exercises can be performed in any or all of these developmental positions. The need to develop proximal stability (e.g., truncal) as a base for distal mobility (e.g., superimposing movement of the extremities) is a key concept in the sequencing of exercises.[41,50] Ultimately the patient must develop the skill to control movement of the spine during complex, total body movements. Many options are employed to strengthen the trunk and extremity musculature through this developmental sequence.

Exercises usually begin in a hook-lying position (see Fig. 15-10). Once the

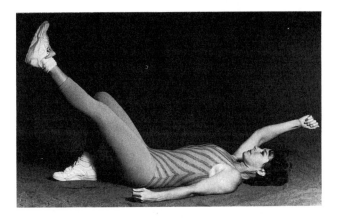

**Fig. 15-15.**   Modified deadbug exercise.

patient is able to actively preposition and control the spine in the hook-lying position, arm movements and lower extremity movements are added to challenge the patient's ability to maintain the SFP. To facilitate coordination while maintaining an SFP, contralateral arm/leg movements are used (Fig. 15-15). The further the patient extends the upper or lower extremities (Fig. 15-16) the more difficult it is to maintain the SFP. The addition of cuff weights on ankles/ wrists further challenges the patient in terms of truncal strength (Fig. 15-17). An increase in the number of repetitions of the "deadbug" exercise facilitates endurance and enhances learning through repetition. An advanced patient may be able to perform difficult truncal stability exercises, such as the one depicted in Fig. 15-18. These exercises require a significant amount of lower abdominal strength to maintain the SFP.

Other exercises for the abdominals traditionally include abdominal curls (refer to Fig. 15-5). Patients can start supine with the feet on a ball. We instruct them to push the feet into the ball (Fig. 15-19) to facilitate the gluteals and

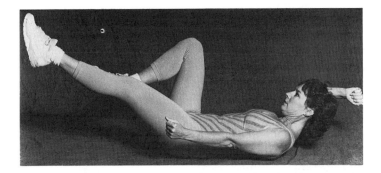

**Fig. 15-16.**   Advanced deadbug exercise: bicycling-like action of the lower extremities with alternating shoulder flexion.

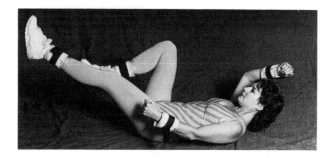

**Fig. 15-17.**    Deadbug with cuff weights to increase the vigor of the exercise.

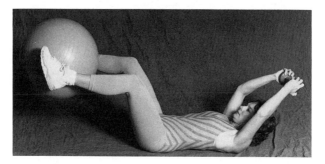

**Fig. 15-18.**    Gym ball between legs with weights in hands moving in opposite directions.

hamstrings and inhibit iliopsoas.[51] Straight-forward and abdominal oblique curls can be performed while maintaining this position. As the patient advances, the performance of abdominal curls on a gym ball further challenges balance and increases the range through which the abdominals must contract (Fig. 20A & B).

   To begin exercising spinal extensors, gluteals, and hamstrings, the bridging position (Fig. 15-21) is used initially. The same principles of maintaining a pain-

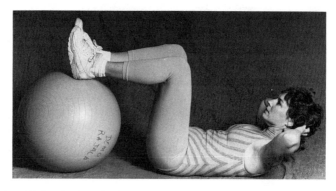

**Fig. 15-19.**    Abdominal curl with feet pushing into ball to inhibit the iliopsoas.

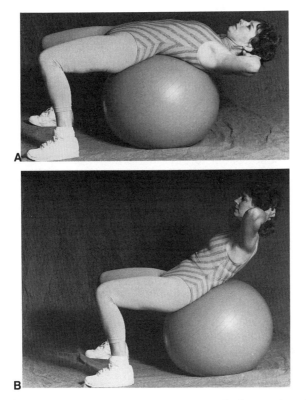

**Fig. 15-20.** **(A)** Abdominal curl on the ball starting in spinal extension. **(B)** End position for abdominal curl on the gym ball.

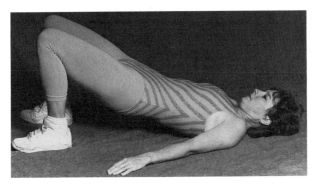

**Fig. 15-21.** Bridge position to strengthen spinal extensors, gluteals, and hamstrings.

less SFP or ROM are encouraged. The patient may begin with simple gluteal sets and progress to the point where the bridge position is maintained while superimposing leg movements (Fig. 15-22) or arm movements (Fig. 15-23). To exercise upper trunk extensors the patient can lie prone over a ball (Fig. 15-24) and extend the trunk within the pain-free range. A "Roman chair" can also be used for extension exercises (see Fig. 15-7B). Endurance can be facilitated by maintaining the spine in extension and superimposing numerous repetitions of upper extremity movements with weights using the "Roman chair" (Fig. 15-25) or in a bridge position on a ball (Fig. 15-26).

When the patient has mastered bridging activities on the floor, a gym ball can be used to challenge balance and to facilitate recruitment of the spinal stabilizers. By bridging with the feet on the ball (Fig. 15-27) while maintaining an SFP, the patient works the back extensors and gluteals quite vigorously. Bridging with the heels or toes dug into the ball also increases the vigor and balance required of the exercise. To facilitate internal/external obliques and the spinal extensors, the physical therapist can perform rhythmic stabilization techniques[50] (Fig. 15-28). This requires advanced balance, strength, and kinesthetic awareness.

Stabilization training in the hands and knees position (quadriped) requires increased balance and kinesthetic awareness of the spinal position in space. If the patient has difficulty maintaining this position initially, a gym ball can be used to support the trunk (Fig. 15-29). As the patient progresses, arm or leg motions can be superimposed while maintaining the SFP (Fig. 15-30).

The duration of the treatment program is dependent on the chronicity of the spinal dysfunction and whether the treatment regimen is changing treatment goals. For the chronic low-back patient it has been suggested that to affect chronic deconditioning and poor movement patterning, 2 to 3 months of intensive treatment may be required prior to noting positive functional improvement.[16]

## Helpful Equipment

We use very simple equipment in our exercise programs. Gym balls, pulleys or Sportcords, wooden dowels, free weights, foam rollers, and simple weight machines provide enough versatility for a vigorous exercise program.

Gym balls are utilized to either provide increased support of the spine and extremities or to challenge the patient's balance and dynamic stabilization skills. Balls come in several different sizes to fit patients with different body types.

Wooden dowels can be used to provide a sensory cue for patients who have difficulty monitoring changes in their spinal position during flexion (see Functional Training).

Pulleys can be used to provide resistance at a variety of angles (e.g., proprioceptive neuromuscular facilitation[50] [PNF] diagonals, latissimus pull-downs) and to simulate pulling (Fig. 15-31) on hoses or ropes. Sportcords or surgical

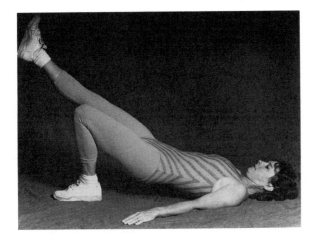

**Fig. 15-22.**    Extending one leg in the bridge position.

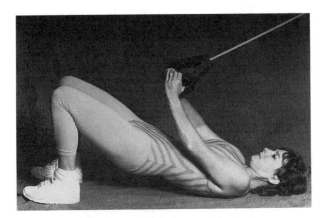

**Fig. 15-23.**    Bridging while using a Sportcord.

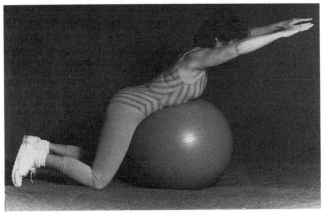

**Fig. 15-24.**    Upper spinal extension over gym ball.

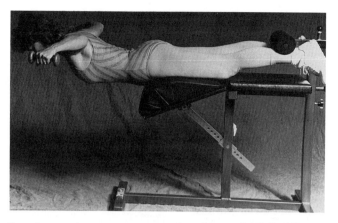

**Fig. 15-25.** Superimposed arm movements when isometrically holding back extension position on ''Roman chair.''

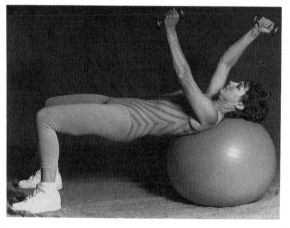

**Fig. 15-26.** Maintaining a bridge position on gym ball, superimposing arm movements with weights.

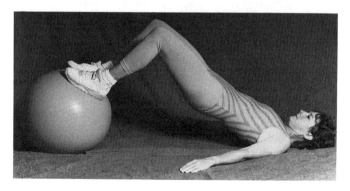

**Fig. 15-27.** Bridging with feet on ball.

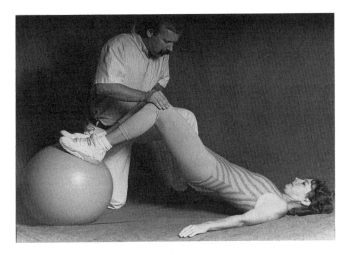

**Fig. 15-28.** Rhythmic stabilization technique in the bridging position with the feet on the ball.

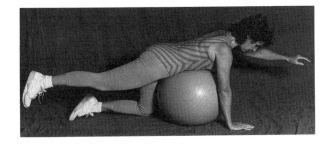

**Fig. 15-29.** Quadriped position with support of the gym ball.

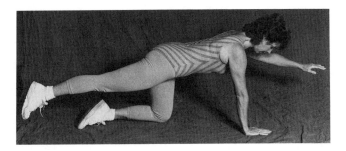

**Fig. 15-30.** Contralateral arm and leg movements in unsupported quadriped position.

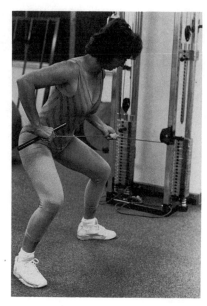

**Fig. 15-31.**   Pulley system used to simulate pulling activity.

tubing are inexpensive items for the patient to use to simulate pulley exercises at home.

Weight training machines can be incorporated to facilitate strengthening of the upper and lower extremities. The patient must be carefully instructed in the use of each machine and monitored for the maintenance of the SFP during exercise. Instruction in the use of various weight training machines is important if the patient will continue to exercise at a gym after discharge from physical therapy.

## Unloading the Spine

Many patients are sensitive to axial loading through the spine during activities of daily living and exercise. When this is the case, an attempt should be made to control the axial load that the spine must bear during exercise or to allow intermittent "unweighting" throughout the day. Various traction devices can be used to provide distraction in supine or in an inclined position before, during, or after exercising. Prone lying over a gym ball also provides gentle distraction. Providing for upper extremity support during upright exercises such as squats, walking, sitting, or cycling will also decrease spinal loading (Fig. 15-32A & B).

When pulley systems or overhead weights are used to provide resistance to the upper extremities during stabilization training, there is a vertical force upward on the spine that helps to counteract the compressive forces generated

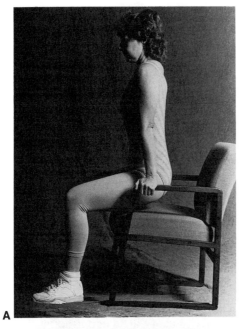

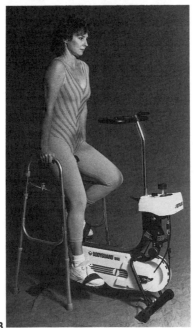

**Fig. 15-32.** **(A)** Unloading the spine while sitting. **(B)** Unloading when riding the bicycle.

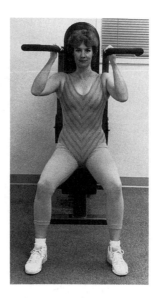

**Fig. 15-33.**   Novak pull-down to unload.

when the abdominals and extensors are cocontracting to stabilize the spine (Fig. 15-33). This type of exercise allows the load-sensitive patient to exercise more vigorously without increasing symptoms.

## Functional Training

Various methods of improving the strength and coordination of truncal muscles have been presented as a precursor to functional training of the patient. Through carefully planned movement training patients are now taught how to perform specific tasks that are pertinent to their daily function. Patients are instructed in how to perform functional activities in a manner that is safe for the spine and that no longer aggravates the symptoms. Repetition of the task (e.g., lifting) helps the patients learn new movement patterns and breaks substitution patterns that put the spine at risk. For example, most back patients need to lean over a sink to shave or wash their faces. Nearly everyone must lift groceries out of a grocery cart. Most patients flex the lumbar spine during these activities. To eliminate the flexion dominated movement patterns, we can teach the patient to maintain an SFP in standing and then advance to transitional movements like half-bending. With the use of a wooden stick and a mirror for visual feedback, the patient is instructed to bend from the hips (hip hinge) while maintaining an SFP (Fig. 15-34). The spine is actively positioned in a pain-free position and the patient is taught to move the spine much like the arm of a crane. More complex spinal control is required to combine the hip hinge with lower extremity movements as in squatting (Fig. 15-35). The squat with the hip

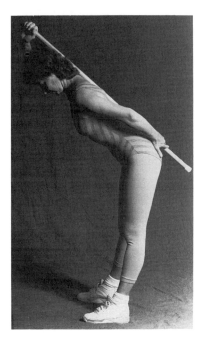

**Fig. 15-34.**    Standing hip hinge.

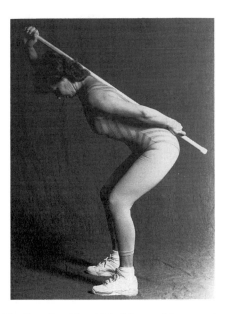

**Fig. 15-35.**    Combined hip hinge with squatting.

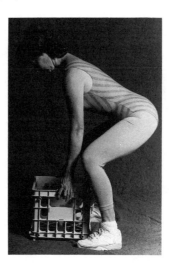

**Fig. 15-36.**    Picking up box using a hip hinge and squat-lift.

hinge allows the patient to pick up a box (Fig. 15-36) or get an object out of a grocery cart (Fig. 15-37).

In preparation for training in lifting the patient can strengthen and improve the endurance of spinal extensors, gluteals, and lower extremities by maintaining the squat position and performing various arm movements with weights (Fig. 15-38). If the goal is to repetitively lift 40-lb boxes, then the patient needs to gradually start lifting loads (e.g., 5 to 10 lb), progressing the weight and

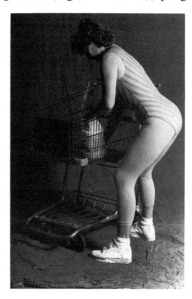

**Fig. 15-37.**    Using a hip hinge to get an object out of shopping cart.

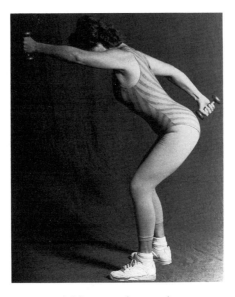

**Fig. 15-38.** Arm activities superimposed on a squat position.

number of lifts toward the demands of the work environment. When patients are able to meet the lifting requirements of their job in the physical therapy gym, then they are ready to return to work.

## Cardiovascular Conditioning

Early in the treatment program aerobic activity is encouraged in a pain-free manner. If walking eases pain, then a walking program is initiated on the treadmill and at home. If the spine is load sensitive, the patient is instructed to walk on the treadmill while taking weight off the spine by using safety rails of the treadmill or the use of a standard walker. This allows the patient to continue with walking in a manner that is painless. We use various equipment such as treadmills, stationary bicycles, cross-country ski machines, and stair climbers to increase the vigor of aerobic training. Ideally, we want to find an aerobic activity that the patient will continue indefinitely when physical therapy is discontinued.

## Flexibility Training

Flexibility training usually begins at the outset of an exercise program. Stretching exercises may be needed to address the mobility of the spine and other joint restrictions. The most common muscle restrictions are found in the length of the hip internal and external rotators, adductors, iliopsoas, rectus

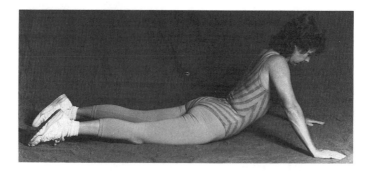

**Fig. 15-39.**   Press-ups to facilitate spinal extension mobility.

femoris, hamstrings, gluteals, gastrocsoleus, and back extensors. The patient is instructed in pre- and post-exercise stretching routines as needed.

Static stretching is easy and safe because the patient is in control of the stretch. The patient positions the body part to be stretched and gradually increases the stretch for 15 to 30 seconds. The duration of stretch has been shown to be as effective at 15 seconds as at 45 to 60 seconds.[52] Proprioceptive neuromuscular facilitation techniques (e.g., hold–relax and contract–relax) have also been shown to be effective methods of muscle stretching.[53]

Exercises such as press-ups (Fig. 15-39), knees to chest (Fig. 15-40), and the cat/camel stretch in the quadriped position help to increase spinal ROM in flexion and extension. It is important to note that many patients will not tolerate direct stretching of the spine during an acute episode of back pain. In these patients, it is best to allow them to exercise and function in a restricted ROM until they have an increased range of their SFP. Continuous reassessment will help the clinician know when it is safe to resume direct spinal stretching exercises. The reader is encouraged to review McKenzie's[10] principles for the application of flexion and extension exercises to different lumbar syndromes.

It should be noted that when stretching muscles of the spine and extremities, nerves and fascia are also being stretched. Breig and Troup[54] have shown

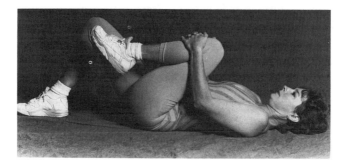

**15-40.**   Knees to chest exercise to facilitate spinal flexion mobility.

that internal rotation and adduction in straight leg raising increases the tension in the lumbosacral nerves. Stretching the hamstrings of back patients in the presence of a "adverse neural tension sign"[34] warrants caution. It is usually safest to begin stretching with the limb in a position that decreases tension on the neural system (e.g., in some hip abduction, external rotation, or spinal lateral–flexion toward the limb that is being stretched). As the neural tension sign decreases then the muscle stretching may be progressed toward hip adduction and internal rotation in order to affect the lateral hamstrings. Because of the effect of stretching on neural structures, the patient's neurologic status should be monitored at regular intervals throughout treatment.

## Home Exercises and Patient Management

Patients usually begin a home exercise program within the first week of treatment. We want to instill in the patient as soon as possible the importance of taking an active part in rehabilitation. We carefully instruct patients in the number of repetitions and sets of each exercise as well as the amount of weight to use. When patients are discharged, they should understand the role of exercise in the ongoing management of spinal pain. They should also be able to apply principles of ergonomics to new tasks they will encounter in the work, home, or recreational environments. We aim to provide our patients with the skills to manage their spinal dysfunction through their lifetime.

We always inform our patients that they need to continue to exercise indefinitely. Spinal disease is in many respects like a sinus allergy. In other words, symptoms will come and go but the underlying problem rarely goes away. If the patient will not be seen again for quite some time we also provide instruction in ways to progress the level of difficulty of the program. Instruction is given in self-treatment techniques and when it is appropriate to seek professional help for an exacerbation of back and/or leg pain. It is suggested to patients with chronic spinal dysfunction that they periodically (e.g., every 3 to 6 months) have their exercise programs re-evaluated to modify the program to meet new goals and to ensure compliance.[55]

## SUMMARY

Therapeutic exercise is one of the most important components in the rehabilitation of the patient with LBP. A thorough evaluation is necessary to identify the patient's unique needs and to set realistic treatment goals. A carefully planned treatment program must be continually assessed to ensure that the treatment goals are being achieved. The exercise and functional training program should be task and/or job specific. It should involve detailed training in spinal kinesthetic awareness, truncal and extremity strengthening, flexibility, endurance, aerobic conditioning, coordination, and specific functional skills. The exercise program should be individualized and challenging to the patient.

The home exercise program should be similar to the program that was performed in the PT gym. Adjunctive exercise equipment such as gym balls, Sportcords, and cuff weights are inexpensive investments that allow patients to perform vigorous exercise programs on an ongoing basis at home.

Finally, a coordinated team effort between the physical therapist, physician, patient, insurance carrier, and other health care providers is necessary for a successful treatment outcome. All team members must communicate consistently to ensure that the rehabilitation program progresses at an optimal rate.

## ACKNOWLEDGMENTS

The authors wish to acknowledge Michael Moore, P.T., Tim McGonigle, P.T., Dennis Morgan, P.T., D.C., and Eileen Vollowitz, P.T., for many conceptual ideas presented in this chapter. In addition, we wish to acknowledge the assistance of Edie Farrell, P.T., and Chris Chenard in producing the photographs. Lastly, we thank Carol Jo Tichenor, M.A., P.T., for her assistance in editing this chapter.

## REFERENCES

1. Bond MB: Low back injuries in industry. Ind Med Surg 39:28, 1970
2. Snook SH, Jensen RC: Occupational Low Back Pain. Praeger Publishers, New York, 1984
3. NIOSH: National Institute for Occupational Safety and Health. Work practices guide for manual lifting. Cincinnati National Institute for Occupational Safety and Health, DHHS Publication No. NIOSH 81, 1981
4. Magora A: Investigation of the relation between low back pain and occupation IV. Physical requirements: bending, rotation, reaching and sudden maximal effort. Scand J Rehabil Med 5:186, 1973
5. Damkot DK, Popi MH, Lord J, Frymoyer JW: The relationship between work history, work environment and low back pain in males. Spine 9:395, 1984
6. Frymoyer JW, Pope MH, Costanza MC et al: Epidemiologic studies of low back pain. Spine 5:419, 1980
7. Manning DP, Shannon HS: Slipping accidents causing low back pain in a gearbox factory. Spine 6:70, 1981
8. Magora A: Investigation of the relationship between low back pain and occupation III. Physical requirements: sitting, standing, and weight lifting. Ind Med Surg 41: 5, 1972
9. Magora A: Investigation of the relation between low back pain and occupation VII. Neurological and orthopedic conditions. Scand J Rehabil Med 7:146, 1975
10. McKenzie R: The lumbar spine. Spinal Publications, Waikanei, New Zealand, 1980
11. McNeill T, Warwick D, Andersson G, Schultz A: Trunk strengths in attempted flexion, extension and lateral bending in healthy subjects and patients with low back disorders. Spine 5:529, 1980
12. Cady LD, Bischoff DP, O'Connell ER et al: Strength and fitness and subsequent back injuries in firefighters. J Occup Med 21:269, 1979

13. Battié MC: Aerobic fitness and its measurement. Spine 16:677, 1991
14. Westin CG: Low back sick-listing. A nonsociological and medical insurance investigation. Acta Sociol Med Scand 2–3:127, 1970
15. Mitchell RI, Carmen GM: Results of a multicenter trial using an intensive active exercise program for the treatment of acute soft tissue and back injuries. Spine 15: 514, 1990
16. Manniche C, Lundberg E, Christensen I et al: Intensive dynamic back exercises for chronic low back pain: a clinical trial. Pain 47:53, 1991
17. Edwards BC, Zusman M, Hardcastle P et al: A physical approach to the rehabilitation of patients disabled by chronic low back pain. Med J Aust 156:167, 1992
18. Lindstrom I, Ohlund C, Ckaes E et al: Mobility, strength and fitness after a graded activity program of patients with subacute low back pain. Spine 17:641, 1992
19. Smith S, Mayer TG, Gatchell RJ, Becker TJ: Quantification of lumbar function. Part 1: isometric and multispeed isokinetic trunk strength measures in sagittal and axial planes in normal subjects. Spine 10:757, 1985
20. Mayer TG, Gatchell RJ, Kishino N et al: A prospective short-term study of chronic low back pain patients utilizing novel objective functional measurement. Pain 25: 53, 1986
21. Saal JS: Flexibility training. Phys Med Rehabil: State of the Art Rev 1:537, 1987
22. Smidt GL, Herring T, Amundsen L et al: Assessment of abdominal and back extensor functions. Spine 11:19, 1983
23. Bogduk N, MacIntosh J: The applied anatomy of the thoracolumbar fusica. Spine 9:164, 1984
24. Gracovetsky S, Farfan H, Hellew C: The abdominal mechanism. Spine 10:317, 1985
25. Saal JA: General principles and guidelines for rehabilitation of the injured athlete. Phys Med Rehabil: State of the Art Rev 1:523, 1987
26. Saal JA, Saal JS. Non operative treatment of herniated lumbar intervertebral disc with radiculopathy. An outcome study. Spine 14:431, 1989
27. Nachemson AL, LaRocca H: Editorial: Spine 1987. Spine 12:427, 1987
28. Maitland GD: Vertebral Manipulation. 5th Ed. Butterworths, London, 1986
29. Schnebel BE, Watkin RG, Dillin W: The role of spinal flexion and extension in changing nerve root compression in disc herniations. Spine 14:835, 1989
30. Vollowitz E: Furniture Prescription. Top Acute Care Rehabil 2:18, 1988
31. Greenough GC, Fraser RD: The effects of compensation on recovery from low back injury. Spine 14:947, 1989
32. Polatin PB, Gatchell RJ, Barnes D et al: A psychosociomedical prediction model of response to treatment by chronically disabled workers with low back pain. Spine 14:956, 1989
33. Mellin G, Hurri H, Harkapaa H, Jarvikoshi N: A controlled study on the outcome of inpatient and outpatient treatment of low back pain. Scand J Rehabil Med 21: 91, 1989
34. Butler D: Mobilization of the Nervous System. Churchill Livingstone, New York, 1991
35. Janda V: Muscle Function Testing. Butterworths, London, 1983
36. Farfan H, Gracovetsky S: The optimum spine. Spine 11:543, 1986
37. Reynolds M. Myofascial trigger points syndromes in the practice of rheumatology. Arch Phys Med Rehabil 62:111, 1981
38. Richardson C, Jull G, Toppenberg R, Comerford M: Techniques for active lumbar stabilisation for spinal protection. A pilot study. Aust J Physiol 38:105, 1992
39. Astrand PE, Rodahl K: Textbook of Work Physiology: Physiological Bases of Exercise. 3rd Ed. McGraw-Hill, New York, 1986

40. American College of Sports Medicine: Guidelines for exercise testing and prescription. 4th Ed. Lea & Febiger, Philadelphia, 1991
41. Morgan D: Concepts in functional training and postural stabilization for the low back injured. Top Acute Care Trauma Rehabil 2:8, 1988
42. Porterfield JA: Dynamic stabilization of the trunk. J Orthop Sports Phys Ther 6: 271, 1985
43. Harris FA: Facilitation techniques and technological adjuncts in therapeutic exercise. p. 110. In Basmajian JV (ed): Therapeutic Exercise. 4th Ed. Williams & Wilkins, Baltimore, 1984
44. Saal JA: The new back school prescription: Stabilization training II. Occup Med State of the Art Rev 7:33, 1992
45. Porterfield JA, DeRosa C: Mechanical Low Back Pain: Perspective in Functional Anatomy. WB Saunders, Philadelphia, 1990
46. Beiring–Sorensen F: Physical measurements as risk indicators for low back trouble over a one year period. Spine 9:106, 1984
47. Estlander A, Mellin G, VanHaranta H, Hupli M. Effects and follow-up of a multi model treatment program including intensive physical training for low low back patients. Scand J Rehabil Med 23:97, 1991
48. Sim–Williams H, Jayson MIV, Young SMS et al: Controlled trial of mobilisation and manipulation for low back pain in general practice. Br Med J 2:1338, 1978
49. Farrell J, Twomey L: Acute low back pain, comparison of two conservative approaches. Med J Aust 1:160, 1982
50. Knott J, Voss DE: Proprioceptive Neuromuscular Facilitation. 2nd Ed. Harper & Row, New York, 1968
51. Janda V, Schmid HJA: Muscles as a pathogenic factor in back pain: p. 17. In: Proceedings of the Fourth Conference of the International Federation of Orthopaedic Manipulative Therapist. Christchurch, New Zealand, February 18–22, 1980.
52. Medeiros J, Madding SW: Effect of duration of passive stretch on hip abduction range of motion. Orthop J Sports Phys Ther 8:409, 1987
53. Sody S, Wortman M, Blanke D: Flexibility training: Ballistic, static or proprioceptive neuromuscular facilitation. Arch Phys Med Rehabil 63:261, 1982
54. Breig A, Troup J: Biomechanical considerations in the straight leg raising test. Spine 4:242, 1979
55. Reilly K, Lovejoy B, Williams R, Roth H: Differences between a supervised and independent strength and conditioning program with chronic low back syndromes. J Occup Med 31:547, 1989

# 16 | Back and Joint Pain: A Rationale for Treatment by Manual Therapy*

*Lance T. Twomey*
*James R. Taylor*

The manual therapist is concerned with the prevention and treatment of musculoskeletal pain and dysfunction by the application of primary physical modalities incorporating exercise, passive joint movement (including mobilization and manipulation), traction, and massage.[1-3] Today, most manual therapists have usually received additional training in pathology, diagnosis, and skills beyond that traditional obtained at the undergraduate level and have had an extended period of supervised clinical practice.[1] Although the historical focus of manual therapy has been directed toward the treatment of back and peripheral joint pain and dysfunction, a survey of Grieve's *Modern Manual Therapy of the Vertebral Column*[1] shows that manual therapy now encompasses the whole field of musculoskeletal medicine. *Physical Therapy of the Low Back* has considered the functional anatomy and biomechanics of the lumbar spine in relation to different treatment modalities and the biomechanical effects that manual therapy can have on the musculoskeletal system of the body.

Back pain appears to be an inevitable accompaniment of the human life cycle. Approximately 80 percent of persons in Western society experience back

---

* Parts of this chapter are from Twomey LT: A rationale for the treatment of back pain and joint pain by manual therapy. Phys Ther 72:885, 1992, with permission.

pain at some stage during their life, and this pain is sufficient to cause an alteration in life-style for at least a period of time and drives individuals to seek some form of treatment.[4] Back pain is the single most expensive musculoskeletal ailment in Western society,[5] although only 8 percent of those with back pain or dysfunction account for almost 80 percent of the costs involved.[6] Until recently, it was believed that back pain was not a problem in "underdeveloped countries," but recent evidence clearly shows that its incidence in such countries with predominantly rural economies is similar to that in the "developed," industrial world and that when back pain clinics are made available, local people flock to them for treatment.[7] Backache is as universal as headache, but it is often impossible to be accurate about the source of the pain, as most demonstrable pathology is also visible in the symptom-free population.[8]

Because current knowledge of the pathogenesis of back pain is incomplete, and many of the diagnostic labels attached to patients are unclear, it is little wonder that treatment remains largely empirical.[8] Nevertheless, in recent years fundamental biologic studies have added considerably to the current understanding of age changes, related pathology, and the effects of trauma on spinal structures.[8-11] Although knowledge of basic biologic information is still proceeding, it forms the basis of understanding of the effects of physical and manual therapy on the tissues of the spine and thus on low back pain. Similarly, recent clinical studies have also monitored the response of particular clinical syndromes to a variety of treatment approaches.

Research into the musculoskeletal system of the body as a whole has demonstrated the beneficial effects of movement on all joint tissues, particularly articular cartilage (AC) and ligaments; it has also shown that the stress of exercise is essential, not only for physical fitness but also for the maintenance of muscle bulk and bone mass, and that problems such as back and joint pain respond favorably to movement and activity and adversely to rest.[11-13] Similarly, experience in the physical treatment of athletes who have severe musculoskeletal injuries to many regions of the body has provided the initial stimulus for the development of the highly successful approach to the treatment of chronic back pain by aggressive, intensive physical therapy and work conditioning.[11,13,14] There is now a better knowledge of the effects of movement and exercise on all elements of the musculoskeletal system, which needs to be understood by physical therapists if they wish to optimize the effects of their manual treatment of back pain and dysfunction problems.

A principal purpose of this final chapter is to consider the still developing link between the biologic sciences and physical therapy. Although the previous chapters reflect a diversity of approaches to treatment, there is much in common in them. Each method utilizes a systematic, ordered approach to patient diagnosis and the progression of treatment based on meticulous analysis of signs, symptoms, and responses to treatment. All treatment methods emphasize movement (passive, active, or both) and advocate life-style changes. Very few of the treatments described are based on a knowledge of the pathologies involved.

## DIAGNOSIS AND ASSESSMENT

Because so many physical therapists are now primary contact practitioners, diagnostic skill and technique have become of the utmost importance to them. The ideal situation remains that the referring physician should have a major responsibility in diagnosis, with a close interaction maintained between physician and physical therapist. However, reality dictates that this will not always happen. Whenever possible, and certainly when there is any suspicion that spinal pain or dysfunction may have a nonmechanical origin, the patient must be seen by a physician. Whatever the case, the physical therapist has to assume the full responsibility for all physical treatment procedures used.

Diagnostic skills are required by physical therapists, not only for primary diagnosis, but also for more "refined" diagnosis of the anatomic origin of back pain or dysfunction in patients referred from physicians. It is usual for such physicians to simply exclude the nonmechanical origins in a painful condition and refer the patient as a case of low back pain. An accurate history, good diagnostic skills, and objective clinical observation (see Chs. 5 through 9) are also essential to assess the appropriateness of treatment methods by noting and measuring the patient's response to treatment. This provides the basis for judgment of the appropriateness of particular treatments and for the progression and development of a treatment plan with a particular patient. The process of diagnosis/initial treatment/reassessment/treatment modification is one of the major contributions that Geoffrey Maitland (see Ch. 5) has made to the ordered, logical, physical treatment of low back pain and dysfunction.

## Behavioral Aspects of Chronic Low Back Pain

Since this book is primarily concerned with back pain of mechanical origin, full discussion of behavioral aspects is outside its scope. However, it must be recognized that in chronic low back pain, the reaction of the patient to pain is an important consideration. This is influenced by many developmental, family, social, and environmental factors related to the particular individual's circumstances. The suggestion that the refractory nature of a chronic low-back condition may be due to nonphysical factors is often resented by patients, who may think that they are being accused of hypochondria, or that the doctor or therapist is looking for excuses for failures in diagnosis or treatment. When the stigma attached by many patients to the idea of "behavioral" causes for chronicity of pain disappears, they may be better able to come to terms with their condition. However, a positive rather than a negative attitude should always be taken in seeking solutions to the patient's pain problem.

The psychological effects of chronic pain provide a powerful motivation to health professionals to prevent chronicity wherever possible by effective therapy. Nachemson[4] points out that the chances of successful rehabilitation to work are reduced to 40 percent in patients in whom pain persists for more than 6 months, since persistence of pain for more than 3 months alters the psychological make-up of the patient.

Physical therapists should never have inflexible and narrow diagnostic horizons that consider only mechanical or organic causes for back pain. Conversely, response to treatment may sometimes be attributable not only to the treatment used, but also to the optimism and ebullience of the therapist's personality, inducing confidence and faith in the patient. Finally, it should be acknowledged that the causes of chronic back pain, as a rule, involve both organic and behavioral factors.

## PREVENTION, EDUCATION, LIFE-STYLE, AND RISK FACTORS

### Education

Experience in the management of back pain strongly supports the view that education regarding a healthy life-style can make a vital contribution to back health. By developing an adequate knowledge of the structure and function of the spine, individuals can learn to maintain correct posture in all activities of daily living and develop muscle fitness. This would involve learning efficient and effective lifting techniques, and avoidance of unnecessary hazards in work or sport due to unsound techniques or inadequate preparation for particularly stressful demands on the spine. By improving postural awareness and encouraging better ergonomic techniques, the wear and tear on the spine can be reduced and a normal and useful range of pain-free spinal mobility can be maintained into old age. In the prevailing epidemic of back pain in our society, everyone should have a reasonable understanding of the structure and function of the back and of the age changes to which it is subject throughout the life span. They should understand the vulnerability of the spine to high loads in particular postures (e.g., loading in extreme flexion and rotation or sudden loading in full extension) as in certain work-related or sporting activities (see Ch. 2), and the potential traumatic consequences of such activities.[15] Conversely, the hazards of a sedentary lifestyle in promoting poor muscle tone, lack of aerobic fitness, poor posture, and predisposing to osteoporosis in later life should be understood if they are to be prevented. Information should be provided at a suitable level, to schoolchildren during their formative years, to adults in general, and also to certain occupational and sporting groups who may be at particular risk.

All back education programs (see Ch. 10) should stress these features. Whereas the structure and function of the segmented rod, which is the vertebral column, is necessarily complex to meet the requirements of support, flexibility, and protection of neural structures (see Chs. 1 and 2), it is relatively easy to convey the essential concepts of its structure and function to a lay audience.

There are many common misconceptions about the spine that should be laid to rest. The vertebral column is not inherently weak due to poor adaptation to the erect posture, although the lumbosacral angle involves shearing stresses on the laminae, predisposing it to spondylolysis. Intervertebral discs do not slip, but with repeated trauma or overload, the annulus may be severely damaged and may bulge in a degenerated disc, or the nucleus may prolapse through a ruptured annulus in a young person. There is no evidence that intervertebral joints "go out" or sublux, requiring regular manipulative "replacement," although the muscle spasm that normally accompanies acute back pain is frequently relieved by spinal mobilization. A more informed and intelligent understanding of the normal spine and its reaction to trauma and degenerative change is essential, not only to prevent injury but also both to understand the need for different forms of treatment and to learn to live with an aging or permanently damaged spine.

## Nutrition and Body Weight

Excessive body weight unnecessarily overloads the spine, accelerates wear and tear, and increases the risk of trauma to spinal components.[15,16] It increases the rate and amount of "creep" in the mobile segment, with potentially painful results when poor posture is maintained for relatively long periods. A sensible informed approach to nutrition and regular exercise are appropriate, both in the prevention and treatment of obesity.

Counseling by a psychologist or membership in a group addressing itself to controlled weight loss may help. Many sufferers from chronic low back pain would benefit by weight reduction, but seem unable to achieve this on their own.

## Posture

The importance of good lumbar posture is repeatedly emphasized in this book, highlighting the general view that poor posture is a prelude to back pain. It is vital to maintain good posture in standing, working, sitting, and in bed. The normal lordotic posture of the lumbar spine allows for the efficient transmission of axial loads and provides the most efficient position from which to move the spine. Flattening of the lumbar lordosis has been associated with aging and by some authorities with low back pain.[1,17,18] This flattening process appears to be a part of "normal" aging and may be accentuated by pathologic change such as disc thinning and vertebral osteoporosis. This process is clearly described in Chapter 2. An essential feature of the McKenzie approach to treatment is the maintenance of a normal lumbar lordosis (see Ch. 6). In standing it is important to stress the close relationship between pelvic and lumbar posture.[19] Physical therapists involved in both preventive programs and in treatment of back pain should stress this, help patients develop an awareness of lumbar spinal posture (see Ch. 2), demonstrate how changes in pelvic position change the posture of the lumbar region, and how abdominal and gluteal muscles control pelvic posture. Thus they should ensure that patients understand how they can easily maintain a normal lumbar lordosis. In prolonged sitting, maintenance of good lumbar posture should be assisted by ergonomically designed seating or by the use of a lumbar roll.

In Western societies, many of us spend a considerable time driving a car.

It is well known that professional drivers frequently suffer from chronic low back pain and that long distance drivers are prone to back injuries when lifting after long periods of driving. These particular problems probably relate to lengthy maintenance of bad posture, usually in a forward slumped position, with resultant "creep" of the soft tissues of the lumbar spinal joints into abnormal positions with abnormal states of fluid distribution in the tissues.[15] In addition, stress associated with driving on congested highways may provoke muscle tensions, and vibration may accentuate the effect of axial loading. The stresses placed on the spine by the abnormal posture itself, by continual use of the limbs in steering, gear-changing, and other maneuvers; or by lifting procedures all contribute to pain or trauma to the spine rendered more vulnerable by these postural and creep changes.[15,16] Better seat design and proper ergonomic positioning of the seat in relation to the controls would improve the position of the lumbar spine and its ability to cope with the stresses of driving (see Ch. 10). In addition, regular changes of position (e.g., by stopping, getting out of the car, and doing stretching exercises at regular intervals during a long drive) would help to prevent or reverse creep changes. At the same time, a realization of the vulnerability of the spine after a long drive would alert individuals to the associated dangers of lifting stresses before recovery. Conversely, prolonged standing in individuals with poor abdominal and gluteal muscle tone or with abdominal muscles rendered less effective by abdominal obesity or pregnancy, may creep into excessive lordosis with backache. Lordosis in older individuals with spinal stenosis (see Ch. 10) may provoke claudicatory pain and require a change to a more flexed posture.

## Effect of Movement and Exercise on Back and Joint Pain

There is no reliable evidence that prolonged bed rest or the avoidance of exercise brings about a reduction in back pain; current research clearly demonstrates that, apart from a quite short period of time immediately after injury, bed rest has no effect on the natural history of back pain.[12,13] Similarly, a consideration of current research makes it abundantly clear that physical activity is beneficial and necessary to most patients with musculoskeletal dysfunction (acute and chronic), including joint and back pain, and that the active rehabilitation of those with disorders such as chronic back pain not only restores function (see Ch. 10), but is also associated with a reduction in pain intensity.[8,13–15,20] Indeed, the opposite appears to be true, that is, that prolonged rest or the avoidance of activity increases the duration and severity of the back pain.[21] Despite this evidence, however, it is clear that bed rest, analgesics, corsets, and the avoidance of physical activity are still the most commonly prescribed forms of medical treatment.[12,13] Indeed, one of the main reasons for providing analgesics for initial pain relief should be to facilitate rehabilitation by movement and exercise.

Although patients naturally wish to adopt a posture that alleviates severe pain, they need to be persuaded that inactivity and especially bed rest cause substantial weakness and loss of tissue from all elements of the musculoskeletal system.[22,23] These changes include a loss of bone, muscle, and connective tissues; a reduction in joint range of motion (ROM), muscle strength, and endurance; and a marked decline in physical fitness in all individuals whose activity levels have been considerably reduced.[22,24] This situation applies equally to the elderly, and there is no truth in the older adage that elderly people do not require as much exercise as younger people,[22] that exercise is somehow dangerous to them, and that they have earned their rest after a lifetime of work. The weight of current research evidence reveals that the musculoskeletal system (including the vertebral column) demands the stress of axial load bearing, movement, and activity at all stages of the life cycle, even into extreme old age.[22,23,25,26] Old people with back pain need a strong, ongoing program of physical activity to improve their function with the continuing assurance that this will also reduce their pain levels.[24]

In the spine, the health of the joints is largely dependent on repeated low-stress movements. The intervertebral discs and zygapophyseal (facet) joints require movement for the effective transfer of fluid and nutrients across joint surfaces.[27,28] Movement and active exercise are unlikely to reduce the number of episodes of back pain that a person suffers, but they will ensure that those affected will be better able to cope with the problem, to recover from it more rapidly, to remain at or return to productive work more quickly, and to have a much improved quality of life.[13]

## Manual Therapy and the Musculoskeletal System

The manual therapist primarily uses movement and exercise as the principal tools in the treatment of musculoskeletal joint dysfunction and low back pain. In recent years, there has been abundant research showing the value of movement to the joints[29] and the musculoskeletal system[30] and supporting the success of manual and physical therapy for back pain.[13] Much of the evidence will be considered and applied in this chapter.

### Joints

The function of AC is to facilitate free movement and load bearing in joints, and it is particularly well adapted to meet its dual tasks of reducing friction and attenuating loadbearing on subchondral bone.[31] Widespread cartilage degeneration is associated with disease processes, whereas localized damage to AC surfaces and to the ligaments and capsule of spinal joints may result from trauma, particularly if repetitive in nature. Pathologic changes need to be clearly distinguished from the "normal" process of aging[8] if manual therapy is to be effective. Aging is characterized by a slow process of AC dehydration, by surface fibrillation characterized by fatigue and splitting of collagen bundles, and by a gradual loss of proteoglycans from the matrix.[31,32] These changes are reflected by a decreased resilience in the response of AC to pressure and a reduction in cartilage thickness in old age in all weight-bearing joints.[33,34] The cartilage changes are accompanied by reductions in the volume of synovial fluid and in its osmolarity, usually with atrophic changes in underlying bone.[29,35] Similarly, age changes (which may be primarily due to disuse) and repetitive minor trauma bring about substantial atrophy of the joint capsule and ligaments; increasing age also causes ligament "stiffening" as the numbers of cross-linkages between adjacent collagen fibrils increase substantially, making the fibers less compliant.[30,36] The principal findings from animal studies show that early lesions in joints occur not where the joint is maximally loaded, but at their periphery where it is not loaded.[32] The softening and fibrillation of AC is indicative of a tissue disintegrating from inactivity, not from overuse.[32,37,38] Many of the joint changes associated with aging are more likely to be due to disuse than to any genetic predisposition of AC and collagen to degenerate with time.[28,38]

The physical therapist using manual therapy continually works with joints affected by age and pathologic change, and attempts to improve movement and reduce pain by passive and active movement techniques. It is therefore important for the physical therapist to understand the physiologic effects that movement has on the various elements of synovial joints. All collagenous tissues rely heavily on movement to ensure adequate nutrition.[28,39] AC demands regular alternate mechanical loading and unloading to remain healthy.[37] Exercise and movement ensure the passage of synovial fluid over its surface, and together with the alternate compression and relaxation of AC that occur during movement, enable the synovial fluid to be expressed and then "sucked back" into the AC as the areas of pressure changes over the surface.[11,27,28,34] The regular physical loading and unloading of joint cartilage that occurs with movement during manual therapy facilitates this process. Although cartilage responds very favorably to movement, it responds poorly to prolonged rest and immobilization, particularly under loading.[34] There is overwhelming evidence showing atrophy and degeneration of AC and underlying subchondral bone during immobilization and especially under conditions of constant loading.

Similarly, ligaments, as dynamic collagenous structures, undergo hypertrophy with exercise and considerable atrophy with disuse. Systematic exercise results in thicker, stronger ligaments that maintain their compliance and flexibility and that also become stronger at the bone–ligament–bone complex.[27]

In the same way, the intervertebral discs, which are the largest avascular collagenous structures in the adult, gain their nutrition by the diffusion of nutrients from a distance, primarily via the vertebral end-plate and secondarily by diffusion through the annulus.[9,39] Disc nutrition is heavily dependent on movement, and recent studies[40,41] show that movements in the sagittal plane bring about the greatest transfer of fluid into and out of the disc. These studies indicate the importance of regular, large-range spinal movements so that adequate intervertebral disc nutrition is ensured. Similarly, other recent studies[8,16] demonstrate that sustained disc loading in one position (e.g., at the limit of flexion) is associated with advanced disc degeneration and low back pain. Movement therapy in all of its forms considerably assists disc nutrition and health.

All of the cartilaginous structures of the body respond adversely to disuse and to conditions of prolonged loading and positively to movement and exercise. Physical therapy procedures, including passive mobilization techniques, utilize both the "stirring" and movement of synovial fluid and the compression and relaxation of cartilage. In addition, movements through the full ROM reduce the tendency toward the adaptive shortening of connective tissues and muscles around the joints and minimize the tendency toward stiffening with age.[8] Recent research has also shown that long-duration, high-mileage walking or running is not associated with premature joint degeneration or osteoarthritis, but is strongly associated with increased bone mineral content in the lower limbs and back.[8,42,43] This evidence is clearly at odds with the often expressed clinical view that repetitive exercise, and particularly running, is associated with the "wearing out" of AC because of the constant stresses of impaction and loading. Current research, however, shows that the old concept of "wear and tear" cartilage loss and osteoarthritis was usually incorrect and that osteoarthritic joint changes begin in areas where collagen is not often stressed by movement and pressure.[32,37] This knowledge reinforces and vindicates the value of exercise and movement in the physical therapy of joint and back problems.

## Bone and Muscle

Bone and muscle are both dynamic structures that respond positively to exercise and adversely to disuse. A strong inverse relationship exists between muscle mass and osteoporosis such that a decline in muscle mass is matched by an increasing fragility of bone.[44] Much of the reduction in muscle mass that occurs with increasing age in Western society is due to disuse and can be substantially reversed by a program of activity.[22,30] This knowledge is fundamentally important for the manual therapist because it focuses attention on the need for both specific and general exercise to be prescribed, particularly for the middle-aged and elderly, as an essential part of treatment programs for most individuals. In this regard, Pardini[24] has demonstrated that most elderly Americans can show up to 50 percent improvement in muscle strength after a relatively short exercise program. High activity levels are essential, particularly to the elderly, if independence is to be valued and if the quality of life is to be maintained into old age.

Numerous controlled studies[41-50] have demonstrated the requirements of bone and muscle for exercise throughout the life cycle. Smith et al[45] examined 30 elderly women with a mean age of 84 years. The women were placed in two groups that were matched for age, weight, and degree of ambulation. The experimental group participated in a 30-minute exercise program, 3 days a week for 3 years. At the end of this period, there was a 5.6 percent difference in bone mineral content between the groups, consisting of a 2.3 percent gain in the experimental group and a 3.3 percent loss in the control group. These results support the findings of Aloia et al,[46] who reported a significant increase in total body calcium in postmenopausal women who exercised regularly for 1 year, in contrast with a fall in total body calcium in a matched sedentary group. Similarly, Ayalon et al,[47] in a study of the effects of dynamic loading exercises for the forearms of postmenopausal women (53 to 74 years of age), showed an increase of 3.8 percent in bone density of the radius and ulna after 5 months of exercise compared with controls, who continued to show a decline in bone density. Other recent studies have demonstrated that bone gain after exercise is both site specific and exercise-type specific. Thus Aisenbrey[51] has shown that among athletes, weight lifters have the greatest bone density and swimmers have the least. Nevertheless, there are some recent indicators showing that habitual swimmers also have greater bone mass than do sedentary individuals.[52] These studies are a small part of an increasing body of evidence supporting the value of high levels of regular exercise in preserving skeletal health. This is true for both genders, but is particularly the case for women after menopause, when hormonal deprivation adds considerably to involutional bone loss.

Similarly, other studies show that it is possible to increase muscle strength, endurance, and hypertrophy into old age.[48,50] Aniansson et al,[49] in a controlled study of the effects of exercise in old men, showed a significant increase in muscle power and increased aerobic capacity after a 12-week program of dynamic and static exercise. Walker,[48] in a review article on exercise and aging, demonstrated that muscles in older individuals responded favorably to exercise programs, particularly if the strengthening programs are individualized and consistent with personal goals.

It is not only the middle-aged and elderly who can benefit from increased levels of activity. It has been found that young people who are immobilized for long periods of time also show alterations usually attributable to muscle and bone aging. It is clear that many of the changes attributed to aging are due to disuse.[30,53] Exercise, properly prescribed and applied in the early stages, can reverse most of these changes.

Based on the understanding of the needs that all elements of the human musculoskeletal system have for movement and exercise throughout life, manual therapists have the responsibility to include exercise as an essential part of prophylaxis and treatment in addition to their other more passive treatment modalities such as massage, mobilization, manipulation, and traction.

## Loading at the Limit of Spinal Movement (End Range)

Although sustained postures in spinal extension are rare, there are many occupations and recreational pursuits that involve a position of full lumbar flexion sustained for long periods of time. Where the spine is loaded at end range, creep (movement further into range) occurs because of an internal adjustment of forces within the tissues involving fluid transfer.[16,54,55] This process squeezes fluid out of the compressed intervetebral disks, facet AC, and the stretched spinal ligaments, and also redistributes the remaining fluid within these structures. Thus creep in flexion is observed as an increase in forward movement that takes the spine beyond its usual end range. This prolonged process not only deprives the soft tissues of part of their nutrition,[56] but the natural collagen "crimp," which is a feature of the resting state of collagen, progressively straightens out as the fibrils elongate under the sustained load.[36,57] Recovery from this new position, once the load is removed, takes a considerable period of time.[17] Such situations occur as a usual part of the working pattern of occupational groups such as bricklayers, stonemasons, and sheep shearers, and in all individuals who maintain a sitting posture in full flexion, under the load of their own body weight, for long periods.

The tissue fluid redistribution described changes the shape of the elements of the mobile segments; places the uncrimped collagen in the disks, facet joints, and ligaments under sustained load (to which it reacts adversely); increases intradiscal pressure; and leaves the lumbar spine literally "hanging" on its facet joints.[34,58] This situation progressively brings about deleterious changes to all the collagenous structures thus placed under loading,[15] and makes those individuals particularly vulnerable to injury after periods of sustained flexion loading. It is for this reason that individuals should avoid lifting heavy loads after long periods of driving.[8]

Physical therapy procedures of active and passive lumbar movement aid nutrition of the discs and facet joints, help and reserve full ranges of movements, and ensure strong ligaments and tendons.[27,34] Lumbar sagittal movements in particular, aid nutrition by bringing about the largest fluid exchange between the discs and the interstitial fluid surrounding the spine.[40,41,59]

This concept of spinal function indicates the need to prescribe large-range trunk movement in the sagittal plane in the early stages of disc and facet joint degeneration. Movement also prevents the adaptive shortening of ligaments and maintains spinal flexibility.[15] The major problem of spinal flexion creep is best managed by ergonomic advice that emphasizes the need for good static and dynamic postures, by regular "pause" exercises (i.e., short periods of exercise focusing on mobility and relaxation) that encourage spinal movement, and particularly by the use of the extension component of sagittal movement as the most efficient means of "unloading" the previously loaded elements of the spine and of rehydrating discs, AC, and soft tissues. The concept also provides an understanding of why extension postures and movements are an important part of the management of low back pain and why extension movements are so useful as a primary form of manual treatment.

Conversely, back pain associated with prolonged standing involves axial creep, that is, relative movement into lumbar extension, especially in middle-aged and elderly subjects who are obese or whose abdominal and gluteal muscles fail to maintain good lumbar posture.[8] Axial creep is best treated by postures and movements that "unload" those previously "compressed" and stretched structures, that is, by movements that emphasize spinal flexion.

## SPINAL MANIPULATIVE THERAPY

### The Spinal Lesion

The nature of the spinal lesion causing back pain remains, in most circumstances, unknown. The mechanism by which spinal manipulatory therapy (SMT) achieves pain relief or accelerates recovery of function[8,60] also remains a mystery. SMT is most unlikely to work by "reducing subluxation," correcting "vertebral alignment," "reducing nuclear herniation," or "tearing joint adhesions," although all of these unsubstantiated hypotheses still have strong advocates.[60-63] There are only a few particular circumstances (e.g., acute locked back), where the mechanical effects of SMT are relatively clear.

Early discussion of common back syndromes led to the use of subjective diagnostic labels based on palpations, such as the "osteopathic lesion," "vertebral blockage," "stiff segments," and the like, but the nature of these hypothetical lesions has never been scientifically established.[60]

Cyriax[61] asserted that nuclear herniation was reducible by specific manipulative procedures, but there is no research data to justify this. Indeed, current knowledge of nuclear herniation or prolapse suggests that it is much less common than previously supposed.[9,64] It is also extremely unlikely that SMT could possibly reduce extruded nuclear material back into its envelope.[8]

Other explanations of the apparent success of SMT encompass neurophysiologic mechanisms, most of which are beyond the scope of this chapter. Useful hypotheses, however, are provided by Haldeman,[61] Paris,[62] and Zusman.[63] In particular, Zusman[63] refers to physiologic mechanisms by which SMT is likely to have an inhibitory effect on reflex muscle contraction (spasm). Zusman also provides an interesting explanation concerning a hysteresis or delayed effect for neural discharge in joint afferents after repetitive end range passive movement. More recently, Butler[65] has linked the neurophysiologic concepts related to a mechanical compromise of neural tissue and axoplasmic flow to provide a challenging explanation for the effects of manipulative therapy.

## Acute, Painful Locked Back

Although this chapter has shown that physiologic processes can help explain the direct effect that repetitive passive or active movement can have on synovial joints and intervertebral discs, it has proved to be more difficult to explain how movement or manipulation can be so effective in the case of acute, painful locked back. This syndrome refers to acute low back pain that is often attributed to a particular movement and that is sometimes associated with a "click" or noise from the back. Patients with this syndrome are usually flexed and rotated, unable to extend, complain of constant severe back pain, and sometimes experience referred pain down one or both legs. On examination, there appears to be a mechanical block to movement, particularly into extension. Such patients often respond favorably to a specific lumbar manipulation or mobilization or to some form of active-assisted movement. The response to a single manipulation is often dramatic, with a sudden reduction of back and leg pain and a full restoration of movement and function.

In attempting to explain the nature of this condition and the mechanism of its response to SMT, a number of alternative ideas have been proposed. Although in the past a few clinicians and researchers have implicated the intervertebral disc,[61] most writers currently believe that it is highly unlikely (given present knowledge of the structure, function, and pathology of the lumbar disc), and consider the facet joints to be the primary source of the problem.[8,66] The two most usual explanations provided as to the facet joint structures likely to be involved are (1) nipping of a synovial joint fringe from the capsule or from a polar recess and (2) entrapment of a meniscus. Although both the capsule and its synovial folds or "menisci" are well innervated,[67,68] they are small, "slippery" structures that are unlikely to be entrapped. Bogduk and Engel[66] proposed a hypothetical mechanism by which a "meniscus" might be so involved.

In Chapter 1, we describe the presence of "joint inclusions" of partially detached flaps of AC at the posterolateral margins of the facet joints in some individuals. The continuity of these firm cartilaginous inclusions with a well-innervated capsule presents a situation that is analogous to a torn meniscus in the knee joint and has the capacity to "block" movement. Separation of the joint surfaces (gapping) by manipulation or movement would allow the piece of firm AC to return to its normal position, take the load off the capsule, and result in the restoration of normal movement and a reduction in pain. This remains a hypothesis, but offers a reasonable explanation for the dramatic effects, often of a single manipulation, in the case of acute, painful locked back.[69]

## SUMMARY

Movement and exercise are essential for the development, maintenance, and continuing strength of the musculoskeletal system throughout life and should form a vital part of any treatment directed toward improving musculoskeletal function. They are also frequently successful in reducing pain from the musculoskeletal system after inactivity, trauma, or disease.[12,13,27,34,63,65] The techniques of manual therapy described in this book all use movement, stretch, and loading to the body and are directed toward functional improvement and pain reduction.[60] Although many of the effects of mobilization and manipulation on joint pain and mobility (particularly for the vertebral column) remain largely speculative, there is a growing body of evidence that suggests a useful biomechanical model to explain the dramatic relief that often follows such procedures.[60,62,69] Nevertheless, over the last decade, the major advances made in the area of back-pain treatment and the management of other musculoskeletal disorders have been based on intensive, aggressive, active physical treatment.[12–14] In addition, recent research has demonstrated that habitual and working postures are important factors in back and regional pain problems.[40,41] Sustained postures near or at the limit of joint ROM, and especially when under loading (of body weight or external objects), substantially reduce the hydration of tissues and the ability of an individual to respond rapidly to environment change.[15]

The other important message for physical therapists is that it is essential to never lose sight of the importance of basic science and its logical application in the diagnosis and treatment of patients. Physical therapists, much more than the average physician, acquire "hands-on" anatomic knowledge that enables them to accurately localize the joint or structure that is dysfunctional or the source of pain. This information is of vital importance in the design of logical treatment, to all members of the health-care team managing a patient. It is also equally important for physical therapists to be aware of the most likely pathology causing pain and dysfunction. Physical therapists arrive at the same conclusion as specialist physicians and surgeons, usually by less invasive means; for example, passive movement and palpatory techniques may yield the same information as discography requiring a painful injection and the costly use of high-technology radiographic equipment. The contribution that the logical, careful, well-trained physical therapist can make to the diagnosis of low back pain should not be underestimated.

## REFERENCES

1. Grieve GP: Modern Manual Therapy of the Vertebral Column. Churchill Livingstone, Edinburgh, 1986
2. Maitland GD: Vertebral Manipulation. 4th Ed. Butterworths, London, 1977
3. Bourdillon JF: Spinal Manipulation. 3rd Ed. William Heinemann Medical Books Ltd., London, 1982
4. Nachemson AL: The lumbar spine: an orthopaedic challenge. Spine 1:59, 1976
5. Kelsey J, White AA: Epidemiology and impact of low back pain. Spine 5:133, 1980
6. Le Blanc FE, Cruess RL, DuPuis M et al: The Quebec Task Force on Spinal Disorders monograph. Spine, suppl. 75:8, 1987
7. Frymoyer JW, Cats-Baril WC: An overview of the incidences and costs of low back pain. Orthop Clin North Am 22:263, 1991
8. Twomey LT, Taylor JR: Physical Therapy of the Low Back. Churchill Livingstone, New York, 1987
9. Bogduk N, Twomey LT: Clinical Anatomy of the Lumbar Spine. Longman Cheshire Pty Ltd., Victoria, Australia, 1987
10. Crock HV: Internal disc disruption: a challenge to disc prolapse fifty years on. Spine 11:650, 1986
11. Twomey LT, Taylor JR: Age related changes of the lumbar spine and spinal rehabilitation. Crit Rev Phys Rehabil Med 2:153, 1991
12. Deyo RA, Diehl AK, Rosenthal M et al: How many days of bed rest for acute low back pain? N Engl J Med 315:1064, 1986
13. Waddell G: A new clinical model for the treatment of low back pain. Spine 12:632, 1987
14. Mayer TG, Gatchell RJ, Kishino N et al: A prospective short-term study of chronic low back pain patients utilizing novel objective function measurement. Pain 25:53, 1986
15. Twomey LT, Taylor JR, Oliver M: Sustained flexion loading, rapid extension, loading of the lumbar spine and the physical therapy of related injuries. Physiother Pract 4:129, 1988
16. Twomey LT, Taylor JR: Flexion creep deformation and hysteresis in the lumbar vertebral column. Spine 7:116, 1982
17. McKenzie RA: The Lumbar Spine: Mechanical Diagnosis and Therapy. Spinal Publications, Waikanae, New Zealand, 1981

18. Kopp JR, Alexander AH, Turocy RH et al: The use of lumbar extension in the evaluation and treatment of patients with acute herniated nucleus pulposis. A preliminary report. Clin Orthop Relat Res 202:211, 1986
19. Twomey LT: Age changes in the human lumbar spine. Doctoral Thesis, University of Western Australia, Perth, Western Australia, 1981
20. Ganora A: Rehabilitation of work related back injury. Aust Fam Phys 15:430, 1986
21. Deyo RA, Tsui-Wu YR: Descriptive epidemiology of low back pain and its related medical care in the United States. Spine 12:264, 1987
22. Shephard RJ: Management of exercise in the elderly. Appl Sports Sci 9:109, 1984
23. Twomey LT: Physical activity and ageing bones. Patient Management 13:27, 1989
24. Pardini A: Exercise, vitality and aging. Aging 344:19, 1984
25. Smith EL, Gilligan C: Effects of inactivity and exercise on bone. Phys Sports Med 15:91, 1987
26. Shephard RJ: Exercise for the elderly: cardiovascular function and aging. Patient Management 12:103, 1988
27. Frank C, Akesow WH, Woo SL-Y et al: Physiology and therapeutic value of passive joint motion. Clin Orthop 185:113, 1984
28. Lowther D: The Effect of Compression and Tension on the Behaviour of Connective Tissues in Aspects of Manipulative Therapy. Longman Cheshire Pty Ltd, Melbourne, Victoria, 1985
29. Salter RB, Field P: The effects of continuous compression on living articular cartilage. J Bone Joint Surg 42A:31, 1960
30. Menard D, Stanish WD: The aging athlete. Am J Sports Med 17:187, 1991
31. Stockwell RA: Biology of Cartilage Cells. Cambridge University Press, Cambridge, England, 1979
32. Bullough PG: Osteoarthritis: pathogenesis and aetiology. Br J Rheumatol 23:166, 1984
33. Bayliss MT, Johnstone B, O'Brien JP: Proteoglycan synthesis in the human intervertebral disc: variation with age, region and pathology. Spine 13:972, 1988
34. Salter RB: The biologic concept of continuous passive motion of synovial joints. Clin Orthop 242:12, 1989
35. Baumgarten M, Bloebaum RD, Ross SD et al: Normal human synovial fluid: osmolarity and exercise-induced changes. J Bone Joint Surg 67A:1336, 1985
36. Broom ND, Marra DL: Ultrastructural evidence for fiber to fiber associations in articular cartilage and their functional implication. J Anat 146:185, 1986
37. Dieppe P: Osteoarthritis: are we asking the wrong questions? Br J Rheumatol 23:161, 1984
38. Eichner EE: Does running cause osteoarthritis? Phys Sports Med 17:147, 1989
39. Maroudas A: Nutrition and metabolism of the intervertebral disc. p. 38. In Gosh P (ed): Biology of the Intervertebral Disc. Vol. 2. CRC Press, Boca Raton, FL, 1988
40. Adams MA, Hutton WC: The effects of posture on diffusion into the lumbar intervertebral discs. J Anat 147:121, 1986
41. Tyrrell AR, Reilly T, Troup JDG: Circadian variation in stature and the effects of spinal loading. Spine 10:161, 1985
42. Lane NG, Block DA, Jones HH et al: Long distance running, bone density and osteoporosis. JAMA 255:1147, 1986
43. Panush RS, Schmidt C, Caldwell JR et al: Is running associated with degenerative joint disease? JAMA 255:1152, 1986
44. Wooton R, Bryson E, Elasser U et al: Risk factors for fractured neck of femur in the elderly. Age Ageing 11:160, 1982

45. Smith EL, Reddin N, Smith PE: Physical activity and calcium modalities for bone mineral increase in aged women. Med Sci Sports Exerc 13:60, 1981
46. Aloia JF, Cohn SH, Cane R et al: Prevention of bone loss by exercise. J Clin Endocrinol Metab 43:992, 1978
47. Ayalon J, Simkin A, Leichter I et al: Dynamic bone exercises for postmenopausal women: effect on the density on the distal radius. Arch Phys Med Rehabil 68:280, 1987
48. Walker J: Exercise and aging. NZJ Phys 14:8, 1986
49. Aniansson A, Grimby G, Rundgren A et al: Physical training in old men. Age Ageing, 9:186, 1980
50. Recker RR: Continuous treatment of osteoporosis: current status. Orthop Clin North Am 12:611, 1981
51. Aisenbrey JA: Exercise in the prevention and management of osteoporosis. Phys Ther 67:1100, 1987
52. Orwoll ES, Ferar JL, Ovlatt SK et al: The effect of swimming on bone mineral content. Clin Res 35:194, 1987
53. St Pierre D, Gardiner PF: The effect of immobilisation and exercise on muscle function. A review. Physiother Can 39:24, 1987
54. Koreska J, Robertson D, Mills RH et al: Biomechanics of the lumbar spine and its clinical significance. Orthop Clin North Am 8:121, 1977
55. Kazarian LE: Creep characteristics of the human spinal column. Orthop Clin North Am 6:3, 1975
56. Adams MA, Hutton WC: Gradual disc prolapse. Spine 10:524, 1985
57. Shah JS, Hampson WGJ, Jayson MIV: The distribution of surface strain in the cadaveric lumbar spine. J Bone Joint Surg 60B:246, 1978
58. Twomey LT, Taylor JR: Sagittal movements of the human lumbar vertebral column: a quantitative study of the role of the posterior vertebral elements. Arch Phys Med Rehabil 64:322, 1983
59. Adams MA, Hutton WC: The effect of posture on the lumbar spine. J Bone Joint Surg 67B:625, 1985
60. Haldeman S: Spinal manipulative therapy: a status report. Clin Orthop 179:62, 1983
61. Cyriax JH: Textbook of Orthopaedic Medicine. Vol. I: Diagnosis and Soft Tissue Lesion. 7th Ed. Ballière Tindall, London, 1978
62. Paris SV: Spinal manipulative therapy. Clin Orthop 179:55, 1983
63. Zusman M: Re-appraisal of a proposed neurological mechanism for the relief of joint pain with passive movements. Physiother Pract 1:64, 1986
64. Stoddard A: Manual of Osteopathic Technique. Hutchinson Books Ltd., London, 1959
65. Butler D: Axoplasmic flow and manipulative physiotherapy. Presented at the Seventh Biennial Conference of the Manipulative Physiotherapists Association of Australia, Leura, New South Wales, 1984
66. Bogduk N, Engel R: The menisci of the lumbar zygapophyseal joints: a review of their anatomy and clinical significance. Spine 9:454, 1984
67. Bogduk N: The innervation of the lumbar spine. Spine 8:286, 1983
68. Giles LGF, Taylor JR: Innervation of lumbar zygapophyseal joint synovial folds. Acta Orthop Scand 58:43, 1987
69. Taylor JR, Twomey LT: Age changes in lumbar zygapophyseal joints: observations on structure and function. Spine 11:739, 1986

# Index

*Page numbers followed by f indicate figures; those followed by t indicate tables.*